Preconception Health and Care: A Life Course Approach

AF167548

Jill Shawe · Eric A. P. Steegers
Sarah Verbiest
Editors

Preconception Health and Care: A Life Course Approach

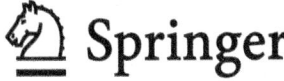 Springer

Editors
Jill Shawe
Faculty of Health
University of Plymouth
Plymouth
Devon
UK

Eric A. P. Steegers
Department of Obstetrics and Gynaecology
Erasmus University Medical Center,
Erasmus MC
Rotterdam
The Netherlands

Sarah Verbiest
Center for Maternal and Infant Health
Jordan Institute for Families,
University of North Carolina at Chapel Hill
Chapel Hill
NC
USA

ISBN 978-3-030-31752-2   ISBN 978-3-030-31753-9   (eBook)
https://doi.org/10.1007/978-3-030-31753-9

This Springer imprint is published by the registered company Springer Nature Switzerland AG
The registered company address is: Gewerbestrasse 11, 6330 Cham, Switzerland

Foreword

How do paradigms shift? Not easily, not smoothly, not without refinement, expansions, and retrenchment, and not without pushback and champions. At least 40 years ago, a movement began to rethink traditional efforts for addressing the major causes of infant mortality and morbidity in industrialized nations: congenital anomalies and low birth weight. Review of observational studies in Europe and basic embryology caused the venerable adage, "prevention in order to be truly preventive must be antenatal" (Ballantyne 1902) to be questioned.

The need for a new approach to impact healthy pregnancy outcomes came with recognition that women enter into prenatal care too late to prevent congenital anomalies and the impact of numerous antecedents to low birth weight including intendedness of the conception, interpregnancy intervals, maternal age, maternal pregravid weight status, prepregnancy chronic disease control, exposures to medications and other drugs, and timing of entry into prenatal care. With recognition of these limitations, a new approach to benefit pregnancy outcomes emerged which was designed to reach women with prevention opportunities before conception. In doing so, women and couples would be able to enter into pregnancy informed about risks to their own health and to the health of their pregnancies and offspring and to have taken any preventive steps that made sense to them and their circumstances. The potential significance of this shift can be appreciated by comparing the tradition of prescribing folic acid through multivitamins for its preventive benefits at the first prenatal visit (by which time the window for preventing neural tube defects has closed) versus educating women about the benefits of adequate folic acid exposure prior to entry into prenatal care and providing them with strategies for achieving the recommendation.

Original efforts to include a preconception emphasis in reproductive health care were vested with obstetricians as they represent the usual gateway to pregnancy-related care at least in the USA and have the most power in defining its parameters. Their acceptance of a paradigm shift was judged essential to successfully prevent common threats to healthy pregnancy outcomes.

The earliest known prepregnancy clinic was established in London in 1978 as a hospital-based service. The clinic largely served an interconceptional population of women who were referred because of previous poor pregnancy outcomes including maternal, fetal, and neonatal complications; occasionally a woman referred herself. The founder of the clinic noted that rarely was a physical exam performed; rather, "opinion" was usually based on a combination of the woman's own history, her past medical records (if available), and a careful assessment of the woman's current fears and future worries (Chamberlain 1980). Engagement of obstetrical providers in the paradigm change was echoed in the USA with the 1987 article, Preconception Health Promotion: A Focus for Obstetric Care (Moos and Cefalo 1987). This article introduced the benefits of systematic assessment in exploring preconceptional issues for women contemplating pregnancy and reaching women not considering pregnancy in the immediate future in nontraditional settings such as family planning clinics.

Shortly thereafter, the first known call to reach *all* women of childbearing potential with preconception information was put forth (Moos 1989).

"Until the health care community incorporates prepregnancy counseling into the routine services available to all women of childbearing age ... the rights of women to exercise personal choices about their reproductive futures will not be realized and opportunities for primary prevention will be lost" (p. 67).

The article posited that the primary purpose of preconception care is education: providing women with the information they need to make informed decisions about their reproductive futures and risks they may want to address prior to conception: in other words, the agenda is about empowerment.

Engaging women directly without the initial information gateway being managed through a clinical encounter is one way to shift power. To introduce and reinforce the idea that the weeks around conception are at least as important as the later weeks of pregnancy in impacting some pregnancy outcome requires repeated exposure to this information. With the goal of introducing the importance of the earliest weeks of pregnancy to as many people as possible, numerous programs were created including school curriculum, health fair exhibits, brochures written at low reading levels, work place strategies, innovative and interactive health appraisals, and eventually internet-based health education strategies.

Initially, these approaches resulted in many women arriving at their annual gynecologic exam or a specifically scheduled obstetrical visit with prepregnancy questions only to be confronted with provider confusions or a perceived patronizing response that the woman should not worry—the questions would be addressed fully at their first prenatal visit. The dissonance in messages created frustration for patients and providers, alike—perhaps an unavoidable conflict when venerable traditions are disrupted. Hoping to create a bridge between women's expectations and providers' preparation, the first comprehensive book for health-care providers (not just physicians or obstetricians) to understand the hows and whys of preconception health care, including literature-based recommendations for specific prepregnancy conditions, was published (Cefalo and Moos 1988, 1995).

All of these initiatives stimulated increasing enthusiasm about the promise of preconception health promotion among governmental agencies, professional and advocacy groups, scientific advisory bodies and regulatory agencies in both the USA and the European Union and the World Health Organization, and thus the way clinical care frames the prevention window around pregnancy began to change.

The unintended consequences of well-intentioned actions must be considered with any paradigm shift: Who might be hurt? Who could be left out? How might the new emphasis be misunderstood? Is it feasible, fundable, effective? Recognizing that preconception interactions around pregnancy risks could easily veer toward paternalism, disempowerment, or biases about who should or should not become pregnant, the intent of preconception counseling was deliberately promoted by pioneers in the field as egalitarian and woman-centered (Cefalo and Moos 1988).

> The intent of preconception programs should not be to make reproductive decisions for women; it should not be to encourage reproduction in one group and discourage it in another. The intent ... should be to provide enough information so that *all* women can make informed decisions about conception, life style and choices in medical care. Care-givers have a legal obligation to provide patients with accurate information on which to base decisions; they do not have the right to make those decisions for them. (p. 7)

The preconception initiative was the first to identify that the traditional silos of reproductive care make little sense and provide less than the maximal benefit to outcomes: the prepregnancy, prenatal, postpartum and interconceptional periods should and can be approached as an integrated pathway of understanding and care for each woman. It is a small leap from the concept of integration to appreciating that healthy women have healthier pregnancy outcomes and that, for the most part, there is little that can be recommended in preconception care that would not benefit women of similar age who are not considering pregnancy. Examples include recommendations about healthy weight, tobacco cessation, no more than moderate alcohol exposure, depression identification and treatment, screening for and addressing intimate partner violence, and many more. Thus, the preconception care paradigm shift is, in reality, a call for better prevention efforts throughout the life span. From this appreciation, the life course concept takes shape. Should primary prevention influences and efforts start with one's own conception, childhood exposures, adolescent health choices, and adult health status or with prenatal and intrapartum experiences? Ultimately, the goal for preventive services should be that all people achieve the highest level of wellness possible, whatever stage of life they are in—calling for a true life course approach.

As should occur with all new paradigms that impact multiple interest groups, the work should be constantly interrogated and be able to shift and evolve. The first wave of the preconception agenda has been fairly critiqued noting important concerns around pronatalism, a focus on the individual instead of the social determinants of health and health equity, implicit biases toward the LGBTQ population, paternalism, accessibility of related vocabulary, lack of engagement of men, women of color, people with low incomes, and others. Reproductive justice leaders and women of color have called for expanded conversations around historic trauma, bodily autonomy, and centering communities in creating their own solutions. As the new decade begins, collaborative steps and plans on how to move forward are a necessity.

With this new volume, Shawe, Steegers, and Verbiest take an important and needed step to move the preconception initiative forward using a collaborative, international perspective; they look to the "what next" and address the evolving frame of preconception care, always mindful that this work should fully engage women, couples, men, and communities, and respect people's values, interests, and needs. Importantly, they provide the current scientific underpinnings for specific recommendations that might be directed to people seeking preconception information. Shawe, Steegers, and Verbiest give us reason to believe that Ballantyne's adage of nearly 120 years ago is being rewritten: "Prevention, in order to be preventive, must start **before** pregnancy." The results will be healthier women throughout their lifetimes, healthier pregnancies should a woman become pregnant and healthier fetuses and neonates—all of this centered with a life course perspective that recognizes the necessity of grounding the work in a healthy community. Could there be a more far-reaching impact?

Center for Maternal and Infant Health Women's Health Care   Merry-K. Moos
University of North Carolina at Chapel Hill,
Chapel Hill, NC, USA

References

1. Chamberlain G. The prepregnancy clinic. Br Med J. 1980;281:29. https://doi.org/10.1136/bmj.281.6232.29.
2. Moos MK, Cefalo RC. Preconception health promotion: a focus for obstetric care: Am J Perinatol. 1987;49(1):63–7.
3. Moos MK. Preconceptional health Promotion: a health education opportunity for all women. Women Health. 1989;15(3):55–68.
4. Cefalo RC, Moos MK. Preconceptional health promotion: a practical guide. Rockville: Aspen Publication; 1988.
5. Cefalo RC, Moos MK. Preconception health care: a practical guide (2nd ed). St Louis: Mosby—Year Book, Inc.; 1995.

Contents

Introduction

1

Jill Shawe, Eric A. P. Steegers, and Sarah Verbiest

Many people hope to become parents and welcome children into their lives. The joy of bringing a new baby into the world and watching that child grow and develop is one sought out across the earth. The desire to have a healthy pregnancy and baby becomes paramount for most families upon conception. However, in spite of the growth of technology, global connectivity, and medical advances, maternal and infant mortality and morbidity are either stagnant or growing across the globe, with disparities in outcomes continuing to widen. Too many young adults don't have the services and support they need to live their best life, laying a foundation for healthy aging and well-being over time. Too many women lose their lives giving birth or suffer severe morbidity in the process of becoming mothers. Too many couples find their hopes of having a healthy child unrealized.

Research has found that while interventions during pregnancy and childbirth are essential for improving outcomes, they are inadequate for realizing ongoing international improvements in perinatal health and achieving equitable outcomes for all people. The shift toward preconception health was put into motion over a decade ago to challenge this paradigm and focus attention, intervention, and support on the person before pregnancy. New insights regarding the importance of embryonic and

J. Shawe (✉)
Faculty of Health, School of Nursing and Midwifery, University of Plymouth, Plymouth, UK
e-mail: jill.shawe@plymouth.ac.uk

E. A. P. Steegers
Department of Obstetrics and Gynaecology, Erasmus MC - Sophia Children's Hospital, Rotterdam, The Netherlands

S. Verbiest
Center for Maternal and Infant Health, UNC School of Medicine, Chapel Hill, NC, USA

Jordan Institute for Families, School of Social Work, University of North Carolina at Chapel Hill, Chapel Hill, NC, USA

© Springer Nature Switzerland AG 2020
J. Shawe et al. (eds.), *Preconception Health and Care: A Life Course Approach*,
https://doi.org/10.1007/978-3-030-31753-9_1

early placental health across the life course as well as the recognition that current pregnancy-related care, starting at the of the first trimester or later, is not sufficient point toward a need to broaden the timeframe in which intervention and services are provided. As described in Chapter 1 by Verbiest, the word itself—"preconception"—has been both narrowly and broadly defined over the past two decades. While the concept of preconception has had some controversy, the underlying premise that people's health matters in and of itself, regardless of pregnancy intention, represents an important paradigm shift.

This work is also built on the construct of life course theory, which centers a person in the context of their family, friends, neighborhood, community, country, and history. Life course approaches recognize a person's key stages of development from birth to old age and seek opportunities across this continuum to intervene, shifting the life trajectory in the best direction possible. This approach elevates the interconnected nature of relationships, experiences, and opportunities and the impact of those factors on well-being and health over time. Life course forces attention on the many factors that can influence an individual's behavior, underscoring the need for multifactorial, multi-sector approaches to complex issues such as nutrition, weight, stress, and violence. Efforts to just "inform" a person about what they should do to change a behavior have long been shown to be inadequate without aligning that information with actionable strategies within a supportive environment.

This book is grounded on values of equity and reproductive justice. Sister Song, Women of Color Reproductive Justice Collective (SisterSong n.d.), defines reproductive justice as *the human right to maintain personal bodily autonomy, have children, not have children, and parent the children we have in safe and sustainable communities.* Equity is intrinsic in reproductive justice underscoring the fact that indigenous women, women of color, transgender people, and women in minority groups across the globe have and continue to experience discrimination and marginalization leading to unacceptable differences in health and well-being for themselves and families. A rights framework underscores that people should have full access to all methods around reproduction—from infertility treatment to contraceptive methods, abortion, and safe and respectful birth. This means that preventive services should be offered to everyone, not just in the context of pregnancy, and that people have the full ability to act as they wish in response to the health information they receive. Finally, this framework highlights the stress of giving birth to a child who by the color or his/her skin or ethnicity of family is at risk for violence and unfair treatment.

Preconception health, when broadly defined and applied with an equity lens, has the potential to remediate past inequity and model a new path. Likewise, preconception care, if not approached carefully and in partnership with the people described above, also holds the potential to cause greater harm and widen disparities. Women should be trusted to make their own decisions and have the autonomy and needed resources to act on their own best interests, as they see them to be. In times of scarce resources, a focus on equity also means shifting programs and supports to center and serve the people with the poorest outcomes and least access.

Over time science has begun to identify the role of men's health in that of their future offspring. This is critical work as it disrupts thinking that may place "blame" on women alone for reproductive outcomes and provides an opportunity for men to also receive preventive services. While still incomplete, this book seeks to describe the research that is available. Men's role in healthy reproductive is important as is the role they play in lifting up the health and well-being of the women in their lives. Chapter 11 by Waelput and de Graaf on the impact of violence on women's well-being underscores the importance of engaging men in addressing and preventing harm.

Language is very important, and this book tries to shift away from the use of "maternal" and "paternal" to "woman" and "man" where possible. This focus on male and female, however, neglects the experience of gender non-binary and transgender individuals. As much as we have worked on language, we recognize imperfections and aim to continually transform this work.

With this backdrop in mind, this collective work aims to provide an update on the most current preconception research and care recommendations. Each chapter was constructed to provide the basic epidemiology of the particular aspect of preconception health and care it is addressing, followed by information about the latest recommendations and strategies for practice. While authors focus primarily on the information that is known, they also elevate areas that require further exploration and investment. The contributing authors bring a wealth of diverse experience and training to this work, representing expertise from eight countries. We are grateful for the considerable time and effort they committed to this collective project.

Chapter 1 by Verbiest begins the book with an overview of preconception health, including the contents of care, a brief history of the movement, and the challenges and opportunities therein. Walani and Moley continue the conversation in Chapter 12 by discussing strategies from across the globe for addressing preconception health. Chapter 13 by Verbiest, Shawe, and Steegers offers a series of directions for consideration in collectively advancing this work.

Chapter 2 by Hoek, Schonemakers, Steegers-Theunissen, and Sinclair takes a cellular look at epigenetics and the influence of exposures on early fetal development. Cornel, Goodman, and Henneman expand the discussion in Chapter 3 to genetics and the importance of providing people with information as they contemplate reproduction. Chapter 4 by Delbaere deepens the discussion by focusing on key issues around fertility, family planning, and reproductive life planning.

Chapters 5–10 focus on different components of preconception health and care. Steegers-Theunissen spotlights the role of nutrition in supporting healthy development for women and men as well as for future children in Chapter 5. This discussion is continued by Bogaerts and Devlieger in Chapter 6 which focuses on the intersection of weight and health across two generations. Chapter 7 by Shawe takes on the challenging topics of tobacco use, alcohol consumption, misuse of prescription medications, use of other substances that are illegal and unregulated (e.g., street drugs), and behavioral health. Neff and Hunt then move the content to consider prevention of, assessment for, and management of chronic diseases and their influence on the health of young adults and future children. Coonrad and Bailey describe a variety of infectious diseases and their potential impact on the health of adults and infants. Chapter 10 shifts to a review of occupational and environmental exposures that should be considered in the context of health equity and intergenerational transmission.

The challenge and opportunity for the field of preconception health/preventive care are the wide range of possible areas for screening, treatment, risk reduction, and social change! As this movement has grown from a simplistic approach to the recognition of the many complexities, we hope that practitioners, policy makers, researchers, community leaders, activities, and young adults own and build this work to achieve a collective higher goal of advancing healthy life courses for people at all stages of life.

Reference

SisterSong. Reproductive justice. n.d. https://www.sistersong.net/reproductive-justice

Preconception Health: An Overview

Sarah Verbiest

2.1 Introduction

Preconception health recognizes that the health and well-being of a woman is foundational to her life course as well as to that of any children she may have. Growing evidence is expanding this understanding to include the role that men's health plays in birth outcomes as well. For many people, becoming a parent is an important life goal. Preconception health science and programs create an important opportunity for couples to maximize the likelihood that they can realize this dream and that their child will be healthy. Seen as an intergenerational benefit, the content of preconception health is comprehensive, the messaging can be difficult, and some of the needed interventions are complex. However, opportunities with a potential two-generation benefit deserve attention from health-care providers, public health advocates, community leaders, funders, researchers, families, and local and national governments and policy-makers.

According to the World Health Organization (2013a), the Centers for Disease Control and Prevention (Robbins et al. 2014) preconception health is an important opportunity for primary prevention of maternal and infant mortality and morbidity, including unwanted pregnancies, pregnancy complications, infertility, stillbirths, birth defects, low birth weight, underweight and stunting, vertical transmission of sexually transmitted infections, lower risk of some forms of childhood cancer, and lower risk of type 2 diabetes and cardiovascular disease later in life. For many years, prenatal care was considered to be the antidote for poor perinatal outcomes. As time continued, however, it became clear that a 9-month antenatal window for

S. Verbiest (✉)
Center for Maternal and Infant Health, UNC School of Medicine, Chapel Hill, NC, USA

Jordan Institute for Families, School of Social Work, University of North Carolina at Chapel Hill, Chapel Hill, NC, USA
e-mail: sarah_verbiest@med.unc.edu

© Springer Nature Switzerland AG 2020
J. Shawe et al. (eds.), *Preconception Health and Care: A Life Course Approach*,
https://doi.org/10.1007/978-3-030-31753-9_2

intervention (which is often only 6 months by the time a woman begins care) while important is inadequate for ameliorating factors that influence fetal growth and development and healthy maternal outcomes.

As discourse on the topic of preconception has evolved, advocates have expanded the conversation to consider care in the context of the larger community and policy environment, to identify the underlying roots of disparities, and to highlight the critical interplay of autonomy, true choice, and the social determinants of health and equity. Life course theory was introduced in 2003 by Lu and Halfon (Lu and Halfon 2003) as a framework for the field of maternal and child health to structure understanding and interventions. This theory describes the interconnections, interdependence, and dynamic interactions across time and space of persons and their environments (Verbeist n.d.). Life course identifies sensitive periods of time in development where attention to protective factors and reduction of risks can have a significant impact. In this model, preconception health is such a period where the well-being of the woman and her future child become interwoven. Equally important, life course can be used to demonstrate the way disparities in health outcomes and life trajectories happen as some people experience barriers to well-being that are carried forward into the next generation.

This chapter will set the stage for readers in understanding the various dimensions of preconception health. Content includes a discussion about definitions, a brief review of the history of the movement, an overview of the components of preconception care, and a discussion about the challenges and opportunities inherent in this work.

2.2   Definitions

The most commonly used meaning of the word preconception is a woman's health before she becomes pregnant. Preconception care is usually defined as a set of interventions that aim to identify and modify biomedical, behavioral, and social risks to a woman's health or pregnancy outcome through prevention and management (Johnson et al. 2006). Table 2.1 provides a number of terms and their definitions that are used by different groups in the context of talking about this topic. The word "preconception" itself presents challenges to the work and larger movement. Language matters, as does the way in which words are interpreted and used. This word has been applied in ways that are both precise and expansive. Some professionals and advocates may use the term as a focus specifically on steps taken 3 months prior to conception to improve fetal development, while others may use the term synonymously with women's health. For example, the Centers for Disease Control and Prevention highlights that "Preconception health and health care focuses on taking steps now to protect the health of a baby in the future. However, preconception health is important for all women and men, whether or not they plan to have a baby one day." (Centers for Disease Control and Prevention 2019a) The field struggles with the cognitive dissonance between the use of a word that by definition connotes a connection with pregnancy and yet by its use is meant to imply a full array of care for women.

Table 2.1 Key definitions

Preconception	The period of time before the fertilization of an ovum
Pre-pregnancy	This is a term that is sometimes used in place of preconception as it is considered to be easier for the general public to understand. It refers to the period of time before a person becomes pregnant
Preconception health (Centers for Disease Control and Prevention 2019b)	The health of women and men during their reproductive years, which are the years they can become pregnant. All women and men can benefit from preconception health, whether or not they plan to have a baby 1 day. Part of preconception health is about people getting and staying healthy overall, throughout their lives
Interconception	This is the provision of preconception care in between the birth of one child and the conception of the next child
Preconception care (Johnson et al. 2006; Centers for Disease Control and Prevention 2019b; World Health Organization 2013b)	The provision of biomedical, behavioral, and social health interventions to women and couples before conception occurs, aimed at improving their health status and reducing behaviors and individual and environmental factors that could contribute to poor maternal and child health outcomes Preconception care is defined as a set of interventions that aim to identify and modify biomedical, behavioral, and social risks to a woman's health or pregnancy outcome through prevention and management *Preconception health care* is the medical care a woman or man receives from the doctor or other health professionals that focuses on the parts of health that have been shown to increase the chance of having a healthy baby Preconception education includes information for the general population about reproductive and the influences on early fetal development as well as information for people about their own health and care prior to conception
Women's health (Gale Encyclopedia of Medicine n.d.; MedlinePlus 2018)	Women's health refers to the branch of medicine that focuses on the treatment and diagnosis of diseases and conditions that affect a woman's physical and emotional well-being Women's health is the effect of gender on disease and health that encompasses a broad range of biological and psychosocial issues
Reproductive health (United Nation Population Fund 2016)	Reproductive health refers to the diseases, disorders, and conditions that affect the functioning of the male and female reproductive systems during childbearing years Good sexual and reproductive health is a state of complete physical, mental, and social well-being in all matters relating to the reproductive system. It implies that people are able to have a satisfying and safe sex life, the capability to reproduce, and the freedom to decide if, when, and how often to do so
Reproductive justice (SisterSong n.d.)	The human right to maintain personal bodily autonomy, have children, not have children, and parent the children we have in safe sustainable communities

(continued)

Table 2.1 (continued)

Health equity (World Health Organization n.d.)	Equity is the absence of avoidable, unfair, or remediable differences among groups of people, whether those groups are defined socially, economically, demographically, or geographically or by other means of stratification "Health equity" or "equity in health" implies that ideally everyone should have a fair opportunity to attain their full health potential and that no one should be disadvantaged from achieving this potential Providing equal care, the same care to everyone, does not always lead to equity as some groups may need additional support and resources to achieve the same outcomes as those who may be more privileged
Health disparity (Orgera and Artiga 2020)	A health disparity refers to a higher burden of illness, injury, disability, or mortality experienced by one group relative to another. This measures the difference in outcomes or experiences across different groups
Women's health equity	This has the same meaning as health equity with a particular emphasis on closing disparities for women, especially marginalized women

A further complication is the lack of resonance that the word "preconception" has among women. Some women simply do not understand what it means, while others take offense at the notion that their health may only matter in the context of a conception! The term pre-pregnancy is clear in its intent, but does not resonate with women who do not want to become pregnant but would benefit from preconception health-related interventions. On the other hand, for people who are trying to conceive and want to have a child, the idea of pre-pregnancy may offer a window of opportunity for extra motivation to make positive lifestyle changes, which may have lifelong benefits for them as well as future offspring.

In 2018, the Lancet published a series of articles about preconception health. In this work, the authors offered three concepts of preconception health, each offering different approaches to interventions. This work offers another way of considering language in this space.

> First, the biological perspective of preconception ranges from weeks to days before embryo development. Second, the individual perspective is linked to the intention to conceive and has a timeframe of weeks to months before pregnancy. And third, the public health perspective includes all women of childbearing age and their partners. Interventions at a public health level will usually take months to years to have an effect. (Barker et al. 2018)

The word preconception and the messages around may be interpreted as a pronatalist or pro baby movement—women seen as vessels instead of as important in and of themselves. While the work since its inception has repeatedly highlighted the importance of women's health, the word "preconception" and the construct can feel suspicious or patriarchal. This can be particularly true for marginalized women whose fertility and reproduction has been subjected to external control in the past (and sometimes present). The World Health Organization's 2012 report cautioned:

Preconception care could be misused to limit the autonomy of women and to undermine their rights. A strong focus on preconception care could run the risk of defining girls as being in a preconception state even before their menarche, and women as being in a preconception state for the entire duration of their fertile period. This could lead to women being: barred from participating in situations and taking up work in some areas on the grounds that it would increase the risk of adverse maternal and child health outcomes; vilified or even prosecuted for their conduct, such as for smoking or drinking alcohol.

Further, an emphasis on preconception care could reinforce the notion that the focus of all efforts to improve the health of girls and women should be at improving maternal and child health outcomes rather than at improving the health of girls and women as individuals in their own right. In addition, blanket approaches to preconception care could be seen to imply that all girls and women will inevitably become mothers. Every effort must be made to prevent preconception care efforts from harming girls and women. (World Health Organization 2013a)

Currently, there is energy in moving toward embracing the larger vision of women's health or reproductive health or justice as a better term as these words seem more aligned with a life course and equity focus. At the same time, clinicians underscore that some recommendations particularly around medications and treatments differ in the context of the woman's desire to become pregnant. Many of the contributing authors for this book have focused their recommendations more specifically on the impact of certain conditions, risks, and treatments within the context of providing care to a woman or couple who may be interested in becoming pregnant.

2.3 History

The push to shift the perinatal paradigm from a singular focus on pregnancy to a broader approach that encompasses a woman and man's health before conception has been underway for decades. Freda, Moos, and Curtis (Freda et al. 2006) published an excellent summary of the history of the movement in the United States in 2006. They note that the first federal position paper to reference the concept of pre-pregnancy care was published in 1979, with a focus on interconceptional care (US Department of Health, Education and Welfare (PHS) HAS/BCHS 1979). Six years later, in 1985, the Institute of Medicine (IOM) published a report on *Preventing Low Birthweight* and emphasized the importance of pre-pregnancy risk identification, counseling and risk reduction, and health education (Institute of Medicine 1985). In this report, the IOM advocated that family planning services should be considered central to this care. They also recommended that the content of reproductive health education, particularly in schools and family planning settings, be expanded to introduce concepts of pre-pregnancy wellness. The third recommendation of the Committee was to develop the idea of preconception consultation to identify and reduce risks associated with poor pregnancy outcomes, particularly for women who had already experienced a poor outcome.

The first Guidelines for Perinatal Care published in 1983 indicated that *when pregnancy is contemplated, the preconception visit should be part of a comprehensive gynecologic examination, and the history should include a detailed family history including ethnic background as well as investigation of lifestyle issues, religion, the home and work environments, hobbies, pets, immunizations, medications and dietary habits* (Brann and Cefalo 1983). In 1985 Moos and Cefalo developed and tested the first preconception health appraisal. They also co-authored several editions of the first clinical textbook on preconception care.

In 1989, another US federally appointed committee, The Expert Panel on the Content of Prenatal Care, gave a strong endorsement to preconception health when it noted that the preconception visit may be the single most important health-care visit when viewed in the context of its effect on pregnancy (Rosen 1989).

Healthy People 2000 the National Health Promotion and Disease Prevention Objectives for the United States published in 1990 moved preconception care into a category of standard of care by setting the objective "Increase to at least 60% the proportion of primary care providers who provide age-appropriate preconception care and counseling" (p. 199). Unfortunately, the Healthy People 2010 objectives eliminated preconception health as a specific objective, focusing only on increasing the percent of women entering pregnancy with optimum levels of folic acid (National Center for Health Statistics 2012).

In 1993, the March of Dimes Birth Defects Foundation published *Toward Improving the Outcome of Pregnancy: The 90s and Beyond* which introduced the concept of "reproductive awareness" as the basic health promotion strategy needed to improve pregnancy outcomes (Berns 2011). The American College of Obstetricians and Gynecologists (ACOG) published their first professional guidelines on preconception health in 1995 (American College of Obstetricians and Gynecologists 1995). These guidelines importantly noted that focusing only on women planning a pregnancy would leave women with unintended pregnancies at risk, highlighting that these women were already at a higher risk for poor outcomes than women who planned a pregnancy. This work recommended that routine visits by women of reproductive age was important. This point was underscored in the 2002 fifth edition of their Guidelines for Perinatal Care, which emphasized the integration of preconception health promotion into all health encounters during a woman's reproductive years (American Academy of Pediatrics 2002). An ACOG Committee Opinion on The Importance of Preconception Care in the Continuum of Women's Health Care was created in September 2005 and reaffirmed in 2017. ACOG published new pre-pregnancy guidelines in 2018. Over the past several years, other organizations in the United States have established guidelines and consensus statements, including guidelines from the American Academy of Family Physicians (Wilkes 2016). In 2015 the federal Maternal and Child Health Block Grant Program (Title V) issued a National Performance Measure focused on increased the percent of women of reproductive age who received a preventive visit in the past year. This represented a monumental shift in approach to focusing one priority on women outside of pregnancy.

There have been a number of meetings globally on the topic of preconception health. There have been three National Summits in the United States and a reconvening of the Select Panel on Preconception Health in 2014. There have been four

European Congresses on Preconception Health, the most recent in September 2019. A key publication in the Netherlands was published in 2007 by the Health Council of the Netherlands which highlighted preconception care as an important part of preventive practice (Health Council of the Netherlands 2007). In 1992 in the United Kingdom, the National Health Service created guidelines promoting 400 μg of folic acid but did not include other preconception health topics. In 2015, Shawe et al. published preconception care policy, guidelines, and recommendations across six European countries, a publication that provided an important foundation for the expansion of this work. The World Health Organization organized a Summit in 2012, and there have been a series of National Birth Defects and Developmental Disabilities Conferences in Low- and Middle-Income Countries (Shawe et al. 2015). These groups have come together to share research findings, set standards, and offer recommendations to the field for advancing this work.

Life Course Theory was introduced to the maternal and child health community in 2003. While a foundational theory to fields such as social work, this was a new concept in public health. As the idea of a life course approach caught the attention of leaders across the United States, the conversations around preconception health and equity also expanded. In 2016 Verbiest, Malin, Drummonds, and Kotelchuck published a challenge to the field (Verbiest et al. 2016) suggesting four key areas for action. These include access to quality health care for all and the need to facilitate change through critical conversations about challenging issues such as poverty, racism, sexism, and immigration; the relevance of evidence-based practice in disenfranchised communities; and how institutions perpetuate inequities. The authors also suggested the importance of developing collaborative spaces in which leaders across diverse sectors can see their roles in creating equitable neighborhood conditions that ensure optimal reproductive choices and outcomes for women and their families. They also suggested that leaders engage in dialogue and action about local and national policies that address the social determinants of health and how these policies influence reproductive and early childhood outcomes (Verbiest et al. 2016). The later launch of the MCH Life Course Research Network and the publication of *Making Change Happen, Moving Life Course Theory into Action* (Verbiest 2018) provided tools and supports to leaders to lean into this approach.

The life course approach similarly gained popularity in other parts of the world with the concept of social obstetrics. Leaders at Erasmus University in the Netherlands have fully embraced this concept, building new programs on this construct. They believe that a life course approach is indispensable to advancing the preconception health movement. They reflect on the work of Lu and others by underscoring that the biological continuum starts during parental preconception gametogenesis and subsequent embryonic and fetal development and manifests throughout life. The different life course stages of each individual consecutively prepare and determine health outcomes and well-being. Intrinsically, this is not limited to a person's own lifetime as the reproductive health of couples also affects the health of future generations. Such a life course approach in obstetric and gynecological patient care provides a path toward healthy aging, with specific attention for lifestyle, prevention, and the social context. This requires a change in mindset of women's health-care providers to feel responsible not only for managing disease but also for managing health (Steegers et al. 2019).

Emerging threats such as the Zika virus brought global attention to the concept of preconception health, this time highlighting the fact that men who were exposed to the virus could transmit that to a fetus prior to conception. Zika forced the Centers for Disease Control and Prevention and other groups to provide recommendations about preconception prevention of Zika and to fund messaging and research as to how to inform couples of the potential risks of exposure and travel. Likewise, the virus illustrated the social determinants of health as it highlighted the increased risk for the virus among communities that might not have access to screens, air conditioning, and mosquito nets.

More recently attention in the United States and other countries has focused on maternal morbidity and mortality. The Global Summit on Maternal Mortality sponsored by the Health Resources and Services Administration (HRSA) in June 2018 included a focus on preconception health along with recommendations in its full 2019 report (Health Resources and Services Administration 2019), highlighting the importance of providing continuous team-based, quality, equity aligned support and use a life course model of care for women before, during, and after pregnancies. Recent calls to action to address the increasing rates of maternal mortality and morbidity, particularly for women of color, have led to a renewed focus on preconception health, this time in the context of protecting the mother from poor birth outcomes.

2.4 Key Components of Preconception Care

The World Health Organization (WHO) convened a group of global experts in 2012 to develop an evidence-based package of preconception care interventions. The basic contents of the package are described below with a few specifics from each item listed for context (World Health Organization 2013a). The full descriptions are available in the report from the 2013 Meeting to Develop a Global Consensus on Preconception Care to Reduce Maternal and Childhood Mortality and Morbidity (World Health Organization 2013b).

- **Nutritional conditions**: Screen for anemia and diabetes, iron and folic acid supplementation, salt iodization, and energy and nutrient-dense food supplementation.
- **Tobacco use**: Screen for tobacco use at all clinical visits, advising about the harm of secondhand smoke and providing advice, pharmacotherapy, and behavioral counseling services for people who wish to quit.
- **Genetic conditions**: Family history, carrier screening and testing, and appropriate treatment of genetic conditions.
- **Environmental health**: Protection from unnecessary radiation exposure in occupational, environmental, and medical settings and lead exposure. Informing women about levels of methyl mercury in fish, promoting use of improved stoves, and avoiding unnecessary pesticides.

- **Infertility/sub-fertility**: Defuse stigmatization of infertility, provide counseling for individuals/couples with unpreventable causes of infertility/subfertility, and create awareness and understanding of fertility and infertility.
- **Interpersonal violence**: Health promotion to prevent dating violence; provide age-appropriate comprehensive sexuality education that addresses gender equality, human rights, and sexual relations; and provide health-care services (including post-rape care), referral, and psychosocial support to victims of violence.
- **Too-early, unwanted, and rapid successive pregnancies**: Keep girls in school, influence cultural norms that support early marriage and coerced sex, engage men and boys to critically assess norms and practices regarding gender-based violence, and educate women and couples about the danger of short birth intervals.
- **Sexually transmitted infections**: Promote safe sex practices through individual, group, and community-based behavioral interventions, promote condom use for dual protection against STIs and unwanted pregnancies, and screen and treat STIs.
- **HIV**: Family planning, HIV counseling and testing, and provide antiretroviral therapy for prevention and pre-exposure prophylaxis.
- **Mental health**: Assess psychosocial problems; counsel, treat, and manage depression in women planning pregnancy and other women of childbearing age; and reduce economic insecurity of women.
- **Psychoactive substance use**: Screen for substance use and provide brief interventions and treatment when needed.
- **Vaccine-preventable diseases**: Vaccination against rubella, tetanus, diphtheria, and hepatitis B.
- **Female genital mutilation**: Screen women and girls for FGM to detect complications, discuss and discourage the practice, and inform women and couples about complications of FGM and access to treatment (World Health Organization 2013b).

In December 2018, the American College of Obstetricians and Gynecologists (ACOG) together with the American Society for Reproductive Medicine released a Committee Opinion on Pre-pregnancy Care (American College of Obstetricians and Gynecologists 2019). Their Pre-Pregnancy Care Guidelines are similar to those of the WHO and include:

- Pre-pregnancy counseling and services should be recognized as a core component of women's health care.
- Family planning and spacing.
- Review of medical, surgical, and psychiatric histories.
- Review of current medications.
- Review of family and genetic history.
- Immunizations.
- Infectious disease screening.
- Focus on individuals with HIV.
- Substance use assessment.

- Exposure to violence, intimate partner violence, and reproductive and sexual coercion.
- Assess nutritional status.
- Achieving and maintaining a healthy body weight.
- Assess exercise and physical activity.
- Assess for teratogens and environmental and occupational exposures.

ACOG also encourages providers to work with women to create a reproductive health plan that should be discussed in a nondirective way at each visit and should include conversations about contraception, fertility, and thoughts about future pregnancy as appropriate (American College of Obstetricians and Gynecologists 2005). Guidelines established by other groups are in alignment with those described above. In Europe, Shawe et al. identified and reviewed the preconception health recommendations across six countries. They found that all of the countries had guidelines for women with chronic diseases but fragmented and inconsistent guidelines for health women and men (Shawe et al. 2015).

Paying attention to emerging threats such as the Zika virus is also critical. Overall, the content of preconception care is comprehensive and includes preventive care that is important overall for the health, well-being, and productivity of young adults. Specialist care is important for people with chronic conditions and health risks. The following chapters in this book will describe the epidemiology, evidence, and recommendations across these various topics.

2.5   Challenges

While there is general agreement about the content of care, there are a number of challenges, which have made it difficult for countries and health-care systems to realize the benefits of this care. None of these barriers are insurmountable—recognizing the challenges paves the way for the development of better strategies to achieve population health goals.

First, as described above, there are many potential risks and interventions to be addressed. This may be a daunting list to cover in a single visit and can be overwhelming to providers and patients. Grouping topics into categories is one proposed strategy. Screening instruments and assessments (electronic and paper) have been used to help women (and men in the future) consider their own needs and identify areas where they would like additional advice and services. More research is needed to develop best practice approaches to screening, including how to circumvent potential provider and system bias. Ideally, health-care systems would be designed so young adults would have consistent preventive care from childhood through old age so that their providers have good records and can therefore be better prepared to support them across the life course, including as they begin thinking about becoming parents.

Public health messaging and campaigns on preconception health are challenged by the need to educate women and men about a wide range of topics many of which may not be relevant to particular people (e.g., tobacco messages are important but irrelevant to people who don't smoke). Further, women's fertility can cover over three decades of life. Marketing strategies that reach women who are 18 are often different from those that work for women who are in their 30s. Women's needs and health change over time as the consider parenthood. Layer this with the importance of creating actionable messages that are culturally and linguistically relevant to a wide audience and the scope of work is considerable. Further, messages that point out potential risks, such as environmental exposures, but do not offer resources and supports to address them may create stress that is harmful and not productive. Finally, just telling people to "do this" or "don't do that" is not effective. Some people may not have the resources to follow the instructions, and others need to hear the messages from providers who understand trauma and have skills such as motivational interviewing. More work is needed to identify best practices and to redesign health-care encounters and related community supports to enable young adults to access their healthiest lives.

Preconception health messages also run the potential of making women feel ashamed, blamed, and guilty, particularly in the context of a poor pregnancy outcome and/or child health problems. Mother guilt is rampant being both self-imposed and reinforced wittingly or not by messages that imply oversimplistic connections between a woman's actions and her child's well-being. An easy conception and a healthy pregnancy and child are never a guarantee. The vast majority of parents would do whatever they could for their child's well-being. People with chronic conditions and risks also deserve the right to have a family. As such, messages must be carefully crafted and tested to build on a person's strengths and provide information that is grounded in the reality of people's lives. In fact, if health information is to be heard and acted upon, attention should be paid to how it makes people feel, with a focus on strengths and the acknowledgement that poor birth outcomes are often the result of multiple factors that may not be in a person's control. Further, professionals should continually work to strengthen the environments in which people work, eat, sleep, play, and pray so that everyone is well.

Some of the service, messaging, and even billing concerns would be easier to address if the majority of couples planned for pregnancy. Preconception health-care visits and even "get ready to get pregnant" programs would be available to help couples who would be likely motivated by a desire for a healthy child. For the couples who are thinking ahead about starting a family, there is a need to have evidence-based programs to support them in their goals. Since preconception-specific visits are not common, many providers may not be adequately prepared to provide this care. Further, couples with limited access to resources may be frustrated in their desire to follow recommendations absent other community supports.

While a simple concept—pregnancy planning—almost half of all pregnancies globally are considered unintended. In reality, the idea of planning for a pregnancy is very complex as described in Chap. 4. As such, programs that only focus on people planning a pregnancy will miss important audiences and could increase disparities in health outcomes if not done carefully. Further, the population of couples trying to achieve pregnancy can be difficult to reach for preconception care. First, most people are not aware that their health status before pregnancy can influence the health of the woman and baby during and after pregnancy. As such, they do not know to seek such care. For other couples, the top priority is getting and staying pregnant. Anxiety related to possible risks, the desire for privacy, and the feeling of a kind of taboo on being outspoken on their pregnancy wish can serve as barriers to seeking services. More research is needed to identify the reasons couples do or do not access preconception care use and to understand facilitators and barriers to care. There is still a lack of knowledge on the efficacy of outreach strategies.

2.6   Opportunities

While the work ahead is not simple, the potential rewards for improving the health and well-being of young adults are significant—for both current and future generations. The cost savings of averting future chronic disease alone make a strong case for investing in preventive care for people of reproductive age. Preconception health provides an opportunity for a system paradigm shift from episodic and sick care to preventive care across the life course. Currently, health-care programs tend to focus on providing care to children, particularly from birth through grade school years, young adults when they seek family planning services or care for sickness or injuries, prenatal care, chronic disease, and cancer care, with a significant investment in care for the elderly. In its essence, in order to improve birth outcomes from generation to generation, people need access to quality care and services across all stages of development.

Traditionally, reproductive care is focused on women largely in the context of pregnancy (or prevention of pregnancy). As a pregnancy advances so does the number of health-care visits followed by significant attention at labor and delivery. Support for new mothers then fall off significantly in some countries such as the United States, where women are not seen again until 6–8 weeks after giving birth. Many women receive intermittent health care during their reproductive years, largely seeking services due to illness. Movements around preconception, postpartum, and interconception care offer a sort of patchwork to the system that demands that women receive care outside of the context of being pregnant. To fully realize population health, there is a need for consistent preventive services across the life course with potentially more intensive care for people who have greater health needs.

Research and programs that approach this topic from a life course perspective can shift the narrative from basic cause and effect thinking to more complex and realistic systems thinking that consider the person in the context of their family, community, and country. Recognizing that each stage of life lays the building blocks for the next stage supports a focus on prevention and wellness. Further, life course approaches consider the role that education, economic mobility, healthy relationships, the environment, and safe communities play in young adult well-being and productivity, the health of their children, and even longer-term chronic disease trajectories for both parent and child. As public health and health-care professionals are recognizing the impact that the social determinants of health have on a person or population's ability to be well, resources and attention should be focused on the conditions that support well-being.

An intentional approach to preconception health holds the potential to significantly reduce health disparities (Fleur et al. 2016) and remediate past harms (Verbiest et al. 2016). Life course models how different risk and protective factors can lead to some groups to benefiting over others over time. Centering the experiences of people who experience health disparities and prioritizing research and resource allocation accordingly while attending to provider and community bias and racism can shift population health trajectories. The life course model calls for building evidence-based community interventions that create healthier living environments, including access to safe places to exercise and play, affordable healthy food, toxic-free homes and workplaces, access to education, and economic opportunity. This shifts some of the responsibility for health from the individual to communities and the larger systems within which they are nested.

Finally, identifying the role that men's health and the quality of their sperm plays in reproductive outcomes offers an emerging opportunity for shifting away from a singular focus on women's behaviors. This is long overdue as men's participation in fatherhood and parenting is essential. The chapter authors in this book describe the current science as it pertains to men's preconception health—more research is needed in this arena.

2.7   Conclusion

At its simplest construct, preconception health expands the point of interventions to improve birth outcomes from a laser focus on (and investment in) pregnancy to a broader understanding of the contributors to healthy outcomes for women and their babies—a couple's health before conception plays a role in the health of the child they hope to have. This simple fact is one that all people have a right to know. Reproductive justice underscores that people both have a right to know the factors that could influence the health of their future child and the right to act on those factors, or not. As described, preconception health can also be a politically charged, complex topic. Figure 2.1 offers a snapshot of the many ways people may view this topic.

Regardless of the complexity, preconception health is a frontier that deserves continued exploration. The 2012 World Health Organization report offers a succinct summary of the potential that preconception health holds:

> From the perspective of health outcomes, in the short-term preconception care could reduce pregnancies that are too early, pregnancies that are too close, and unplanned pregnancies. Preconception care could contribute to reducing the risk of genetic disorders and environmental exposure, to reducing maternal and childhood mortality, and to improving maternal and child health outcomes. It could also contribute to improving the health and well-being of women in other areas of public health, such as nutrition, infertility and subfertility, mental health, intimate partner and sexual violence, and substance use.

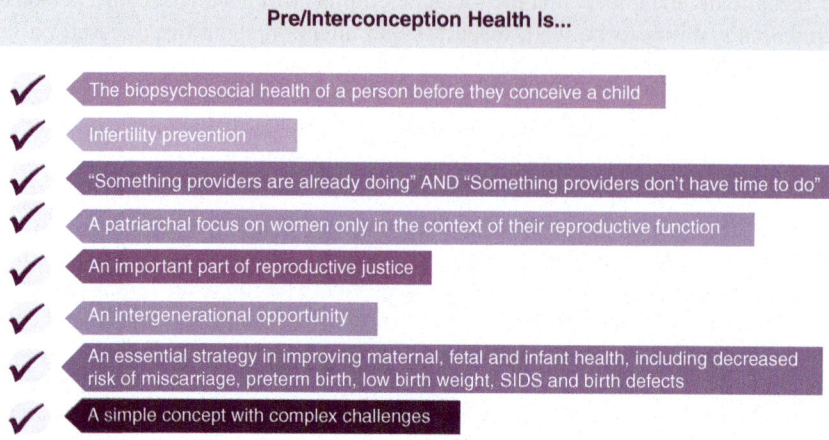

Fig. 2.1 The complexities and opportunities of preconception health

In the long term, preconception care could contribute to improving the health of babies and children as they grow into adolescence and adulthood. By supporting women to make well-informed and well-considered decisions about their fertility and their health, preconception care could contribute to the social and economic development of families and communities. By creating awareness of the importance of men's health and men's behaviours on maternal and child health outcomes, and by promoting male involvement, preconception care could result in additional benefits. From the programmatic perspective, preconception care provides a window to include interventions that have not traditionally been included in maternal, newborn and child health programmes, such as reduction in use of and exposure to tobacco. (World Health Organization 2013b)

Preconception and interpregnancy care are components of a larger health-care goal—optimizing the health of every person of reproductive age and the communities where they live—to assure intergenerational benefits and a healthier society.

References

American Academy of Pediatrics. American College of Obstetricians and Gynecologists. Guidelines for perinatal care. 5th ed. Elk Grove Village, IL: American Academy of Pediatricians; 2002.

American College of Obstetricians and Gynecologists. ACOG technical bulletin preconception care number 205. Int J Gynaecol Obstet. 1995;50(2):201–7. https://doi.org/10.1016/0020-7292(95)90357-7.

American College of Obstetricians and Gynecologists. ACOG Committee Opinion #313: the importance of preconception care in the continuum of women's health care. Obstet Gynecol. 2005;106(3):665–6. https://doi.org/10.1097/00006250-200509000-00052.

American College of Obstetricians and Gynecologists. ACOG Committee Opinion No. 762: pregnancy counseling. Obstet Gynecol. 2019;133(1):e78–89. https://doi.org/10.1097/AOG.0000000000003013.

Barker M, Dombrowski SU, Colbourn T, Fall CHD, Kriznik NM, Lawrence WT, et al. Intervention strategies to improve nutrition and health behaviors before conception. Lancet. 2018;391:1853–18. https://doi.org/10.1016/S0140-6736(18)30313-1.

Berns SD, editor. Toward improving the outcome of pregnancy III: enhancing perinatal health through quality, safety and performance initiatives. Reissued edition. In: Medical Resources. March of Dimes Foundation. 2011. https://www.marchofdimes.org/professionals/toward-improving-the-outcome-of-pregnancy-iii.aspx. Accessed 12 Oct 2019.

Brann AW, Cefalo RC. American Academy of Pediatrics, American College of Obstetricians and Gynecologists. Guidelines for perinatal care. American Academy of Pediatrics: Evanston, IL; 1983.

Centers for Disease Control and Prevention. Preconception Health and Health Care. In: Before Pregnancy. Centers for Disease Control and Prevention. 2019a. https://www.cdc.gov/preconception/index.html. Accessed 28 Aug 2019.

Centers for Disease Control and Prevention. Overview. In: Before pregnancy. Centers for Disease Control and Prevention. 2019b. https://www.cdc.gov/preconception/overview.html. Accessed 28 Aug 2019.

Fleur M, Damus K, Jack B. The future of preconception care in the United States: multigenerational impact on reproductive outcomes. Ups J Med Sci. 2016;121(4):211–5. https://doi.org/10.1080/03009734.2016.1206152.

Freda MC, Moos M, Curtis M. The history of preconcpetion care: evolving guidelines and standards. Maternal Child Health J. 2006;10:43–52. https://doi.org/10.1007/s10995-006-0087-x.

Gale Encyclopedia of Medicine. Women's health. In: The free dictionary. (n.d.). https://medical-dictionary.thefreedictionary.com/women%27s+health. Accessed 28 Aug 2019.

Health Council of the Netherlands. Preconception care: a good beginning. In: Health Council of the Netherlands. The Hague. 2007. https://www.healthcouncil.nl/documents/advisory-reports/2007/09/20/preconception-care-a-good-beginning. Accessed by 12 Oct 2019.

Health Resources and Services Administration. U.S. Department of Health and Human Services. HRSA Maternal Mortality Summit: Promising Global Practices to Improve Maternal Health Outcomes Technical Report. In: Maternal Health. Health Resources & Services Administration. 2019. https://www.hrsa.gov/sites/default/files/hrsa/maternal-mortality/Maternal-Mortality-Technical-Report.pdf. Accessed 28 Aug 2019.

Institute of Medicine. Preventing low birthweight. Washington, DC: The National Academies Press; 1985. https://doi.org/10.17226/511.

Johnson K, Posner SF, Biermann J, Cordero JF, Atrash HK, Parker CS, et al. Recommendations to improve preconception health and health care—United States: a report of the CDC/ATSDR Preconception Care Work Group and the Select Panel on Preconception Care. Recommendation and Reports Vol. 55, No. RR-6. In: Morbidity and Mortality Weekly Report (MMWR). Centers for Disease Control and Prevention. 2006. https://www.cdc.gov/mmwr/pdf/rr/rr5506.pdf. Accessed 28 Aug 2019.

Lu MC, Halfon N. Racial and ethnic disparities in birth outcomes: a life-course perspective. Maternal Child Health J. 2003;7:13–30. https://doi.org/10.1023/a:1022537516969.

MedlinePlus. Women's health. In: MedlinePlus. National Library of Medicine (US). 2018. https://medlineplus.gov/ency/article/007458.htm. Accessed 28 Aug 2019.

National Center for Health Statistics. Healthy people 2010 final review. In: National Center for Health Statistics. Centers for Disease Control. 2012. https://www.cdc.gov/nchs/data/hpdata2010/hp2010_final_review.pdf. Accessed 12 Oct 2019.

Orgera K, Artiga S. Disparities in health and health care: five key questions and answers. Kasier Family Foundation. 2020. https://www.kff.org/disparities-policy/issue-brief/disparities-in-health-and-health-care-five-key-questions-and-answers/. Accessed 12 Oct 2019.

Robbins CL, Zapata LB, Farr SL, Kroelinger CD, Morrow B, Ahluwalia I et al. Core state preconception health indicators—pregnancy risk assessment monitoring system and behavioral risk factor surveillance system, 2009. Surveillance Summaries Vol. 63, No. 3. In: Morbidity and Mortality Weekly Report (MMWR). Centers for Disease Control and prevention. 2014. http://beforeandbeyond.org/wp-content/uploads/2018/05/ss6303.pdf. Accessed 28 Aug 2019.

Rosen MG. Caring for our future, the content of prenatal care: a report of the Public Health Service Expert Panel on the Content of Prenatal Care. Washington, DC: Public Health Service. Department of Health and Human Services; 1989.

Shawe J, Delbaere I, Ekstrand M, Hegaard HK, Larsson M, Mastroiacovo P, et al. Preconception care policy, guidelines, recommendations and services across six European countries: Belgium (Flanders), Denmark, Italy, the Netherlands, Sweden and the United Kingdom. Eur J Contracept Reprod Health Care. 2015;20(2):77–87. https://doi.org/10.3109/13625187.2014.990088.

SisterSong. Reproductive justice. n.d. https://www.sistersong.net/reproductive-justice. Accessed 28 Aug 2019.

Steegers EAP, Fauser BCJM, Hilders CGJM, Jaddoe VWV, Massuger LFAG, van der Post JAM, et al., editors. Textbook of Obstetrics and Gynecology: a life course approach. 1st ed. Cham: Springer Publishing; 2019.

United Nation Population Fund. Sexual and reproductive health. UNDP. 2016. https://www.unfpa.org/sexual-reproductive-health/. Accessed 28 Aug 2019.

US Department of Health, Education and Welfare (PHS) HAS/BCHS. Primary care effectiveness—an approach to clinical quality assurance in BCHS programs and projects. Washington, DC: US Department of Health, Education and Welfare (PHS) HAS/BCHS; 1979.

Sarah Verbeist. Chapter 1. n.d. p. 1.

Verbiest S., editor. Moving life course theory into action: making change happen. Washington, DC: American Public Health Association; 2018. doi:https://doi.org/10.2105/9780875532967.

Verbiest S, Malin CK, Drummonds M, Kotelchuck M. Catalyzing a reproductive health and social justice movement. Maternal Child Health J. 2016;20:741. https://doi.org/10.1007/s10995-015-1917-5.

Wilkes J. AAFP Releases Position Paper on Preconception Care. In: Practice Guidelines. Am Fam Physician. 2016;94(6):508–10.

World Health Organization. Department of Maternal, Newborn, Child and Adolescent Health. Preconception care: maximizing the gains of maternal and child health. In: Early child development—preconception care. 2013a. https://www.who.int/maternal_child_adolescent/documents/preconception_care_policy_brief.pdf?ua=1. Accessed 28 Aug 2019.

World Health Organization. Meeting to develop a global consensus on preconception care to reduce maternal and childhood mortality and morbidity. In: Maternal, newborn, child and adolescent health. 2013b. https://www.who.int/maternal_child_adolescent/documents/concensus_preconception_care/en/. Accessed 28 Aug 2019.

World Health Organization. Health equity. In: Health topics. n.d. https://www.who.int/topics/health_equity/en/. Accessed 28 Aug 2019.

The Science of Preconception

3

Jeffrey Hoek, Régine Steegers-Theunissen, Kevin Sinclair, and Sam Schoenmakers

3.1 General Preface

The chance of a successful pregnancy and healthy offspring is largely determined by the state of maternal but also paternal health during the periconception period, which starts at least 14 weeks before conception until 10 weeks afterward (12 weeks of gestation). Massive cell multiplication, differentiation, and programming processes of gametes and (extra) embryonic tissues during these 6 months around conception mean that these tissues are particularly sensitive for genetic and/or environmental exposures. Obstetric care mostly starts only at around 8–10 weeks of gestational age with a first ultrasound scan by a midwife or obstetrician, thereby missing the opportunity of prevention and treatment of harmful exposures, in order to optimize periconception health conditions. To emphasize the importance of preconception care, this chapter gives an overview of the biology of gametogenesis, embryogenesis, and placentation as determinants of the success of pregnancy course and outcome and health of the offspring during the life course. Because achieving a healthy lifestyle is one of the most important preventive measures in preconception care, the impact of maternal as well as paternal lifestyle on outcomes largely determined in the periconception period will be discussed.

J. Hoek · R. Steegers-Theunissen · S. Schoenmakers (✉)
Department of Obstetrics and Gynecology, Erasmus MC – University Medical Centre Rotterdam, Rotterdam, The Netherlands

K. Sinclair
School of Biosciences, University of Nottingham, Nottingham, UK

© Springer Nature Switzerland AG 2020
J. Shawe et al. (eds.), *Preconception Health and Care: A Life Course Approach*,
https://doi.org/10.1007/978-3-030-31753-9_3

3.2   Introduction

In the 14 weeks before conception, future parents already contribute to the health of their yet to be conceived baby. During those weeks, the eggs and sperm, which contain hereditary (genetic) material for future offspring, mature in the gonads. Chromosomal aberrations and mutations in this genetic material but also unhealthy nutrition and lifestyle exposures can prevent the fertilization of the egg clinically presented as subfertility. However, when conception is successful, it is known that several maternal pregnancy problems and adverse birth outcomes find their origin during the first 12 weeks of pregnancy. This is important, since during this time window many women are not aware that they are pregnant and outsiders cannot see that she is pregnant. Derangements in biological processes of embryonic and placental development during these first few months of pregnancy very much determine whether the baby will have a congenital malformation and be born too early or too small and whether the mother will develop preeclampsia (high blood pressure) later in pregnancy. The fact that the prenatal environment can influence the health conditions of the offspring also later in life is known as the Developmental Origins of Health and Disease (DOHaD). An intriguing new example of this concept is that the smaller the embryo is during the first trimester of pregnancy, the higher the risk for cardiovascular problems around 6 years of age (Jaddoe et al. 2014). These children exhibit more fat deposition, higher lipid levels in blood, and a higher blood pressure. Furthermore, genes from elderly people who were in the womb during the hunger winter of 1945 in the Netherlands show variations in programming and therefore function differently.

Genetic background and environment factors, determined by external exposures of the milieu and internal maternal conditions, influence the development and growth of the baby and the placenta. Although the future father contributes half of his genes to the baby, the effect on placental and fetal growth and development are less well understood. Compared to the genetic background, general environmental factors such as air pollution and hazardous substances can be modified, as well as nutrition, lifestyle, tobacco and alcohol use, and exposure to teratogenic medications. As an example, low-dose folic acid 0.4 mg per day is recommended to start before pregnancy and to continue during the first trimester of pregnancy for the prevention of congenital malformations, in particular neural tube defects. The effect of folic acid on the development of the egg and sperm cells (gametogenesis) and embryonic and placental development is discussed in more detail below. The chance of having a baby with congenital malformations or developing placenta disorders is mainly due to a combination of genetic factors and environmental exposures. Although the genetic information is stored in the genes of the DNA (Box 3.1), the programming and expression of these genes is influenced by environmental factors. This whole process of interactions between genes and environmental factors is explained in more detail below.

> **Box 3.1 DNA**
> *DNA, which is also known as deoxyribose nucleic acid, is a large molecule composed of two chains that wind around each other to form the well-known double helix. DNA contains all the genetic information needed for development, growth, and reproduction. The specific sequences of the DNA that contain information necessary to produce proteins are called genes. The total DNA is tightly wrapped around each other and divided over several so-called chromosomes. Each nucleus of cells in the human body contains 23 pairs of these chromosomes: 22 pairs autologous chromosome and 1 pair of sex chromosomes (the Y and X chromosome, where women have 2 X chromosomes and men have 1 X chromosome and 1 Y chromosome).*

In general, due to the initial unawareness of pregnancy and relative late uptake of obstetric care, around 10 weeks of gestational age, important opportunities are missed to improve preconception and periconception health of both mothers and fathers to be. Despite current knowledge and medical innovations, the frequency of pregnancy complications for mothers and babies has remained largely the same over the years. Combined with the later health consequences during the life course and even in the next generations, these aspects emphasize the importance of optimizing all aspects of women's and men's health in the period preceding pregnancy and the first few months thereafter.

3.3 Development of the Gametes (Eggs and Sperm), Embryo, Placenta, and Fetus

3.3.1 Development of the Eggs

In women, already in the first few weeks of fetal development in the womb, all early eggs are formed from the stem cells (Fig. 3.1a). At this stage the early eggs are arrested from further cell divisions and are stored in the female gonads, the two ovaries, until they are recruited for growth from menarche onward during reproductive life. Since the eggs are formed during the first few weeks of development in the womb, the need for a healthy environment during the periconceptional phase again is emphasized. Only during the period just before the ovulation under influence of female hormones do these arrested eggs resume their cell division. Recruitment of eggs and ovulation will take place until menopause. The cell division of the eggs is completed after one sperm cell fertilizes the egg.

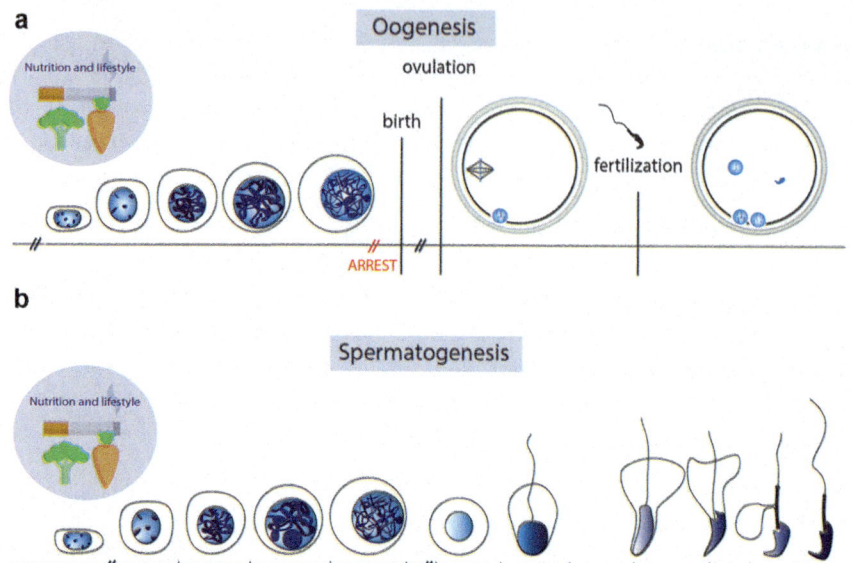

Fig. 3.1 Overview of the development of eggs and sperm. (**a**) *Development of eggs:* The process of egg development starts a couple of weeks after fertilization during the few weeks of development in the womb. At this stage the early eggs are arrested from further cell divisions and are stored in the ovary until they are recruited for growth from menarche onward during reproductive life. (**b**) *Development of sperm:* The development of sperm starts with the activation of the hormonal axis (the hypothalamic-pituitary-adrenal (HPA) axis) and the onset of puberty after which the stem cells are recruited to start their cell divisions

3.3.2 Development of the Sperm

In contrast to the development of the eggs, the cell divisions in male sperm cells do not start during the very early phases of development in the womb but the stem cells that will form the sperm are already present in the first weeks after conception. Sperm cells start to develop when the male hormonal axis becomes activated at the beginning of puberty and continues until death. Importantly, in the context of early embryonic development and paternal health, the whole process of spermatogenesis takes place within a 2- to 3-month period, which means that every 3 months there is a total renewal of sperm cells (Fig. 3.1b). This also emphasizes the need for a healthy environment during the preconception phase for men who wish to have a child, allowing optimal production and development of sperm.

1-cell embryo	2-cell	4-cell	6-cell	8-cell

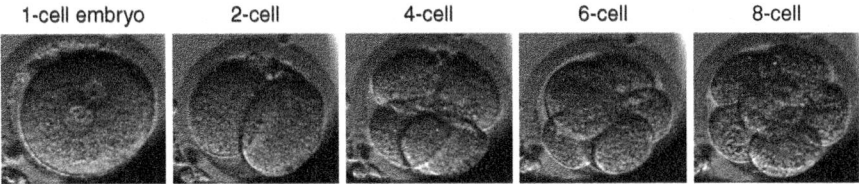

Fig. 3.2 First cell divisions of the embryo a few hours after conception showing the earliest development of the embryo. Derived from the EmbryoScope™, Vitrolife. Embryo images were automatically recorded every 10–20 min until embryo Day 3. In these 3 days, every cell divides twice until an 8-cell embryo is formed

3.3.3 Fertilization

Fertilization of the egg by one sperm cell is the first important step in the process of the development of the embryo. Directly after fertilization, the early embryo starts dividing. Between embryonic Days 3 and 5, the embryo is transported from the ovary through one of the two fallopian tubes to the uterine cavity. Around embryonic Day 5, the developing embryo reaches the uterine cavity, and at embryonic Day 7, the outer layers of the embryo invade the epithelium of the uterus, initiating implantation of the embryo. In vitro morphokinetic techniques allow the visualization of these very early embryonic cell divisions. The EmbryoScope™ is an incubator for embryos resulting from in vitro fertilization (IVF) with or without intracytoplasmic sperm injection (ICSI) and takes pictures every 10–20 min creating a developmental time-lapse movie of the preimplantation embryos (Fig. 3.2).

3.3.4 Endometrium

During each menstrual cycle, the epithelium of the uterus, called endometrium, builds up and sheds in a cyclic manner. For establishment of a viable pregnancy, this epithelium needs to be synchronized with the dividing embryo after fertilization and should be prepared for implantation of the developing embryo; this process is called endometrial receptivity. Endometrial receptivity is a complex process involving many factors such as structural, anatomical, together with a range of nutrition and lifestyle factors.

3.3.5 Development of the Embryo

After arrival in the uterus, the embryo implants and continues to develop and grow. With the advancements in three-dimensional ultrasound techniques, embryonic growth and development according to the Carnegie stages can be monitored more precisely (Rousian et al. 2018). Embryonic growth was believed to be uniform in every pregnancy and embryo, but it is now apparent that many maternal and paternal factors can influence the process of individual embryonic growth (Steegers-Theunissen et al. 2016). These factors are addressed below. Interestingly, being smaller as a baby in the first trimester of pregnancy is associated with an increased risk of being born too early, too small, and with cardiovascular risk factors at the age of 6 (Jaddoe et al. 2014).

3.3.6   Development of the Placenta

The formation of the placenta begins with the implantation of the embryo into the endometrium, a special layer in the uterus of the mother. The outer layer of a 5-day-old embryo is called the trophoblast and invades the endometrium. Blood vessels in the uterus of the mother are formed, and remodeled, due to the invading trophoblast cells. This formation and remodeling makes sure enough blood passes through the placenta, which is necessary for the exchange of gases and nutrients between mother and fetus. Impaired placental development and functioning result in abnormal formation and development of the placenta and is associated with a number of pregnancy complications for mother and baby. The most important complications are preeclampsia, a disease characterized by high blood pressure in pregnancy, preterm birth, and babies too small for gestational age (SGA).

3.3.7   Microbiome

The local environments of the male and female reproductive tracts, including the gonads, harbor an extensive amount of different microbes, which appear to be associated with reproductive success and necessary to maintain health (Koedooder et al. 2019). The relationship between human tissues and local microbes can either be beneficial and symbiotic or disadvantageous and dysbiotic (in which a state of dysbiosis is associated with inflammation and disease). Unfortunately, up until now, it is unknown how to change the local microbiome for the better or which composition of microbes is optimal. However, in women the presence of the bacteria *Lactobacillus* is associated with reproductive health and success.

3.4   Mechanisms Underlying Conception, Embryogenesis, and Placentation

The development of sperm, eggs, embryos, and placentas is influenced by individual genetic variations and aberrations in combination with environmental exposures. The genetic background or predisposition itself is set in the inherited DNA and cannot be changed. However environmental exposures like nutrition and lifestyle can be modified. The prevalence of the most harmful environmental exposures is over- and undernutrition and tobacco and social alcohol use, even in the preconception period.

Smoking is highly prevalent (approximately 25%) in men of reproductive age, whereas this is slightly lower in female population (approximately 20%). The prevalence of alcohol use preconceptionally is even higher with a prevalence of up to 90% in men and 75% of women.

3.4.1 Oogenesis (Egg Production)

The quality of the egg is associated with the future quality of the embryo and pregnancy outcomes. Examples that can influence the quality by inducing DNA damage in the eggs are smoking and alcohol. Tobacco derivatives can accumulate in the intracellular fluid of the egg and cause detrimental and unrepairable effects to DNA and cellular processes. The preconceptional phase is the most active phase of oocyte development, as eggs are recruited and activated from their dormant state. During the development of the egg, essential cellular building blocks are required, which are present in a healthy diet with a balance between micro- and macronutrients. Previous studies also showed that maternal intake of vitamins in the weeks preceding pregnancy can alter the reserve of nutrients within the oocyte (Ashworth et al. 2009). Subsequently, inadequate concentrations of vitamins in women undergoing IVF-ICSI treatment are associated with impaired oocyte quality and ultimately with impaired embryonic quality.

3.4.2 Spermatogenesis (Sperm Production)

Smoking by men of reproductive age is proven to be harmful for the stability of DNA of sperm cells (Wyck et al. 2018). This is reflected in the deterioration of sperm parameters such as concentration, motility, and abnormal morphology among smokers. These parameters determine the quality of the sperm and are therefore strongly associated with pregnancy chance and pregnancy outcomes. Smoking in men also results in a significantly longer time for a couple to achieve pregnancy. Alcohol consumption (particularly >14 units per week) can also deteriorate sperm concentration, motility, and morphology. Importantly, decreased sperm motility due to alcohol intake appears to be dose-dependent. The exact etiology of the association between decreased poor sperm quality and alcohol use is not completely understood. Direct toxicity seems to be a plausibly theory, but alcohol also interacts with, for example, the nutrient, vitamin, and hormonal status of men. Chronic abusive alcohol use is associated with decreased vitamin levels caused by, for example, poor diet and malabsorption in the intestinal system. Multiple studies investigated the effects of the B vitamin folate and trace element zinc on sperm quality (Box 3.2). Besides a decline in sperm quality, different environmental factors can also induce sperm DNA damage and reduce DNA repair and synthesis. Insufficient intake of vitamins, such as with an unhealthy diet, but also alcohol and smoking are detrimental for DNA quality, which is associated with subfertility and miscarriage. Each day millions of sperm cells are produced and then undergo final maturation in

Box 3.2 Folate and Sperm Quality
Multiple studies have shown an association between the vitamin B folate levels in blood and semen and sperm quality. Four separate randomized controlled trials (RCTs) investigated the association between oral folic acid supplement use and sperm quality. One reported a significant increase in the percentage motile sperm from 18.1% to 20.4% after 3 months of 5 mg/day folic acid supplement use. No differences were seen regarding normal morphology and concentration. A 5-month folic acid supplementation resulted in higher folate concentrations in peripheral blood but a non-significant increase in sperm quality.

preparation for ejaculation and fertilization. The production of all these million sperm cells everyday again indicates the possible vulnerable effects of day-to-day interferences and differences in paternal exposure to nutrition and lifestyle factors on spermatogenesis.

3.4.3 Fertilization

Recent research showed that the early stages of embryo development are influenced by parental nutrition and lifestyle behaviors. Smoking and alcohol use but also dieting and excessive consumption of red meat negatively influence very early embryo development, such as implantation. On the other hand, high intakes of cereals, vegetables, and fruits are positively associated with embryonic quality. Since folate and other vitamins are important for egg and sperm health, a logical consequence is that this also impacts on the success of conception, which is the subject of investigation of many studies in patients undergoing IVF-ICSI (Box 3.3).

3.4.4 Endometrium

Correct functioning of the endometrium and properly timed endometrial receptivity is a complex process of interacting hormonal, anatomical, and signaling factors but also anatomical aspects which all can be influence by nutrition and lifestyle behaviors. Smoking, for example, causes the uterine vessels to constrict induced by the presence of nicotine. This hampers optimal blood flow to the endometrium, thereby reducing the chance of embryo implantation. Alcohol use can induce menstrual disorders, decreasing the chance of achieving a pregnancy and an ongoing pregnancy. However, very little is known about the exact role of the vitamins and a healthy diet on endometrial health. Low intake of vitamins and low availability of folate and other vitamins are associated with alterations in hormonal and vascular function which might interfere with normal menstrual cycle physiology, thus affecting implantation and endometrial receptivity (Agarwal et al. 2005).

> **Box 3.3 Nutrition, lifestyle and IVF-ICSI**
> *In couples undergoing IVF-ICSI treatment, associations between folate blood levels and pregnancy rate are demonstrated. Women with folate levels in the highest tertile (>329 ng/mL) have a pregnancy chance of 40%, while women with lower folate levels have a 20% chance of pregnancy. This indicates that adequate folate levels in blood are associated with an odds ratio for pregnancy of 2.6. Furthermore strong adherence to a healthy diet, which consists of fruit, vegetables, fish, whole-wheat products, and vegetable oils and is indicative of a good vitamin status, is associated with an increased pregnancy chance after IVF-ICSI. Also, adhering to a Mediterranean diet, which contains high intakes of vegetable oils, vegetables, fish, and legumes, is strongly associated with higher folate concentrations and vitamin B6 in blood, which in turn is associated with an increased chance of pregnancy of 40%.*

3.4.5   Embryo

3.4.5.1 Maternal Influences

Embryonic growth was believed to be uniform in every pregnancy and embryo, but it is now apparent that many factors can influence individual embryonic growth. Smoking cigarettes during the periconceptional period is associated with smaller embryos in the first trimester of pregnancy in a dose-dependent manner (Van Dijk et al. 2018). Smoking of more than ten cigarettes per day results in a reduced embryonic size of 20.2% at 6 weeks of gestation and a reduction of 6.0% at 12 weeks of gestation. Smoking not only effects embryonic size but also decreases embryonic head volume and head circumference. The same effects, although of lesser magnitude, hold for alcohol use during periconceptional period. Drinking alcohol resulted in a decrease of embryonic size 2.5% at 6 weeks of gestation 2.2% at 12 weeks of gestation compared to women abstaining from alcohol consumption during pregnancy. Periconceptional folate and vitamin status of the mother is associated with first-trimester embryonic growth (van Uitert and Steegers-Theunissen 2013). Importantly, embryonic growth during the first trimester is associated with pregnancy outcomes. There also seems to be an optimum curve regarding maternal folate levels, where both excessively high and low levels are associated with smaller first-trimester embryos (van Uitert et al. 2014). Since folate and other vitamin levels are strongly associated with dietary intake, one can hypothesize that diet influences embryonic health. Indeed, pregnant women with a strong adherence to the healthy Mediterranean diet have a decreased risk of spina bifida, a serious congenital malformation of the spine, in their offspring, as comparable to women who have a low adherence to this diet. On the other hand, women adhering to an unhealthy Western diet, consisting of a high intake of meat, pizza, legumes, and potatoes, with little fruit, have an increased risk of giving rise to offspring with a cleft lip with or without a cleft palate.

3.4.5.2 Paternal Influences

Paternal influences on embryonic growth are more difficult to investigate. Since paternal smoking, for example, not only directly affects sperm quality but usually also indirectly influences the mother through passive smoking, investigations into the direct effect of paternal smoking on the embryo are hampered. Investigation of very early embryonic development before implantation using the EmbryoScope has recently revealed that paternal smoking is associated with decreased preimplantation embryo quality. The role of the paternal vitamin status is less well established, although one study found that paternal folate levels in blood were also associated with embryonic growth (Hoek et al. 2019). These results indicate that the preconceptional paternal folate status can also influence embryonic and fetal well-being and can lead to a transgenerational effect of both parental folate abnormalities.

3.4.6   Placenta

It is largely unknown to what extent periconceptional nutrition and lifestyle influences first-trimester placental development and function. It is hypothesized that the same factors influencing egg and sperm quality, fertilization, and embryonic growth also effect placental development since the placenta develops from the same embryonic origin. Placental development and growth is initiated shortly after the implantation of the embryo. A recent systematic review summarizing the unhealthy effects of diverse aspects of periconceptional maternal lifestyle on placenta development also indicates a role for endometrial quality, since endometrial receptivity is necessary for optimal implantation and trophoblast invasion (Reijnders et al. 2019). Smoking and alcohol consumption are each negatively associated with placental development, and alterations in vitamins are implicated in these effects. Periconceptional vitamin supplement use and adherence to a Mediterranean diet (which is considered highly folate rich) in the second and third trimester of pregnancy are positively associated with a more optimal blood flow to the placenta.

3.4.7   Microbiome

Necessary nutrients such as riboflavin (vitamin B2), folate, and cobalamin are not only are supplied by diet but are also synthesized by gut microbiota, as are choline, thiamin (vitamin B1), nicotinic acid (vitamin B3), pantothenic acid (vitamin B5), pyridoxine (vitamin B6), biotin (vitamin B7), and B12. Especially, certain bacteria such as *Bacteroidetes*, *Fusobacteria*, and *Proteobacteria* produce the vitamins B2, B6, B9, and B12. Beside the production of these essential vitamins, these bacteria also regulate the access to the DNA so genes can be read and aid in other (epi) genetic processes. One of the other roles of the local microbes could be protection against the external environment or invasion of different pathogens. Recent research has identified bacteria in egg fluid in which *Lactobacillus* species prevail.

Importantly, the presence of *Lactobacillus* in egg fluid seems to be associated with better embryo quality. Also, sperm fluid contains bacteria, including *Lactobacillus*. Even now, it is unknown if the microbes in sperm fluid are associated with sperm health or fertility outcome. The presence of *Lactobacillus* bacteria in the endometrial fluid is associated with successful pregnancy outcomes, while the presence of other specific microbes is associated with implantation failure or miscarriage. Generally speaking, the presence of *Lactobacillus* in at least the female urogenital tract seems to be beneficial for pregnancy outcomes.

The beneficial effects of the *Lactobacillus* bacteria could be explained by the fact they possess diverse antimicrobial qualities, such as the ability to produce lactic acid. The main property of lactic acid is to lower the pH of the local environment due to its acidic nature, providing protection against invading pathogens. Environmental factors such as diet, use of antibiotics, vaginal douching, but also geographical location can strongly determine and influence the presence of certain bacteria. Importantly, a change in dietary pattern changes the microbial composition of the gut within 24 hours, which in turn will most likely change the biosynthesis capacity of all abovementioned different and necessary vitamins. However, the effect of environmental, nutritional, and lifestyle behavior on the composition of the microbiome of the parental urogenital tracts is still unknown as are ways of correcting the balance in bacteria.

3.5   Preconception Health Care

The primary goal of preconception care is improvement of preconception health of both parents to achieve a healthy pregnancy with a healthy child. Preferably, preconception counselling should easily be accessible, with generalized individual preconception health care for all couples who are planning a pregnancy (Fig. 3.3). First, couples need to be screened for risk factors preconceptionally. These risk factors include not only the abovementioned nutritional and lifestyle factors but also medical (such as inflammatory bowel diseases), obstetrical (previous preterm birth), and family histories (such as bleeding disorders), hereditary disorders, all intoxications or substance abuse, and (teratogenic) prescription drug regimens. When risk factors are identified in couples, they need to be referred to a medical specialist for personalized preconception care. Once referred to a medical specialist, the identified risks need to be evaluated and when necessary need to be addressed and corrected. Temporary anticonception measures are recommended so risk factors can be addressed and health can be properly promoted before achieving a future pregnancy. When caring for women who have chronic disease states, such as rheumatoid arthritis, women should be counselled about the influence of a pregnancy on their medical condition, the influence of the medical condition on a future pregnancy, and the influence of both on maternal health later in the life course. Teratogenic medications, such as anti-epileptic agents, need to be changed to non-teratogenic regimens. Attention for aspects such as sexual health, gender, and sex also need to be incorporated in preconception care.

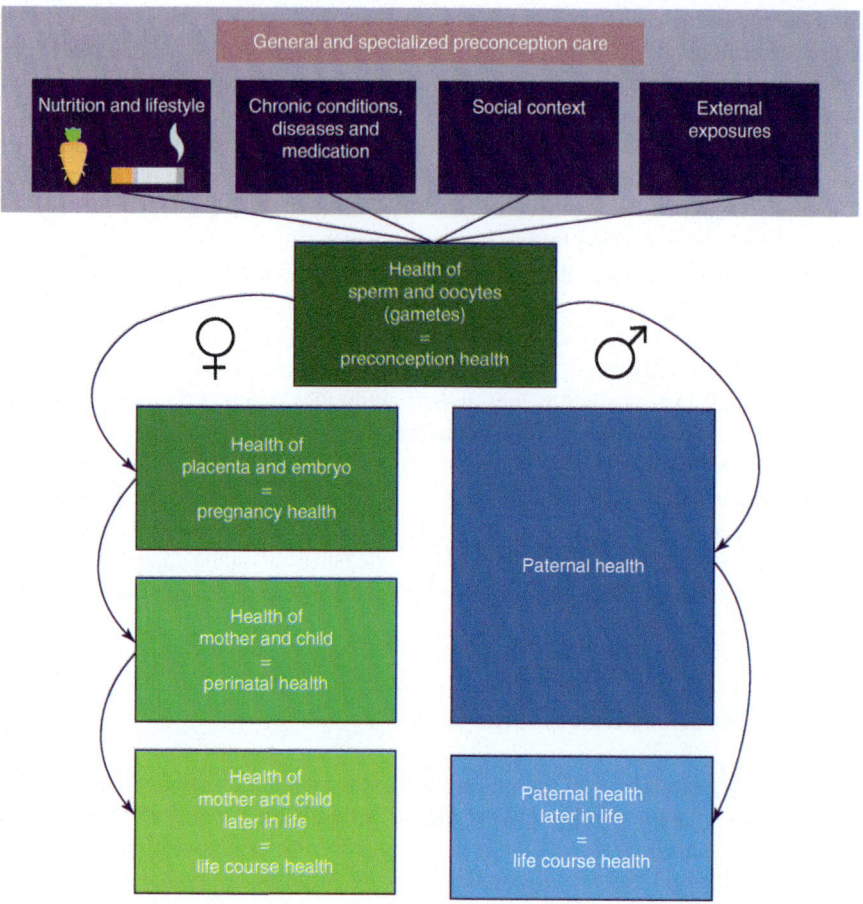

Fig. 3.3 Overview of preconception care and influence on the life course

3.6   General Recommendations for Practice

In this chapter we described the importance of preconception care by giving an overview of the biology of gametogenesis (formation of eggs and sperm), embryo-genesis, and placentation as determinants of the success of pregnancy course and outcome and health of the offspring during the life course. Because achieving a healthy lifestyle is one of the most important preventive measures in preconception care, we addressed the impact on outcomes during the life course of maternal as well as paternal lifestyle aspects during the periconception period. Other important factors that can influence the course and outcome of pregnancy, such as the presence of healthy bacteria, medication use, worksite hazardous exposures, and medical conditions, are briefly mentioned. All these factors can influence the course of preg-nancy, while pregnancy itself can also have an influence on a chronic medical condition, and ultimately these interacting influences affect the life course later in life. Since a multitude of factors are involved, it is important to assess potential risk factors preconceptionally to prevent pregnancy complications in general and aim to achieve a healthy as possible pregnancy. Recommendations for general preconception practice:

1. General nutrition and lifestyle advice should be given to all people and particularly couples who wish to conceive. The main advice should be to stop smoking, stop drinking alcohol, stop using recreational drugs, stop teratogenic and addictive medication, use only medication on prescription, start taking folic acid 0.4–0.5 mg daily, and start with eating at least 250 g of vegetables and 2 pieces of fruit per day.
2. When having to deal with a chronic condition, the woman should be engaged in a conversation about the influence of pregnancy on the condition and the influence of the condition on pregnancy course and the combined effect on health later in the life course for her and her child. Contraception should be offered if more time is needed to improve health and optimally plan a future pregnancy.
3. Teratogenic medication should be changed to non-teratogenic medication preferably during the preconception period.

3.7   Concluding Remark

The most known preconceptional intervention influencing maternal health and pregnancy is folic acid. Daily usage of 0.4 mg in the periconception period has proven to reduce the risk of congenital malformations like neural tube defect and congenital heart defects. This chapter underscores that lifestyle factors like nutrition, alcohol, and smoking as well as also environmental factors such as the local bacteria can influence the formation of sperm and oocytes, embryogenesis, pregnancy chance, placentation, and embryonic growth. Furthermore, more general risk factors such as medication, hazardous substances, and chronic conditions can influence pregnancy course and outcome. This is important since the developmental processes during the first few weeks of pregnancy heavily influence pregnancy course and outcome as well as the health of the newborn during the life course. Identifying and treating but preferable offering effective interventions to prevent modifiable risk factors of both future mother and father in preconception care will possibly increase the chance of a healthy pregnancy and a couple's chance of a healthy live born baby. Preconception care contributes to better health of future parents and their offspring, higher quality of life, and possibly a reduction in health-care and societal costs.

References

Agarwal A, Gupta S, Sharma RK. Role of oxidative stress in female reproduction. Reprod Biol Endocrinol. 2005;3:28.
Ashworth CJ, Toma LM, Hunter MG. Nutritional effects on oocyte and embryo development in mammals: implications for reproductive efficiency and environmental sustainability. Philos Trans R Soc Lond Ser B Biol Sci. 2009;364(1534):3351–61.

Hoek J, Koster MPH, Schoenmakers S, Willemsen SP, Koning AHJ, Steegers EAP, et al. Does the father matter? The association between the periconceptional paternal folate status and embryonic growth. Fertil Steril. 2019;111(2):270–9.

Jaddoe VW, de Jonge LL, Hofman A, Franco OH, Steegers EA, Gaillard R. First trimester fetal growth restriction and cardiovascular risk factors in school age children: population based cohort study. BMJ. 2014;348:g14.

Koedooder R, Mackens S, Budding A, Fares D, Blockeel C, Laven J, et al. Identification and evaluation of the microbiome in the female and male reproductive tracts. Hum Reprod Update. 2019;25(3):298–325.

Reijnders IF, Mulders A, van der Windt M, Steegers EAP, Steegers-Theunissen RPM. The impact of periconceptional maternal lifestyle on clinical features and biomarkers of placental development and function: a systematic review. Hum Reprod Update. 2019;25(1):72–94.

Rousian M, Koster MPH, Mulders A, Koning AHJ, Steegers-Theunissen RPM, Steegers EAP. Virtual reality imaging techniques in the study of embryonic and early placental health. Placenta. 2018;64(Suppl 1):S29–35.

Steegers-Theunissen RP, Verheijden-Paulissen JJ, van Uitert EM, Wildhagen MF, Exalto N, Koning AH, et al. Cohort profile: the Rotterdam Periconceptional Cohort (Predict Study). Int J Epidemiol. 2016;45(2):374–81.

Van Dijk MR, Borggreven NV, Willemsen SP, Koning AHJ, Steegers-Theunissen RPM, Koster MPH. Maternal lifestyle impairs embryonic growth: the Rotterdam periconception cohort. Reprod Sci. 2018;25(6):916–22.

van Uitert EM, Steegers-Theunissen RP. Influence of maternal folate status on human fetal growth parameters. Mol Nutr Food Res. 2013;57(4):582–95.

van Uitert EM, van Ginkel S, Willemsen SP, Lindemans J, Koning AH, Eilers PH, et al. An optimal periconception maternal folate status for embryonic size: the Rotterdam Predict study. BJOG. 2014;121(7):821–9.

Wyck S, Herrera C, Requena CE, Bittner L, Hajkova P, Bollwein H, et al. Oxidative stress in sperm affects the epigenetic reprogramming in early embryonic development. Epigenetics Chromatin. 2018;11(1):60.

Genetic Health Care Before Conception

Martina C. Cornel, Selina Goodman,
and Lidewij Henneman

4.1 Introduction

Every child inherits two copies of their genes, one from each of their biological parents, and in this way genes are passed on to the next generation. Often people do not think about their genes, until they have a child born with a recessive condition. When they might ask the question: 'Could we have known before that we were carrier of this disorder?', the theoretical answer is 'Yes', since they would have been carriers throughout their lives. However, testing for carrier status often is done only after the birth of an affected infant, potentially followed by testing relatives. Medical issues related to genetic factors being passed on are preferably discussed before pregnancy, since the impact of inherited disorders to the lives of parents and their family may be enormous. For some couples, the risk for each child to have an inherited disease is 25%, 50% or, though rarely, even 100%. It is therefore important that time is available for providing information about a possible genetic risk to couples planning a pregnancy.

Most congenital anomalies have a multifactorial aetiology, where several genes and several environmental factors play a role. Some environmental factors can be modified to reduce the risk (e.g. taking folic acid before conception to reduce the

M. C. Cornel (✉)
Department of Clinical Genetics, Amsterdam Public Health Research Institute, Amsterdam UMC, Vrije Universiteit Amsterdam, Amsterdam, The Netherlands
e-mail: mc.cornel@amsterdamumc.nl

S. Goodman
College of Medicine and Health, University of Exeter Medical School, Exeter, UK
e-mail: S.M.Goodman@exeter.ac.uk

L. Henneman
Department of Clinical Genetics, Amsterdam Reproduction and Development Research Institute, Amsterdam UMC, Vrije Universiteit Amsterdam, Amsterdam, The Netherlands
e-mail: l.henneman@amsterdamumc.nl

© Springer Nature Switzerland AG 2020
J. Shawe et al. (eds.), *Preconception Health and Care: A Life Course Approach*,
https://doi.org/10.1007/978-3-030-31753-9_4

risk of neural tube defects), but often neither the genetic factors nor the environmental factors are known. The recurrence risk for multifactorial congenital anomalies is often very low. In this chapter, we will focus on conditions where one gene plays a major role, and the risks are often 25% or more. Preconception knowledge of genetic risk may influence preconception care, prenatal care, mode of delivery and postnatal care and may also inform reproductive choices (Ten Kate 2012).

An accurate family history is an essential part of a preconception consultation (Bennett 2012; Solomon et al. 2008). Family history taking should include known monogenic conditions, that is, genetic conditions caused by mutation (s) in a single gene, for example, cystic fibrosis (CF) or Duchenne muscular dystrophy (DMD), in addition to developmental problems and miscarriages, which may be indicative of balanced chromosome anomalies. If the family history is negative for these conditions, there still may be an increased risk of having a child with an inherited disorder. This may be linked to ancestry and/or consanguinity, leading to an increased risk for autosomal recessive disorders. In autosomal recessive disorders, carrier couples are most often only recognized after the birth of an affected child. In preconception care practices, in the absence of a positive family history, the discussion around carrier testing is, however, often ad hoc and does not commonly occur (Metcalfe et al. 2008).

Issues related to genetic risk can be quite diverse. Sometimes a couple's questions are related to having a relative with developmental delay. If the couple doesn't know or have the relative's formal diagnosis, diagnostic testing will be needed to support appropriate counselling. In other cases, if a genetic disease runs in the family and if couples want this information, DNA testing may need to be done to test for the familial mutation. Sometimes future parents can be reassured that the condition in the family does not lead to a high recurrence risk for their future child(ren). If couples are carriers of a familial mutation and want to conceive using their own sperm and ovum, then prenatal care must be organized where chorionic villi sampling or amniocentesis during pregnancy is suggested; and neonatal care may also have to take into account familial risk factors. An additional consideration to raise is that identifying a high genetic risk in a couple is likely to have consequences for their relatives. Therefore, talking with a couple about how to share this information with family members is also important.

These different situations could apply to any couple, so the issue of genetic risk is relevant to all couples who are planning a pregnancy. To narrow the scope of this chapter, content will focus on the following higher-risk groups:

(a) Couples that come to the genetic clinic with a question about a specific disorder that runs in their family or because they have a child with a genetic disorder
(b) Couples from a specific ancestry group, in whom ancestry-based carrier testing might be discussed (e.g. hemoglobinopathies (HbP) such as sickle cell disease)
(c) Couples where the partners are biologically related, i.e. consanguineous couples

In terms of general issues, we will discuss (1) genetic health care in relation to preconception care (goal, autonomy, informed decision-making); (2) family history and patterns of inheritance, especially recessive conditions; and (3) techniques that are used in the genetic laboratories in 2019 (more or less targeted, from simple high-performance liquid chromatography (HPLC)/electrophoresis for HbP to expanded carrier screening using sequencing techniques or analyses as in whole exome sequencing (WES) for consanguineous couples).

4.2   Genetic Health Care in Relation to Preconception Care

Genetic health care is predicated on the principle that each individual has the right to be informed about the risks to their own health and their options for reproduction in the context of genetic conditions affecting them or their family. Integral to this is that their choices should be well informed and they should be supported through their decision-making (Elwyn et al. 2000). The principle of autonomy is therefore central to this care, where a non-directive approach is used in counselling that promotes self-determination and the couple's ability to make decisions for themselves (Kessler 1997; Skirton 2018). Establishing a professional-client relationship of trust is fundamental as is maintaining the confidentiality of personal information (Arribas-Ayllon and Sarangi 2014). Most of these principles in genetic health care are common to preconception care, with the important distinction that inherited factors influencing a pregnancy cannot be changed by the couple. In choices whether to test and to use reproductive options their self-determination is paramount.

4.3   Counselling Couples about Genetic Risk

Preconception care seeks to provide prospective parents with information and support about the options available to them which will optimize their chance of having a healthy child (Atrash et al. 2008; de Wert et al. 2012). Therefore, identifying both non-genetic and genetic risk factors that could impact on the health of the mother and child is central to this care. This shows the importance of family history taking the importance of family history taking, asking about consanguinity and ancestry and offering carrier screening tests. Risk factors of concern are likely to be established during preconception counselling. As stated previously, in the initial preconception consultation, a key component is the ascertainment of a full medical and family history which helps identify potential genetic risks to the mother and baby (Jack et al. 2008; Ioannides 2017). The issues of consanguinity and ethnicity are particularly relevant to autosomal recessive conditions although evidence suggests that some health professionals can feel reluctant to ask direct questions about how partners might be related (Bishop et al. 2008).

Where environmental risk factors such as smoking or alcohol consumption are likely to impact the pregnancy, couples can be given clear, directive advice about how to reduce those environmental risks. In contrast, if genetic risk factors are found, these need to be discussed with a different, non-directive, approach. This is because individuals do not have a choice over what genes they have and couples may face a range of challenges, both psychological and social, depending on the way the genetic condition is inherited (Riedijk et al. 2012). When clinicians use an empathic, person-centred approach, it enables them to draw out and explore the couple's views and coping strategies while respecting their autonomy (de Wert et al. 2012). Preconception counselling can give the couple a chance to take in information about their situation and consider the options available to them, such as preimplantation genetic diagnosis, prenatal testing or using donor gametes (BenNagi et al. 2016). This non-directive approach is fundamental to genetic counselling but may be less familiar to clinicians working in other areas of health care.

Whatever the route to diagnosis, receiving a genetic diagnosis is likely to have a profound effect on individuals and couples, altering their perception of themselves, their future health and their hope of having a family. Evidence suggests that many people experience a genetic diagnosis as a form of loss (McAllister et al. 2007). Thus loss, where it relates to lost expectations, projected future or sense of self, has been termed 'ambiguous loss' and may not be recognized by friends and family because it is not associated with something tangible like the death of a person (Sobel and Cowan 2003). Consequently, the grief associated with such loss may be complicated by having no socially recognized outward expression. This type of 'disenfranchised grief' (Doka 2002) can happen on many levels; such as when the loss is not recognized as a loss (like a couple's choice to remain childless to avoid passing on a life-limiting genetic condition), alternatively a loss can relate to loss of life but may not be openly acknowledged, such as following the termination of a pregnancy where the foetus is affected by a genetic condition (Whitney 2017).

A genetic diagnosis can also be seen very positively, providing opportunities for reproduction in a couple where the likelihood of illness can be reduced or avoided. Reproductive empowerment has been found to be a key motivation and outcome for individuals who had sought carrier testing for both X-linked and autosomal recessive conditions (Lewis et al. 2012). Quoting from a European guideline on prenatal testing which could also be applied to preconception genetic testing: 'Professionals should ensure prospective parents make an informed choice through provision of accurate, balanced information in a clearly understandable form' (Skirton et al. 2014).

4.4 The Importance of Communication in Families Affected by Genetic Conditions

Unlike other areas of health care which apply only to the individual patient or couple, the issue of sharing information with relatives needs to be discussed with patients either during their preparation for genetic testing or in follow-up. Disclosure of a genetic diagnosis with relatives for whom it may have implications is something that can disrupt family dynamics in the short term. However, evidence suggests that withholding information or keeping secrets is more destructive to family cohesion in the longer term (Metcalfe et al. 2008).

Most patients recognize the importance of informing their family members about a genetic diagnosis (Dheensa et al. 2018), but this may be deferred until such time as the patient themselves has adjusted to their knowledge of the diagnosis (Forrest et al. 2008). When a couple are preparing for a pregnancy, this can be an emotional time; they may consider their decision-making private and be particularly sensitive to the opinions of family members. Consequently, the common barriers to communication in families can also inhibit contact at this time. Typical barriers include the emotional and geographical distance to relatives; family norms of how health issues are discussed; and what is perceived as the right time to disclose information (Chivers Seymour et al. 2010).

It is important to determine the couple's perspectives on all issues pertaining to the planned pregnancy, including communication with the wider family, prior to a genetic diagnosis being made. Otherwise, the ramifications of a diagnosis are unlikely to be fully appreciated. Counselling couples can be problematic because the views and concerns of both individuals need to be balanced and considered. Nonetheless, preconception counselling is valued by both men and women (de Weerd et al. 2001).

When couples are sharing sensitive information with both families, then differences of opinion may emerge; the risk of blaming or fear of stigma is particularly relevant when a genetic diagnosis is made in one partner that seriously effects their chance of having a healthy child. The emotional consequences of a genetic diagnosis in a family may be particularly acute in some cultures or social settings (Oosterwal 2009), but it would be important not to make assumptions about the couple's views because these will be unique to them. Health professionals can try to understand the unique circumstances that their patient is facing and their perspectives. With insight about whether their patient feels ready to pass on information to their family members, and the potential obstacles that they are likely to face, then health professionals are better placed to help them both practically and psychologically (Mendes et al. 2018).

4.5   Family History and Patterns of Inheritance

Taking a family history may start by asking about children, brothers and sisters and parents (first-degree relatives), followed by children of brothers and sisters, brothers and sisters of parents and grandparents (second-degree relatives). Preferably a pedigree is drawn to help gain insight into the family structure and risks for the potential future child and decide whether referral criteria are met (Bennett 2012). While drawing a pedigree, one can discuss whether these relatives are healthy. Some health problems may be asked more specifically, such as developmental delay, miscarriages or any specific health problems the patient has questions about. Ancestry may be the next question, paying special attention to African, Asian or Mediterranean ancestry (HbPs), Jewish ancestry (Tay-Sachs disease amongst others) and other country-specific risk groups and finally, consanguinity should be discussed.

Table 4.1 Classification of genetic disorders

Genotype			Examples (phenotype)
Major categories	Sub-categories		
Monogenic disorders	Autosomal	Recessive	Cystic fibrosis, sickle cell disease
		Dominant	Huntington's disease, hereditary breast cancer
	X-linked	Recessive	Duchenne muscular dystrophy, haemophilia
		Dominant	Rett syndrome
Mitochondrial disorders			Leber hereditary optic neuropathy
Chromosomal disorders			Down syndrome
Multifactorial and complex disorders			Neural tube defects, cleft lip

Source: Based on Ten Kate (2012)

4.6 Patterns of Inheritance

There are different types of genetic disorders (Table 4.1).

4.6.1 Autosomal Recessive Disorders

More than 1100 conditions follow a pattern of autosomal recessive inheritance (Kingsmore 2012). When a child is born with such a condition, it is often not known to the parents because the family history is negative for disease. Yet, both parents are healthy carriers of the condition. If one child in a family has an autosomal recessive disorder, the recurrence risk for future brothers and sisters is 25%. Preimplantation genetic diagnosis (embryo selection) and prenatal diagnosis may be available for serious conditions (BenNagi et al. 2016). Using donor gametes may also be considered. Although both parents are 'obligate carriers', a DNA test before the next pregnancy is needed to determine the variant involved. Brothers and sisters of a carrier have a 50% chance of being a carrier themselves. Particularly, in populations with a high carrier frequency, other relatives may be at increased risk of having a child with the condition, and carrier testing may be available. For example, if a pregnant woman of African descent has a nephew with sickle cell disease (SCD), her risk to be a carrier is 50%, and in some populations, the risk for her partner to be a carrier as well may be more than 10%. Thus the a priori risk for a future child to have SCD might be 1–2%. For consanguineous couples, the risk of autosomal recessive disorders is also increased. A gene variant may 'meet itself' if a rare variant, which was present in one of the common ancestors, was passed on to both cousins, for example. In a cousin-cousin marriage, the inbreeding coefficient (or the likelihood for a rare variant to meet itself) is 1 in 16.

4.6.2 Autosomal Dominant Disorders

Unlike autosomal recessive conditions, autosomal dominant conditions tend to affect more generations. Both men and women can be affected. If one of the prospective parents has an autosomal dominant disorder, the likelihood to pass it on to their offspring is 50%. Some examples of conditions following this pattern of inheritance are Huntington's disease (HD), inherited breast and ovarian cancer (due to *BRCA* mutations), other inherited tumour syndromes, hypertrophic cardiomyopathy, familial hypercholesterolemia, neurofibromatosis and tuberous sclerosis.

All autosomal dominant conditions can be passed on by men and women because the genetic variants determining them are not on either of the sex chromosomes. In some cases, the inherited familial mutation is asymptomatic, but it can still be passed on to the next generation, such as in young relatives in HD families. Prenatal diagnosis (PND) and preimplantation genetic diagnosis (PGD) may be available for serious autosomal dominant disorders, and the use of donor gametes may be considered. Knowing the gene variant is important, so DNA testing before pregnancy is needed to identify the pathogenic variant involved. Should a woman mention that a (distant) relative of hers carries, for instance, a *BRCA* mutation, then it is important to evaluate who in the family was tested and the residual likelihood for the woman to be a carrier as well.

4.6.3 X-Linked Disorders

Some conditions express a more severe phenotype in one of the sexes. For X-linked recessive disorders, such as Duchenne muscular dystrophy (DMD) or haemophilia, boys/men have a severe phenotype, and female carriers have little or no symptoms, but they can pass on the condition. Should DMD be mentioned in the family history, then it is extremely important to evaluate whether the woman planning a pregnancy could be a carrier of the condition, since her future sons might be severely affected. If there is a woman in a pedigree between the client and the affected person, she might be an unaffected carrier. If there is a healthy man between the client and the affected person, he cannot carry the pathogenic variant. If the brother of the healthy father of the client had DMD, she is not at risk; if the brother of the mother of the client had DMD, she is.

4.6.4 Mitochondrial Inherited Disorders

Women pass on their mitochondria to their offspring, but men do not. Therefore, if a woman is a carrier of a mitochondrial disease, she will pass it on to all of her offspring, both sons and daughters. An example of a condition with mitochondrial inheritance is Leber hereditary optic neuropathy (LHON) which results in loss of vision. The severity of the phenotype depends on the relative number of affected mitochondria, so there is a spectrum of more and less severely affected persons.

4.6.5   Disorders due to Chromosome Translocations

While many aneuploidies such as Down syndrome occur 'by chance', in a few percent of cases, there may be an inherited predisposition. In these cases, the chromosomes of the parent are rearranged, so that otherwise separated (parts of) chromosomes are joined. Having several miscarriages as well as infants with severe developmental delay may raise suspicion of a chromosome translocation. Sometimes clients will say that the 'Down syndrome in their family was inherited', referring to a situation where one chromosome 21 is joined to the other chromosome 21 or, for instance, to chromosome 14. Karyotyping would need to take place before a pregnancy, and the recurrence risk of Down syndrome in the family will depend on the rearrangement involved.

4.6.6   New ('De Novo') Mutations

Some developmental problems may be due to mutations that occur for the first time in a family (Deciphering Developmental Disorders Study 2017). In general, this implies a low recurrence risk for brothers and sisters of the affected person, although the mutation may have occurred in the ovarian tissue of the mother or the spermatogonia of the father. If more cells in the ovarian tissue or testis carry the mutation, also a sibling may get the disorder. A new mutation may imply a recurrence risk for sibs of a few percent. Thus, there may be an indication for PND even in women who had a previous child with a 'new' or so-called 'de novo' mutation. In these cases, relatives outside of the nuclear family are not at increased risk.

Greater likelihood of having a child with a de novo mutation has also been found to be associated with increasing paternal age (Girard et al. 2016). Since new mutations may occur anywhere throughout the genome, this means that for any pregnancy there is a small chance of having a child with an autosomal dominant, autosomal recessive, X-linked disorders or chromosome anomaly even without any known family history of a genetic condition.

4.7   Consanguinity

The risk of autosomal recessive disorders in offspring is increased by consanguineous marriage. Cousins who marry are most often first cousins, i.e. the sons and daughters of siblings. Marriage between first cousins roughly doubles the risk of congenital anomalies (~2–6%) when compared to couples who are unrelated (~2–3%). The excess risk is most distinct for rare autosomal recessive diseases, which can be hard to foresee in the preconception phase, as often these disorders have not previously occurred in the family. Actual risks depend on the prevalence of specific recessive disorders, a family history of disorders and/or the occurrence of consanguineous marriage over several generations. For most consanguineous couples, the birth of an affected child is contrary to expectations generally held by them and places a heavy burden on these families.

In clinical genetics, a consanguineous marriage is defined as a union between two individuals who are related as second cousins or closer (Bittles 2001). Whether or not consanguinity is an indication to refer to a clinical genetic centre depends on local resources and protocols. Worldwide the prevalence of consanguineous marriages varies, with high percentages in Northern Africa, the Middle East and West Asia, where intra-familial unions collectively account for 20% to more than 50% of all marriage (Global Prevalence of Consanguinity n.d.; Hamamy 2012). The reasons to favour consanguineous marriages are mainly social, such as stability of the relationship and the compatibility with the wider family (Hamamy 2012). Couples with ancestors from these areas who now live in Western Europe often favour consanguineous marriages. In the Netherlands, for instance, 0.1% of native Dutch mothers of newborns in Rotterdam who were born between 2002 and 2005 have a consanguineous partner vs. 24% in Dutch people of Turkish ancestry and 22% in Dutch people of Moroccan ancestry (Ten Kate et al. 2014). In Bradford, amongst British Pakistani, the rate has found to be even higher and has been sustained in the current childbearing generation (Sheridan et al. 2013), although this may not be extrapolated to Pakistani living in other parts of the United Kingdom (Shaw 2014).

Health-care professionals need to be able to discuss both the (social) advantages and (medical) disadvantages with prospective parents, preferably before conception. Most consanguineous couples are generally positive about the provision of risk information, especially if information is offered either prior to conception or even before marriage (Teeuw et al. 2014). However, as shown in the United Kingdom, many initiatives to address the needs of these couples are restricted to local initiatives (Salway et al. 2016). In primary care, health professionals' perceived difficulties in direct questioning about consanguinity may further prevent determining accurate (family) history, restricting identification of at-risk pregnancies (Bishop et al. 2008; Teeuw et al. 2012). Consequently, most couples are unaware that genetic counselling is available, thus resulting in a low uptake amongst people at risk of recessive disorders. New genetic technologies such as whole exome carrier testing allow for a better risk assessment for consanguineous couples, thereby facilitating informed reproductive decision-making (Sallevelt et al. 2017; Kirk et al. 2019).

4.8   Carrier Status in Relation to Ancestry

The prevalence of autosomal and X-linked recessive disorders, whose symptoms range from very mild to severe, together is estimated to be 30 per 10,000, implying that 1–2 in 100 couples in the general population will be at 1-in-4 risk of having affected offspring (Sankaranarayanan 1998; Ropers 2012). For some people, the risk of having an affected child is higher than average. This accounts for couples having a positive family history of disease and for couples in a consanguineous relationship. Moreover, some subpopulations are at an increased risk of specific diseases based on geographic origin or (common) ancestry. Hemoglobinopathies (HbPs) such as sickle cell disease (SCD) and thalassaemias are more common in people with ancestors coming from Africa, the Caribbean, Asia, the Middle East and the Mediterranean area, while cystic fibrosis (CF) is more frequent in people with ancestors in Europe (Fig. 4.1).

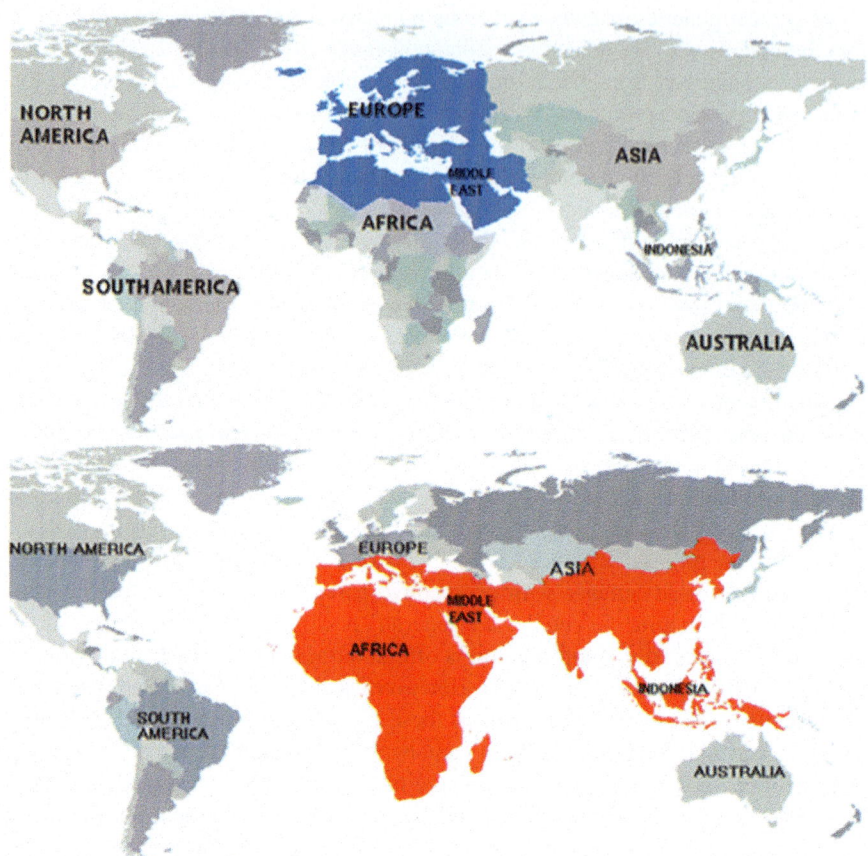

Fig. 4.1 Global distribution according to ancestry of patients and carriers of cystic fibrosis (in *blue*) and the hemoglobinopathies (sickle cell disease and thalassaemias) (in *red*). (Source: Ten Kate (2012). Courtesy of Dr. P. Lakeman, Department of Clinical Genetics, Amsterdam UMC, Amsterdam, the Netherlands) [copy from https://link.springer.com/article/10.1007/s12687-01 1-0066-9/]]

Furthermore, if partners of a couple both originate from a place known for a high frequency of a particular autosomal recessive disease, which is usually rare in the general population, their risk for that disorder may also be increased. In addition, it has been shown that over 40% of Ashkenazi Jews carry recessive mutations for specific diseases, such as Tay-Sachs disease (Lazarin et al. 2013).

In preconception care, the risk for genetic disease may be assessed by either taking a couple's medical and family history or through genetic screening. Carrier screening for recessive disorders is defined as the identification of carrier status in healthy individuals with no a priori increased risk, i.e. without a positive family history (Henneman et al. 2016). It allows couples to find out whether both partners are carriers of the same disorder, thus facing a 1-in-4 risk of having an affected child with that specific disorder in each pregnancy. Screening is preferably done before pregnancy (preconception) as there is less of a time constraint, and it provides couples with the maximum number of reproductive options (de Wert et al. 2012). Available options include preimplantation genetic diagnosis, prenatal diagnosis, use of donor gametes, refraining from pregnancy, adoption or accepting the risk of having an affected child. In the past, as a result of the known higher risk for subpopulations to recessive disease, initiatives to identify carriers of recessive disease have been selectively targeted to certain ethnic groups. This type of screening has often been referred to as ethnicity-based or ancestry-based carrier screening and started with screening programmes focussing on one or few disorders. Well-known examples are carrier screening for β-thalassaemia in Southern European and Middle Eastern countries (Cousens et al. 2010) and carrier screening for Tay-Sachs disease in the Ashkenazi Jewish community. Other screening initiatives are aimed at genetically isolated regions with high prevalence of disease, for example, the Arab and Druze communities in Israel (Zlotogora et al. 2009); the Saguenay-Lac-Saint-Jean region of Quebec, Canada; and a genetically isolated village in the Netherlands, where people are offered screening through a preconception outpatient clinic for several rare disorders (Mathijssen et al. 2015).

The offer of these screening programmes has been largely supported by the communities, who are highly familiar with these genetic diseases (Holtkamp et al. 2017). Through these screening initiatives, the birth prevalence of severe disorders in many of these communities has dramatically decreased, as many identified carrier couples take measures to prevent disease, including preimplantation genetic diagnosis and prenatal diagnosis. As a result of Tay-Sachs disease screening, which started back in the 1970s, the birth prevalence of Tay-Sachs disease in the Jewish community decreased by more than 90% (Kaback 2001). Conversely, there are disadvantages to ancestry-based screening: first, diseases are not limited to specific ethnic groups; second, ancestry-based screening may increase the risk of stigma; and third, that it is increasingly difficult to define who is at risk because of multiethnic backgrounds (Henneman et al. 2016; Edwards et al. 2015).

4.9 From Ancestry-Based Carrier Testing to Universal Screening

We can illustrate this with a possible scenario: *After having two healthy boys, a couple is informed after neonatal screening about their third child, a daughter, has cystic fibrosis (CF). The couple is shocked to hear this message. There is no CF in either side of the family. They are invited for genetic counselling with a clinical geneticist, who explains about autosomal recessive inheritance, the fact that they are a carrier couple with 1-in-4 risk having a child with CF. The couple asks the clinical geneticist: 'Could we have known this beforehand, before (her) birth?'.* Theoretically, this would have been possible, but as carrier screening for CF is not offered in most countries worldwide, the answer would be 'No'.

The standard practice in most countries is to only offer carrier testing to individuals who have a family history of/or partner with a particular recessive disease. In this way, only a minority of carrier couples will be identified, since the majority of affected children are born to couples with no previous known family history, as is the case in this example. Moreover, only a minority of relatives in high-risk families request carrier testing (McClaren et al. 2010). Carriers of autosomal recessive diseases are usually healthy, and thus, most carriers do not know that they are a carrier of a gene variant and they are not aware of their potential risk of having an affected offspring. In most cases, the diagnosis of a child with recessive disease is still highly unexpected. It has therefore been suggested that carrier screening in the general population is warranted, for example, for disorders such as CF.

Over the years, several professional organizations have produced and updated guidelines and recommendations for population-based preconception CF carrier screening (Delatycki et al. 2014; American College of Obstetricians and Gynecologists Committee on Genetics 2011), and CF carrier screening programmes have been established in a number of countries. For example, following the ACGM/ACOG statements, CF carrier screening was introduced into routine care in the United States in 2001, as was screening for spinal muscular atrophy (American College of Obstetricians and Gynecologists 2017). Furthermore, it was stated in 2011 that in the United States CF carrier screening should be offered pan-ethnic as it had become increasingly difficult to assign a single ethnicity to individuals (American College of Obstetricians and Gynecologists Committee on Genetics 2011). In Italy and Australia, CF carrier screening is offered regionally, and in Israel, population screening for CF is offered to all citizens.

Traditionally, carrier screening programmes have been designed and aimed at high-risk populations for a limited number of disorders. Technological developments have altered the screening landscape. With the introduction of high-throughput DNA sequencing approaches, it is now possible to screen for many disorders, genes or sequence variants simultaneously at a faster turnaround time and without significantly increasing costs (Henneman et al. 2016). Carrier screening panels have thus 'expanded' to include many more disorders. Almost everyone is a carrier of an estimated 1 up to 7 recessive disorders (Bell et al. 2011). The availability of these expanded panels encourages the transition of an ancestry-based offer towards screening, regardless of ancestry or geographic origin. Obviously, carrier screening has optimal impact if it is done before pregnancy, so that couples can be informed about their reproductive options at a moment when most options are available. The preconception screening service needed for carrier screening using expanded panels no longer needs to target according to ancestry. Following these developments, recommendations for testing and inclusion of certain disorders have also changed, expanding to screening panels that differ in their severity and treatability of diseases (American College of Obstetricians and Gynecologists 2017). Advantages of expanded screening panels include the increase of equity and the potential decrease of risk of stigma for ethnic groups (Edwards et al. 2015). Medical professionals, including genetics professionals, are also critical of these developments. Concerns include difficulties with selecting specific mutations that should be included in a panel and challenges with counselling and pre- and post-test information (Henneman et al. 2016; Edwards et al. 2015). Ultimately the goal is to enhance reproductive autonomy and to guide pregnancy planning based on couples' personal values. Availability and cost of carrier testing varies between countries (Delatycki et al. 2020). Testing for a single disorder with a high frequency in the population may be cheap, while expanded testing may currently cost hundreds of dollars or euros. It may not be available to everyone based on their income, insurance and where they live (Delatycki et al. 2020).

4.10 Genetic Issues in the Fertility Clinic

When couples are trying to achieve a pregnancy, but do not do so despite regular sexual intercourse for over a year, then they may be seen in a fertility clinic. Infertility is a common issue for many couples, affecting around 8–15% worldwide (Flannigan and Schlegel 2017; Vander Borght and Wyns 2018). Couples who are referred to fertility clinics may already be aware of the underlying cause of their infertility, or alternatively a genetic diagnosis may be made as a result of their investigations. In all cases where a genetic basis to the couple's infertility has been identified, they should be offered referral to specialist services for genetic counselling and genetic risk assessment.

By definition, the likelihood of conception is already reduced when a couple have been seen in the fertility clinic because of their infertility. In common with other circumstances where couples have sought advice about potential genetic risk factors, their respective family histories will provide important information, with the addition of their ages and individual medical histories. There is not scope here to describe the range of possible diagnoses that might arise in this situation, but some examples include:

- Chromosomal abnormalities, such as balanced translocations or microdeletions which may already be known to a family following the birth of an affected child. It should be noted that chromosome abnormalities are regularly identified *only* after a couple have suffered recurrent miscarriages (Hyde and Schust 2015). Chromosome analyses (karyotype) are not routinely performed in men unless a man has severe oligospermia or azoospermia, but of these, 10–15% will be found to have a chromosomal abnormality (Flannigan and Schlegel 2017).
- Klinefelter syndrome (47 XXY) is the most common cause for male infertility, where variation in X inactivation results in reduced androgen production, reduced sensitivity to androgen receptors and increased oestrogen in these men (Flannigan and Schlegel 2017).
- Microdeletions of the Y chromosome are associated with severe male infertility, most specifically deletions within the azoospermia factor (AZF) region on the long arm of the Y chromosome (Flannigan and Schlegel 2017; Carrell et al. 2018).
- Kallmann syndrome (KLS) is a clinical diagnosis where individuals have hypogonadotropic hypogonadism (HH) and anosmia (Flannigan and Schlegel 2017; Oliveira et al. 2001). KLS has a varied aetiology but is most commonly X-linked

due to variants in the KAL-1 gene. In men with KLS, there is insufficient stimulation of the testicle to induce testosterone production and spermatogenesis because of HH, but in some cases, this is amenable to treatment (Flannigan and Schlegel 2017).

- Premature ovarian insufficiency in women (POI) has a varied aetiology (Qin et al. 2015), but possible underlying genetic causes of POI are Turner syndrome (usually 45, X karyotype or a mosaic karyotype with a 45, X cell line) or that a woman is a fragile X pre-mutation carrier (Tucker et al. 2016). Fragile X syndrome is an X-linked condition with developmental delay and behavioural problems in affected males, which would have profound implications for that woman's relatives (European Society for Human Reproduction and Embryology (ESHRE) Guideline Group on POI et al. 2016). A diagnosis of POI is likely to be an extremely distressing diagnosis, particularly if the woman has experienced a delay in diagnosis and she is nulliparous (Milsom and O'Sullivan 2017).
- Congenital bilateral absence of the vas deferens (CBAVD) affects 95% of men with CF and may be a presenting feature of the condition if they are otherwise mildly affected (de Souza et al. 2018).

4.11   Techniques Available for Testing

If a specific monogenic disorder runs in the family, Sanger sequencing may be used to investigate the (absence or presence of the) familial mutation. In cases with a chromosome anomaly, karyotyping may be done to identify a balanced translocation. Historically, beta-hexosaminidase A (HEXA) enzyme analysis has been performed for carrier screening for Tay-Sachs disease. HPLC/electrophoresis has been used to find carriers of sickle cell disease and other HbPs. These tests were targeted to a specific disease running in the family or to a condition that is frequent in a certain population, enzyme analyses, HPLC and electrophoresis being relatively inexpensive. Increasingly, high-throughput DNA testing has become available for less targeted expanded carrier screening using sequencing techniques. Whole exome sequencing (WES) may be used preconception for consanguineous couples (Sallevelt et al. 2017; Kirk et al. 2019) or couples with a child affected by a condition that might be genetic (Vissers et al. 2017). For the latter, the advantage is that WES identifies more conclusive diagnoses than standard care pathways in a relatively short time, so it may even be cost-saving (Vissers et al. 2017). Carrier screening using WES will increase the percentage of at-risk couples being recognized before conception. Equally, these techniques could be applied to benefit couples who have no information about their family history, such as when one member is adopted or has lost touch with their biological family.

4.12   Conclusion

In summary, there are many situations in preconception care where genetics may play a role. Genetic counselling is important for couples who ask about their risk of conceiving a child with a disorder that runs in the family, or in other contexts such as screening for recessive conditions, for consanguineous couples and the diagnostic process in the fertility clinic, amongst others. Screening for recessive conditions can take an expanded approach, without starting from ancestry, although implementation is still emerging. However, the limited availability of resources in some countries may lead to prioritization of conditions of high prevalence, such as for conditions like the hemoglobinopathies. Similarly, resource issues and differences in professional recognition may impact on the availability of genetic counsellors in different countries to contribute their expertise to counselling couples prior to conception (Abacan et al. 2019). Thus, technical possibilities multiply with the increasing availability of high-throughput genomic testing, but counselling remains both vital and challenging, just as it was decades ago (Skirton 2018; Patch and Middleton 2018).

References

Abacan M, Alsubaie L, Barlow-Stewart K, Caanen B, Cordier C, Courtney E, et al. The global state of the genetic counseling profession. Eur J Hum Genet. 2019;27:183–97. https://doi.org/10.1038/s41431-018-0252-x.

American College of Obstetricians and Gynecologists. Committee opinion no. 691: carrier screening for genetic conditions. Obstet Gynecol. 2017;129:597–9. https://doi.org/10.1097/AOG.0000000000001952.

American College of Obstetricians and Gynecologists Committee on Genetics. ACOG Committee opinion no. 486: update on carrier screening for cystic fibrosis. Obstet Gynecol. 2011;117:1028–31. https://doi.org/10.1097/AOG.0b013e31821922c2.

Arribas-Ayllon MS, Sarangi S. Counselling uncertainty: genetics professionals' accounts of (non) directiveness and trust/distrust. Health Risk Soc. 2014;16:171–84. https://doi.org/10.1080/13698575.2014.884545.

Atrash H, Jack BW, Johnson K. Preconception care: a 2008 update. Curr Opin Obstet Gynecol. 2008;20:581–9. https://doi.org/10.1097/GCO.0b013e328317a27c.

Bell CJ, Dinwiddie DL, Miller NA, Hateley SL, Ganusova EE, Mudge J, et al. Carrier testing for severe childhood recessive diseases by next-generation sequencing. Sci Transl Med. 2011;3:65ra4. https://doi.org/10.1126/scitranslmed.3001756.

BenNagi J, Serhal P, SenGupta S, Doye K, Wells D. Preimplantation genetic diagnosis: an overview and recent advances. Obstetric Gynaecol. 2016;18:99–106. https://doi.org/10.1111/tog.12264.

Bennett RL. The family medical history as a tool in preconception consultation. J Community Genet. 2012;3:175–83. https://doi.org/10.1007/s12687-012-0107-z.

Bishop M, Metcalfe S, Gaff C. The missing element: consanguinity as a component of genetic risk assessment. Genet Med. 2008;10:612–20.

Bittles A. Consanguinity and its relevance to clinical genetics. Clin Genet. 2001;60:89–98. https://doi.org/10.1034/j.1399-0004.2001.600201.x.

Carrell DT, Jenkins TG, Emery BR, Hotaling JM, Aston KI. The role of reproductive genetics in modern andrology. In: Palermo G, Sills E, editors. Intracytoplasmic sperm injection. Cham: Springer; 2018. p. 23–38.

Chivers Seymour K, Addington-Hall J, Lucassen AM, Foster CL. What facilitates or impedes family communication following genetic testing for cancer risk? A systematic review and meta-synthesis of primary qualitative research. J Genet Couns. 2010;19:330–42. https://doi.org/10.1007/s10897-010-9296-y.

Cousens NE, Gaff CL, Metcalfe SA, Delatycki MB. Carrier screening for beta-thalassaemia: a review of international practice. Eur J Hum Genet. 2010;18:1077–83. https://doi.org/10.1038/ejhg.2010.90.

de Souza DAS, Faucz FR, Pereira-Ferrari L, Sotomaior VS, Raskin S. Congenital bilateral absence of the vas deferens as an atypical form of cystic fibrosis: reproductive implications and genetic counseling. Andrology. 2018;6:127–35.

de Weerd S, van der Bij AK, Braspenning JC, Cikot RJ, Braat DD, Steegers EA. Psychological impact of preconception counseling: assessment of anxiety before and during pregnancy. Community Genet. 2001;4:129–33. https://doi.org/10.1159/000051172.

de Wert G, Dondorp WJ, Knoppers BM. Preconception care and genetic risk: ethical issues. J Community Genet. 2012;3:221–8. https://doi.org/10.1007/s12687-011-0074-9.

Deciphering Developmental Disorders Study. Prevalence and architecture of de novo mutations in developmental disorders. Nature. 2017;542:433–8. https://doi.org/10.1038/nature21062.

Delatycki MB, Alkuraya F, Archibald A, Castellani C, Cornel M, Grody WW, Henneman L, Ioannides AS, Kirk E, Laing N, Lucassen A, Massie J, Schuurmans J, Thong MK, van Langen I, Zlotogora J. International perspectives on the implementation of reproductive carrier screening. Prenat Diagn. 2020;40(3):301–10. https://doi.org/10.1002/pd.5611.

Delatycki MB, Burke J, Christie L, Collins F, Gabbett M, George P, et al. Human Genetics Society of Australasia position statement: population-based carrier screening for cystic fibrosis. Twin Res Hum Genet. 2014;17:578–83. https://doi.org/10.1017/thg.2014.65.

Dheensa S, Lucassen A, Fenwick A. Limitations and pitfalls of using family letters to communicate genetic risk: a qualitative study with patients and healthcare professionals. J Genet Couns. 2018;27:689–701. https://doi.org/10.1007/s10897-017-0164-x.

Doka KJ. How we die: stigmatized death and disenfranchised grief. In: Doka KJ, editor. Disenfranchised grief: new directions, challenges, and strategies for practice. Champaign, IL: Research Press; 2002. p. 323–36. ISBN-13: 978-0878224272.

Edwards JG, Feldman G, Goldberg J, Gregg AR, Norton ME, Rose NC, et al. Expanded carrier screening in reproductive medicine-points to consider: a joint statement of the American College of Medical Genetics and Genomics, American College of Obstetricians and Gynecologists, National Society of Genetic Counselors, Perinatal Quality Foundation, and Society for Maternal-Fetal Medicine. Obstet Gynecol. 2015;125:653–62. https://doi.org/10.1097/AOG.0000000000000666.

Elwyn G, Gray J, Clarke A. Shared decision making and non-directiveness in genetic counselling. J Med Genet. 2000;37:135–8. https://doi.org/10.1136/jmg.37.2.135.

European Society for Human Reproduction and Embryology (ESHRE) Guideline Group on POI, Webber L, Davies M, Anderson R, Bartlett J, Braat D, Cartwright B, et al. ESHRE Guideline: management of women with premature ovarian insufficiency. Hum Reprod. 2016;31:926–37. https://doi.org/10.1093/humrep/dew027.

Flannigan R, Schlegel PN. Genetic diagnostics of male infertility in clinical practice. Best Pract Res Clin Obstet Gynaecol. 2017;44:26–37. https://doi.org/10.1016/j.bpobgyn.2017.05.002.

Forrest LE, Curnow L, Delatycki MB, Skene L, Aitken M. Health first, genetics second: exploring families' experiences of communicating genetic information. Eur J Hum Genet. 2008;16:1329–35. https://doi.org/10.1038/ejhg.2008.104.

Girard SL, Bourassa CV, Lemieux Perreault LP, Legault MA, Barhdadi A, Ambalavanan A, et al. Paternal age explains a major portion of de novo germline mutation rate variability in healthy individuals. PLoS One. 2016;11:e0164212. https://doi.org/10.1371/journal.pone.0164212.

Global Prevalence of Consanguinity. n.d. http://consang.net/index.php/Global_prevalence. Accessed 7 Sept 2019.

Hamamy H. Consanguineous marriages: preconception consultation in primary health care settings. J Community Genet. 2012;3:185–92. https://doi.org/10.1007/s12687-011-0072-y.

Henneman L, Borry P, Chokoshvili D, Cornel MC, van El CG, Forzano F, et al. Responsible implementation of expanded carrier screening. Eur J Hum Genet. 2016;24:e1–e12. https://doi.org/10.1038/ejhg.2015.271.

Holtkamp KCA, Mathijssen IB, Lakeman P, van Maarle MC, Dondorp WJ, Henneman L, Cornel MC. Factors for successful implementation of population-based expanded carrier screening: learning from existing initiatives. Eur J Pub Health. 2017;27:372–7. https://doi.org/10.1093/eurpub/ckw110.

Hyde KJ, Schust DJ. Genetic considerations in recurrent pregnancy loss. Cold Spring Harb Perspect Med. 2015;5:a023119. https://doi.org/10.1101/cshperspect.a023119.

Ioannides AS. Preconception and prenatal genetic counselling. Best Pract Res Clin Obstet Gynaecol. 2017;42:2–10. https://doi.org/10.1016/j.bpobgyn.2017.04.003.

Jack BW, Atrash H, Coonrod DV, Moos MK, O'Donnell J, Johnson K. The clinical content of preconception care: an overview and preparation of this supplement. Am J Obstet Gynecol. 2008;199(Suppl 2):S266–79. https://doi.org/10.1016/j.ajog.2008.07.067.

Kaback MM. Screening and prevention in Tay-Sachs disease: origins, update, and impact. Adv Genet. 2001;44:253–65. https://doi.org/10.1016/S0065-2660(01)44084-3.

Kessler S. Psychological aspects of genetic counseling. XI. Nondirectiveness revisited. Am J Med Genet. 1997;72:164–71. https://doi.org/10.1002/(sici)1096-8628(19971017)72:2<164::aid-ajmg8>3.0.co;2-v.

Kingsmore S. Comprehensive carrier screening and molecular diagnostic testing for recessive childhood diseases. PLoS Curr. 2012:e4f9877ab8ffa9. https://doi.org/10.1371/4f9877ab8ffa9.

Kirk EP, Barlow-Stewart K, Selvanathan A, Josephi-Taylor S, Worgan L, Rajagopalan S, Cowley MJ, Gayevskiy V, Bittles A, Burnett L, Elakis G, Lo W, Buckley M, Colley A, Roscioli T. Beyond the panel: preconception screening in consanguineous couples using the TruSight one "clinical exome". Genet Med. 2019;21:608–12. https://doi.org/10.1038/s41436-018-0082-9.

Lazarin GA, Haque IS, Nazareth S, Iori K, Patterson AS, Jacobson JL, Marshall JR, Seltzer WK, Patrizio P, Evans EA, Srinivasan BS. An empirical estimate of carrier frequencies for 400+ causal Mendelian variants: results from an ethnically diverse clinical sample of 23,453 individuals. Genet Med. 2013;15:178–86. https://doi.org/10.1038/gim.2012.114.

Lewis C, Skirton H, Jones R. Reproductive empowerment: the main motivator and outcome of carrier testing. J Health Psychol. 2012;17:567–78. https://doi.org/10.1177/1359105311417193.

Mathijssen IB, Henneman L, Van Eeten-Nijman JM, et al. Targeted carrier screening for four recessive disorders: high detection rate within a founder population. Eur J Med Genet. 2015;58:123–8. https://doi.org/10.1016/j.ejmg.2015.01.004.

McAllister M, Davies L, Payne K, Nicholls S, Donnai D, MacLeod R. The emotional effects of genetic diseases: implications for clinical genetics. Am J Med Genet A. 2007;143A:2651–61. https://doi.org/10.1002/ajmg.a.32013.

McClaren BJ, Metcalfe SA, Aitken M, Massie RJ, Ukoumunne OC, Amor DJ. Uptake of carrier testing in families after cystic fibrosis diagnosis through newborn screening. Eur J Hum Genet. 2010;18:1084–9. https://doi.org/10.1038/ejhg.2010.78.

Mendes Á, Metcalfe A, Paneque M, Sousa L, Clarke AJ, Sequeiros J. Communication of information about genetic risks: putting families at the center. Fam Process. 2018;57:836–46. https://doi.org/10.1111/famp.12306.

Metcalfe A, Coad J, Plumridge GM, Gill P, Farndon P. Family communication between children and their parents about inherited genetic conditions: a meta-synthesis of the research. Eur J Hum Genet. 2008;16:1193–200. https://doi.org/10.1038/ejhg.2008.84.

Milsom S, O'Sullivan S. Premature ovarian insufficiency. O&G Magazine. 2017;19(1). https://www.ogmagazine.org.au/19/1-19/premature-ovarian-insufficiency/. Accessed 1 May 2019.

Oliveira LM, Seminara SB, Beranova M, Hayes FJ, Valkenburgh SB, Schipani E, Costa EM, Latronico AC, Crowley WF Jr, Vallejo M. The importance of autosomal genes in Kallmann syndrome: genotype-phenotype correlations and neuroendocrine characteristics. J Clin Endocrinol Metab. 2001;86:1532–8. https://doi.org/10.1210/jcem.86.4.7420.

Oosterwal G. Multicultural counseling. In: Uhlmann WR, Schuette JL, Yashar B, editors. A guide to genetic counseling. Hoboken, NJ: John Wiley & Sons; 2009. p. 331–61. ISBN: 978-0-470-17965-9.

Patch C, Middleton A. Genetic counselling in the era of genomic medicine. Br Med Bull. 2018;126:27–36. https://doi.org/10.1093/bmb/ldy008.

Qin Y, Jiao X, Simpson JL, Chen ZJ. Genetics of primary ovarian insufficiency: new developments and opportunities. Hum Reprod Update. 2015;21:787–808. https://doi.org/10.1093/humupd/dmv036.

Riedijk S, Oudesluijs G, Tibben A. Psychosocial aspects of preconception consultation in primary care: lessons from our experience in clinical genetics. J Community Genet. 2012;3:213–9. https://doi.org/10.1007/s12687-012-0095-z.

Ropers HH. On the future of genetic risk assessment. J Community Genet. 2012;3:229–36. https://doi.org/10.1007/s12687-012-0092-2.

Sallevelt SCEH, de Koning B, Szklarczyk R, Paulussen ADC, de Die-Smulders CEM, Smeets HJM. A comprehensive strategy for exome-based preconception carrier screening. Genet Med. 2017;19:583–92. https://doi.org/10.1038/gim.2016.153.

Salway S, Ali P, Ratcliffe G, Such E, Khan N, Kingston H, Quarrell O. Responding to the increased genetic risk associated with customary consanguineous marriage among minority ethnic populations: lessons from local innovations in England. J Community Genet. 2016;7:215–28. https://doi.org/10.1007/s12687-016-0269-1.

Sankaranarayanan K. Ionizing radiation and genetic risks IX. Estimates of the frequencies of mendelian diseases and spontaneous mutation rates in human populations: a 1998 perspective. Mutat Res. 1998;411:129–78. https://doi.org/10.1016/S1383-5742(98)00012-X.

Shaw A. Drivers of cousin marriage among British Pakistanis. Hum Hered. 2014;77:26–36. https://doi.org/10.1159/000358011.

Sheridan E, Wright J, Small N, Corry PC, Oddie S, Whibley C, Petherick ES, Malik T, Pawson N, McKinney PA, Parslow RC. Risk factors for congenital anomaly in a multiethnic birth cohort: an analysis of the Born in Bradford study. Lancet. 2013;382(9901):1350–9. https://doi.org/10.1016/S0140-6736(13)61132-0.

Skirton H. More than an information service: are counselling skills needed by genetics professionals in the genomic era? Eur J Hum Genet. 2018;26:1239–40. https://doi.org/10.1038/s41431-018-0133-3.

Skirton H, Goldsmith L, Jackson L, Lewis C, Chitty L. Offering prenatal diagnostic tests: European guidelines for clinical practice. Eur J Hum Genet. 2014;22:580–6. https://doi.org/10.1038/ejhg.2013.205.

Sobel S, Cowan CB. Ambiguous loss and disenfranchised grief: the impact of DNA predictive testing on the family as a system. Fam Process. 2003;42:47–57. https://doi.org/10.1111/j.1545-5300.2003.00047.x.

Solomon BD, Jack BW, Feero WG. The clinical content of preconception care: genetics and genomics. Am J Obstet Gynecol. 2008;199:S340–4. https://doi.org/10.1016/j.ajog.2008.09.870.

Teeuw ME, Hagelaar A, Ten Kate LP, Cornel MC, Henneman L. Challenges in the care for consanguineous couples: an exploratory interview study among general practitioners and midwives. BMC Fam Pract. 2012;13:105. https://doi.org/10.1186/1471-2296-13-105.

Teeuw ME, Loukili G, Bartels EA, Ten Kate LP, Cornel MC, Henneman L. Consanguineous marriage and reproductive risk: attitudes and understanding of ethnic groups practising consanguinity in Western society. Eur J Hum Genet. 2014;22:452–7. https://doi.org/10.1038/ejhg.2013.167.

Ten Kate LP. Genetic risk. J Community Genet. 2012;3:159–66. https://doi.org/10.1007/s12687-011-0066-9.

Ten Kate LP, Teeuw ME, Henneman L, Cornel MC. Consanguinity and endogamy in the Netherlands: demographic and medical genetic aspects. Hum Hered. 2014;77:161–6. https://doi.org/10.1159/000360761.

Tucker EJ, Grover SR, Bachelot A, Touraine P, Sinclair AH. Premature ovarian insufficiency: new perspectives on genetic cause and phenotypic spectrum. Endocr Rev. 2016;37:609–35. https://doi.org/10.1210/er.2016-1047.

Vander Borght M, Wyns C. Fertility and infertility: definition and epidemiology. Clin Biochem. 2018;62:2–10. https://doi.org/10.1016/j.clinbiochem.2018.03.012.

Vissers LELM, van Nimwegen KJM, Schieving JH, Kamsteeg EJ, Kleefstra T, Yntema HG, et al. A clinical utility study of exome sequencing versus conventional genetic testing in pediatric neurology. Genet Med. 2017;19:1055–63. https://doi.org/10.1038/gim.2017.1.

Whitney DK. Emotional sequelae of elective abortion: the role of guilt and shame. J Pastoral Care Counsel. 2017;71:98–105. https://doi.org/10.1177/1542305017708159.

Zlotogora J, Carmi R, Lev B, Shalev SA. A targeted population carrier screening program for severe and frequent genetic diseases in Israel. Eur J Hum Genet. 2009;17:591–7. https://doi.org/10.1038/ejhg.2008.241.

Fertility

5

Ilse Delbaere and Jenny Stern

The topic of planning or preparing for pregnancy is complex. Words such as 'planning' and 'pregnancy intention' have different meanings for different communities. The ability to 'plan' a pregnancy assumes that women have access to resources, power over decisions about their reproductive health, and the ability to control their own future and raise their children in a safe environment (Ross 2017). Planning for a pregnancy may be a Western middle-class concept that doesn't fit different cultures or religious perspectives. This chapter recognizes these complexities and aims to describe people's general motivations to have children and the extent to which people understand human reproduction and lifts up critical issues around fertility that can impact a couple's ability to achieve pregnancy. The chapter highlights age as one of the most important determinants of female fertility and a leading contributor to the higher need of assisted reproduction within the population. Female and male conditions requiring medical assistance to conceive are also described. Assisted reproductive techniques have their limitations but are currently efficient and still evolving rapidly with some very evolutionary procedures to come. Understanding fertility is important for all young adults. Health-care providers have a responsibility for educating people about their fertility and providing unbiased information and reproductive care

I. Delbaere (✉)
Vives University of Applied Sciences, Kortrijk, Belgium
e-mail: Ilse.Delbaere@vives.be

J. Stern
Sophiahemmet University, Stockholm, Sweden

Uppsala University, Uppsala, Sweden
e-mail: Jenny.Stern@kbh.uu.se

© Springer Nature Switzerland AG 2020
J. Shawe et al. (eds.), *Preconception Health and Care: A Life Course Approach*,
https://doi.org/10.1007/978-3-030-31753-9_5

5.1   Family Planning and Size

With the introduction of effective contraception, the question as to whether people want to have children or not became relevant. The answer to this question is generally 'yes'. In almost all studies in Western countries on this subject, more than 90% of respondents said they wanted to have children at some point in their lives (Lampic et al. 2006; Virtala et al. 2011; Peterson et al. 2012; Sørensen et al. 2016). The ideal number of children per family in European countries is one or two (Almeida-Santos et al. 2017; Lampic et al. 2006). The most reported reasons for having children are 'because of the contribution to life satisfaction' (Almeida-Santos et al. 2017) 'developing as a person' and 'giving and receiving love' (Lampic et al. 2006; Tydén et al. 2006). The former is true for Western countries and middle- to high-income situations. Although all societies value having children very highly, in non-Western countries and low-income situations, there may be differences in the decision to have children, the ideal number of children and the gender preference. In some countries, women are subordinated when not having children; also access to contraception, governmental decisions (e.g. the former one-child policy in China) and cultural and religious aspects (e.g. encouragement to have children at a young age) have an impact on family planning (Bos and Van Rooij 2007). In low-income settings, children may contribute to the financial security of the family. Nonetheless, the global fertility rate halved worldwide over the last 50 years, due to empowerment of women, increased level of education and the availability of contraception for an increasing proportion of women (Max 2017).

Contraception provides women with the opportunity to control their fertility and, as such, helps to achieve the desired number of children. Nowadays, a growing number of couples experience difficulties in obtaining the desired number of children. The difference between the mean intended and realized family size is called the *fertility gap*. The fertility gap in Europe is 0.34 children per women (0.25 in Germany and Austria to 0.71 in Scandinavian countries) (Sobotka and Lutz 2010). There are various reasons why people cannot fulfil their ideal family size: not having a suitable partner, financial constraints or competition with educational, professional or personal ambitions. In general, such a fertility gap (fewer children born than intended) is observed in high-income countries. In low and middle-income countries, women still tend to have more children than intended (Channon and Harper 2019).

A great deal of young people consider their late twenties to be the ideal time to have children. In reality, a significant part of women postpone their motherhood until their early thirties and men until their mid-thirties (Daniluk et al. 2012). In 2017, the mean age of Flemish first time mothers was 29 years (Devlieger et al. 2018); this is comparable with the mean age of primiparae in other European countries (Eurostat 2015). In the United States, the mean age of primiparae was 26.8 years (Hamilton et al. 2018), but in this country, there are significantly more older, first time mothers in cities. According to Mills et al. (2011), there are a variety of reasons for couples to postpone parenthood: women have access to effective contraception and there are a lot of opportunities to pursue personal fulfilment for women (educationally and professionally) (Mills et al. 2011; Waldenström 2016). Furthermore, changing partners, economic uncertainties, professional aspirations and absence of a supportive social network may contribute to the decision to delay parenthood.

Since a great deal of couples tend to delay parenthood, one could ask which prerequisites are seen for starting a family. In literature on delayed parenthood, educational and professional aspirations of women are often put forward as the main reason to postpone a first pregnancy. Nevertheless, studies show that also emotional aspects contribute to the readiness of parenthood. Relationship stability is often cited as a prerequisite, more than financial stability (Sørensen et al. 2016; Almeida-Santos et al. 2017; Lampic et al. 2006; Chan et al. 2015). Studies using the Swedish Fertility Awareness Questionnaire reported the following issues as most important for men and women in Swedish populations: 'having a partner to share responsibility', 'feeling sufficiently mature' and 'having a stable relationship' (Lampic et al. 2006; Tydén et al. 2006; Skoog Svanberg et al. 2006). However, in the study by Alfaraj et al. (2019), 'completing my studies' and 'not being too old' are most commonly cited as important before having children (Alfaraj et al. 2019).

Although emotional aspects tend to contribute to a great extent to the decision to start having children, Van Bavel (2010) assessed a discrepancy in maternal age at first pregnancy according to discipline of study/career in Western situations (Van Bavel 2010). Women who have a career in more male-dominated disciplines tend to postpone more. Aspirations to become a mother and to be able to combine motherhood with a job may be the reason why women are still overrepresented in fields of education and humanities and underrepresented in powerful or technological jobs, even though these jobs are more lucrative. The results of this study suggest that women who want to have children at a relatively young age (motherhood on top of the agenda) may choose their field of study and profession according to this future perspective.

5.2 Unintended Pregnancy

Although 90% of European women who wish to avoid having children use contraception, unintended pregnancy remains high in Western countries: 34% in Western Europe to 54% in Eastern Europe (Baird et al. 2018). In the United States, unintended pregnancies declined from 51% in 2008 to 45% in 2011 (Finer and Zolna 2016). Since most people in Western countries have their first sexual intercourse at age 15–18 and most of these women have their first child at age 30 or later, there are many years where women are 'at risk' to conceive unintendedly. Other determinants for unintended pregnancies are desired number of children (each desired child means approximately 2 years less exposure to unintended pregnancy), effective contraception use (Baird et al. 2018) and economic conditions (more desire for pregnancy and less unintendedness when conditions are good) (Finer and Zolna 2016).

Indeed, easy access to effective contraceptive methods is the most important determinant to reduce unintended pregnancy. Although the use of contraception is high in Western countries, an important number of unintended pregnancies have been found in couples using no contraception at all. Lack of knowledge, fear of risks and side effects and religious beliefs may deter couples from using contraception. Worldwide, governmental interventions to improve access to contraception and qualitative sex education in school may be helpful to improve unintended pregnancy rates.

Unplanned pregnancy has been associated with a number of adverse pregnancy outcomes, such as spontaneous abortion, preterm birth and low birth weight (Goossens et al. 2016). Furthermore, an unplanned pregnancy has an impact on the physical and psychological wellbeing of both mother and child. Postpartum depression is, for example, more common among women with unplanned pregnancies (Mercier et al. 2013). As such, prevention of unplanned pregnancies is a major topic of global health priority (United Nations 2015).

In studies assessing unwanted, unintended and unplanned pregnancies, the question wording is very important (Moreau et al. 2014), and different measurements and wordings are used in different studies making comparisons of prevalence of unplanned pregnancies precarious. An 'unplanned' pregnancy is more socially accepted for women than an 'unwanted' pregnancy. Categorization of pregnancy intention and planning in a dichotomous manner, intended versus unintended and planned versus unplanned, is an oversimplification of a very complex construct in that some women experience conflicting attitudes and feelings towards a future pregnancy, which can result in inadequate contraceptive use. As such, it is very important to use accurate measures in order to assess unwanted and unintended pregnancies. In order to measure the prevalence of unplanned pregnancies in a population, it is necessary to use an instrument that takes this complexity of pregnancy planning into account. The London Measure of Unplanned Pregnancy (LMUP) and the Swedish Pregnancy Planning Scales are such valid and reliable instruments (Barrett et al. 2004; Drevin et al. 2017; Goossens et al. 2018). With the use of these instruments, ambivalent feelings about becoming pregnant can be captured.

5.3 Age as a Predictive Factor for Fertility: Women and Men

The trend to postpone motherhood also impacts fertility rates, in that female fertility decreases after the age of 25 and this is even more prominent after the age of 30 (Delbaere et al. 2007) (see Fig. 5.1). Success of assisted reproduction strongly depends on age (Leridon 2004). There are an increased risk of comorbidity with age and a cumulative effect of possible exposure to disadvantageous lifestyle factors such as obesity. As advanced maternal age is associated with prolonged time needed to conceive, postponed parenthood may affect the desired family size of couples (Schmidt et al. 2012).

Habbema et al. (2015) conducted a computer simulation in order to calculate the recommended age to start a family for women, depending on the number of children wanted and whether they are prepared to undergo fertility treatment or not. They

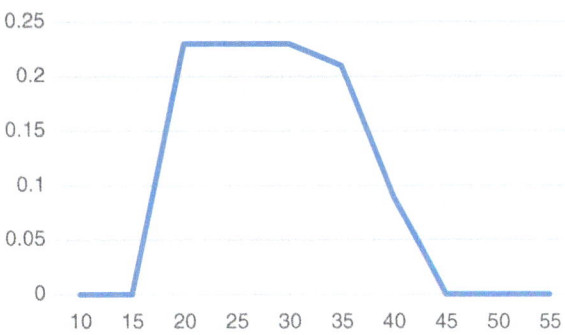

Fig. 5.1 Probability of being pregnant in a single menstrual cycle in function of women's age

found that couples who desire a one-child family have a 90% chance to realize this when they start at the age of 32 (at latest) for the female partner. When in vitro fertilization (IVF) is an option for this couple, they should start at female age 35 at latest. When the couple desires a two-child family, they should start to conceive when the woman is 27 years old (31 years when IVF is an option), and when the couples want three children, they should start at female age of 23 years (28 in the case that IVF is an option). Couples can start 4–11 years later in the case that they accept 75% or lower chances to complete their desired families (Habbema et al. 2015).

In previous research, Leridon (2004) also used a computer simulation to assess whether assisted reproduction can compensate for the effect of age on fertility. This is not the case. With advancing age, a woman's chances of getting pregnant decrease and the chances of miscarriage increase (Davies et al. 2009).

It is said that women have a biological clock in that they are born with their lifetime's supply of follicles within their ovaries. No extra eggs are produced during the lifetime of a woman. When women approach the age of 40, there is an effect of ageing on the ovary and the eggs, which explains a higher risk of having a baby with Down syndrome and miscarriages and a lower chance of getting pregnant. The higher number of miscarriages in older women also indicates a higher degree of genetic defects in these pregnancies. Down syndrome occurs 1/200 at age 38, 1/100 at age 40 and 1/30 at age 45. In theory, preimplantation genetic screening can be offered to older women going through assisted reproductive technology (ART). With this technique, embryos can be screened for Down syndrome or other conditions before embryo transfer (Davies et al. 2009).

Women younger than 30 years have a chance of one in five to have a miscarriage; when they are 40, the chance of having a miscarriage is 50%. Women aged 35–39 years are half as fertile as when they are 25, and at age 40, women are half as fertile as when they are 35, as depicted in Fig. 5.1 (Davies et al. 2009). At age 37, women usually have around 25,000 oocytes left, but oocyte loss goes faster in the late thirties and forties. Only 1000 oocytes are left at age 50 (which is the mean age for menopause in women living in Western countries).

Couples trying to conceive have 85% chance to conceive within a year when the woman is aged less than 30. At the age of 30 it is 75%, at age 35 it is 66%, and at age 40 it is 44%. Usually couples are advised to try to conceive for 1 year before seeking medical help; however, when the woman is 35, some authors suggest they should consult a specialist already after 6 months in order not to waste precious time at this age (Davies et al. 2009).

Men don't have a biological clock, since they produce sperm within the testicles throughout their lifetime. They can father children into old age. Nevertheless, some studies point out that age has an effect on semen quality (Brahem et al. 2011). In a sample of 140 infertile patients, an increase of diploidy and a decline in semen volume and sperm vitality were found (Dain et al. 2011).

While individuals in same-sex relationships have the same reproductive functions as others, they often need to use the services of fertility clinics when they want to become pregnant.

With regard to same-sex male couples, it is important that egg donation and surrogacy are regulated and that cooperating women are fully informed (Mackenzie et al. 2019). Same-sex couples, as in all people who seek fertility services, should receive non-judgmental, unbiased, quality care (Mackenzie et al. 2019).

5.4   Methods to Monitor the Window of Fertility

In this chapter, the term 'fertility awareness' is used to depict the knowledge about fertility-related issues in the population. However, 'fertility awareness' is more often used in order to describe insight into the menstrual cycle and practices to use this knowledge for the purpose of family planning (natural family planning). Although these fertility awareness-based methods can be less effective as an alternative for contraception (Urrutia et al. 2018), some of these methods may be effective to monitor the window of fertility for women planning a pregnancy.

The cervical mucus method or Billings ovulation test is one common approach. A few days before ovulation, vaginal secretion is wetter, clearer and more slippery (comparable with egg white). This highly fertile kind of mucus encourages sperm penetration through the cervix. Infertile secretions are generally dry, sticky, cloudy and less stretchable. Menstruation should be considered as fertile, because menses mask the aspects of cervical secretion. This is also the case for sexual fluids; as such, secretion signs should not be interpreted during menstruation and in the first day after having sex. If women learn to recognize this kind of secretion, they can better assess their fertility window [www.fertility.org].

The TwoDay Method® is a variation of the cervical mucus method: any cervical mucus observed that day or the prior day indicates a fertile day. Each day two questions should be asked: First: did the woman note any secretions that day? Second: did the woman note any secretions the day before? If the answer is yes to at least one of these questions, she can be considered fertile. If the answer is no to both of these questions, she is probably not fertile. The advantage of cervical mucus methods is that it is compatible with cycles of any length.

The basal body temperature method uses temperature charts for monitoring fertility, based on the principle that waking temperature rises immediately after ovulation. This home test is of limited value for women trying to conceive and is no longer advised for planning pregnancy. Although recording temperature on waking may confirm ovulation has occurred, it is only detected retrospectively when the most fertile time may have passed. In addition, temperature may be subject to other body changes than ovulation alone.

The symptothermal method combines BBT, cervical methods and cervical position data to identify the window of fertility. Two signs are used to 'double-check' each phase as confirmation for the couple that the woman is fertile, and together with training from a qualified practitioner, this is more reliable if fertility awareness is to be used for contraception. For those planning a pregnancy, monitoring cervical secretions alone is suggested to be least intrusive and a good prospective marker in order to identify the best time for timing of sexual intercourse.

Ovulation kits are available to predict ovulation by measuring luteinizing hormone level and/or estrogen metabolites. Kits can be expensive but are used by some women to identify their fertile time.

5.5 Subfertility and Infertility

A pregnancy that takes place within the first year of trying to conceive with regular intercourse indicates normal or average fertility. For some couples without medical conditions, it may take 2 years to conceive. Young women with a regular cycle and no previous gynaecological problems can wait for 2 years to conceive before seeking medical help. Women with anovulation or women who have experienced previous gynaecological problems, such as endometriosis, ectopic pregnancy or pelvic infection, should contact medical help without delay. One in seven couples experiences difficulties in getting pregnant. While many benefit from medical intervention, this is not true for everyone. The process of trying to become pregnant can be very challenging for couples.

5.5.1 Female Subfertility

An average menstrual cycle takes 28 days. The first day of the cycle is the first day of the period; the last day is the day before the subsequent period. Ovulation takes place on average on day 14 (Fig. 5.2). When the menstrual cycle is longer, ovulation comes later (e.g. in a cycle of 30 days, the ovulation will likely take place on day 16) and vice versa. Since there is a rise in luteinizing hormone (LH) at the time of ovulation, a urine test detecting this hormone can be used to assess ovulation. Once the egg is released, it can be fertilized for 24 h. Sperm, on the contrary, can stay alive and active for several subsequent days. As a consequence, sexual intercourse before ovulation is advised. As such, the sperm is ready and 'at place' at the time of ovulation. The fertility window is considered to be a few days before ovulation and 1 or 2 days after ovulation where fertilization is possible. There are a number of conditions which may challenge female fertility. Some of the most important will be discussed in the next sections.

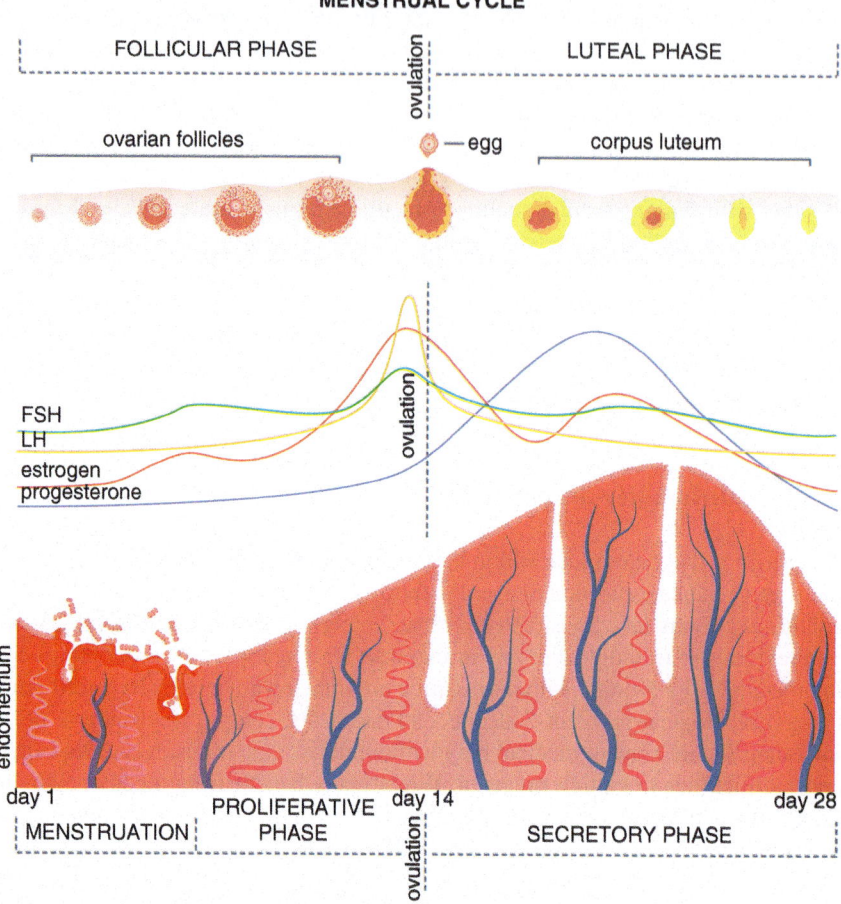

Fig. 5.2 The menstrual cycle (Marochkina Anastasiia/Shutterstock.com)

Polycystic ovary syndrome or PCOS is the most common hormonal disorder in women of reproductive age; 7% of women suffer from this condition. As the name indicates, the ovaries contain an increased number of follicles which are observable by ultrasound; however, there is a lack of regular ovulation which causes infertility in most women with PCOS. Moreover, an increased level of androgens is produced which can cause hirsutism and acne (Davies et al. 2009).

Anovulation occurs when a woman ovulates not at all. When this is the case, menstrual cycles may be irregular (gaps of 2 months in between periods or less than 26 days), and periods may be prolonged. Polycystic ovary syndrome is one of the most common causes of anovulation. As this is an abnormality of the ovary, coordination of production of hormones is disordered (Davies et al. 2009).

When the ovarian reserve is depleted under the age of 40, it is termed **premature ovarian failure** or insufficiency. Normal follicle development does not longer occur and there is anovulation. Oocyte donation is recommended with this condition.

Endometriosis is a disease with presence of functional endometrial glands outside the uterine cavity, most commonly in the ovaries, the fossa ovarica, the uterosacral ligaments and the posterior cul-de-sac. It features chronic inflammation, and endometriosis is similar to malignancies in that it is characterized by both progressive, invasive growth and estrogen-dependent growth. Endometriosis has been classified in four stages based on the severity, amount, location, depth and size of growths, those stages being stage I (minimal disease), stage II (mild disease), stage III (moderate disease) and stage IV (severe disease), depending on the extent of affection of the pelvis (Olive 2005).

Fertility is dependent on the grade of endometriosis; only women with moderate and severe endometriosis usually experience fertility problems. Medication is only useful for pain relief, not to improve pregnancy rates. In order to improve fertility, surgical treatment is applied in order to destroy nodules of endometriosis and liberate adhesions around the ovaries and fallopian tubes. After surgery, fertility may be boosted by the combination of ovarian stimulation and intrauterine insemination. After four unsuccessful cycles, IVF may be advised (Davies et al. 2009).

Tubal disease is the limitation of the tubal function due to pelvic adhesions or tubal damage. Because of this tubal damage, effective transport of gametes is affected, and tubal disease is thus an important cause of infertility. Diagnosis of pelvic disease is made laparoscopically, often in combination with hysterosalpingography, hysterocontrast sonography, fertiloscopy and salpingoscopy (Akande 2007).

Management of tubal disease would benefit from a classification system to distinguish infertile patients with tubal disease into favourable and unfavourable groups for surgery in order to reconstruct occluded fallopian tubes. Because of the accessibility of IVF, this technique is most often used when women with tubal disease want to become pregnant. Nonetheless, this is not a real therapy for the disease (Akande 2007).

5.5.2 Male Subfertility

Sperm quality may interfere with the accomplishment of pregnancy. Normal semen analysis depicts a volume greater than 1.5 mL, a total sperm number of more than 39 million per ejaculate and a sperm concentration of more than 15 million sperm per millilitre, more than 40% of sperm should be motile, and 32% of sperm should move with progressive motion; finally more than 4% of the sperm should have a normal shape (WHO 2010).

When a **low volume of semen** is found, it may be indicative for **retrograde ejaculation** where the sperm moves backwards into the bladder. This may be the case after prostate or abdominal surgery and in men with diabetes, multiple sclerosis or spinal cord problems. On the other hand, a low volume may also be due to a blockage in the ejaculatory ducts at the level of the prostate.

Oligozoospermia occurs when there are too few sperm within the ejaculate (less than 15 million per mL). This is related with too many abnormal forms (*teratozoospermia*, normal morphology <4%) or reduced numbers of motile sperm (*asthenozoospermia*, less than 40% motile sperm). Oligoasthenoteratozoospermia (or OATS) is the term used when all three are present. There are numerous potential causes of OATS, including varicoceles, chemotherapy, hormonal problems, partial ejaculatory duct obstruction or genetic causes.

The term **azoospermia** is used when there is no sperm at all in the semen analysis. This can be due to a block in the tubes from the testes or to testicular failure. The latter may be due to drug use, radiotherapy, trauma or infections, undescended testicles or genetic reasons (Davies et al. 2009).

Men with retrograde ejaculation (and thus a low volume of semen) can be treated with ephedrine or imipramine, which contract the bladder neck muscle in order to prevent semen backflow. Moreover, sperm can be recovered from the urine or retrieved from the testicle and be used for ICSI. When the lower volume of semen is due to a blockage in the ejaculatory ducts, unblocking surgery may be successful. In the case of OATS or azoospermia, sperm can be retrieved from the testis and can be used for IVF/ICSI treatment. This is done by *MESA* (*micro-epididymal sperm aspiration*) or *TESE* (*testicular sperm extraction*) (Davies et al. 2009).

5.5.3 Combined Subfertility and Infertility

The term combined subfertility is used when both the male and female partner have a condition that impacts their fertility. Combined infertility is a term used when there is a diagnosis of both male and female infertility in a couple.

Unexplained infertility occurs when all tests have been performed and all major causes of infertility can be excluded. One in four couples with fertility problems gets this diagnosis. When this is the case, intrauterine insemination or controlled ovarian hyperstimulation is used as therapy or the combination of both.

5.5.4 Fertility Investigation

Ovulation tests are available over the counter and are a good place to start. They can assess the luteinizing hormone (LH) in the urine, which peaks right before ovulation. A positive result predicts ovulation within 24–36 h. These tests can be helpful in regular cycles. In women with high basic LH or women with PCOS or early menopause, these tests may give false results. More sophisticated home tests can measure both LH and oestradiol in order to indicate the fertility window (5 days). A laboratory test for the hormone progesterone may assess whether ovulation has occurred. There is a peak in progesterone a week after ovulation (and thus a week before the next period). Furthermore, ultrasound scanning can be used to monitor the development and release of the egg (Davies et al. 2009).

The ovarian reserve is the amount of eggs stored in the ovaries. This declines when women get older, but even some young women can have low reserves. It is important to test the ovarian reserve, in that it predicts the response to fertility drugs and thus chances of successful treatment. Assessment of ovarian reserve includes a blood test to measure anti-Müllerian hormone (AMH) or ultrasound scanning to measure the size of ovaries and the number of visible follicles, which is an indicator for the ovarian reserve.

Before a **semen analysis**, men are asked not to ejaculate for 3 days. The sample should then be produced by masturbation into a sterile container, kept warm and handed into the laboratory within an hour. Laboratory analysis will assess the quantity of semen, the appearance, the quantity and the proportion. The sample will also be tested for infection and antibodies. When the sample has poor quality, a new test will be analysed after a few weeks, in that sperm quality may vary from time to time. When there are subsequent poor tests, a blood test will be performed to check hormone levels and any genetic cause of poor sperm quality. Furthermore, blockage of the vas deferens can be assessed or a biopsy from the testis may be taken (Davies et al. 2009).

A tubal assessment studies the passageway from the sperm to the egg and involves different tests:

- Ultrasound to scan blocked or swollen fallopian tubes.
- Hysterosalpingography (HSG) is a radiographic test using contrast agent to picture the passage through the uterus and tubes.
- Laparoscopy (in combination with hysteroscopy) can picture the uterus and tubes as well (Davies et al. 2009).

5.5.5 Assisted Reproductive Techniques (ART)

Since a couple of decades, a large number of fertility problems can be handled medically with a variety of techniques. Couples who were due to remain childless 40 years ago can now fulfil their desire to start a family.

Many studies assessing fertility awareness have also registered men and women's attitudes towards assisted human reproduction. Daniluk et al. (2012) found in a Canadian population that men and women had a positive attitude towards assisted reproduction in the case of subfertility. Men were significantly more open to consider using egg and embryo donation, gestational surrogacy and fertility preservation. Women were significantly more open for home fertility testing, IVF, ICSI and donor sperm. These results indicate that both men and women desire to have their own genetic offspring. A study by Lampic (2006) depicts that women are likely to turn to IVF in case of infertility (73% women versus 65% men).

Intrauterine insemination (IUI) is a form of fertility treatment in which a sample is prepared in the laboratory to extract and concentrate healthy sperm. Consequently, the small volume of fluid (0.5 mL) with fertile sperm is passed through the cervix and released in the uterus. This procedure only takes a few minutes and is done without anaesthetic on the day of ovulation or the day before. IUI is often performed when there is a mild male infertility, in that sperm washing before IUI can remove anti-sperm antibodies. Fresh sperm from the partner, frozen-thawed sperm from the partner (e.g. stored samples before cancer therapy) or donor sperm can be used with IUI. Furthermore, IUI is often the first-line treatment for unexplained infertility, for infertility associated with mild endometriosis and for women whose infertility can be due to cervical problems (e.g. in reduced production of cervical mucus after cone biopsy) (Davies et al. 2009).

Controlled ovarian hyperstimulation or superovulation means that medication (most often clomiphene or gonadotrophin) is used to stimulate the growth and ovulation of more than one egg. This increases the chance of pregnancy. In the case of unexplained infertility, the chance of pregnancy is doubled when clomiphene is administered. There is also a higher chance for multi-foetal gestations and ovarian hyperstimulation. The drugs are given by means of daily intake, starting early in the menstrual cycle. The cycle is monitored by ultrasound in order to check the number of developing oocytes.

The combination of controlled ovarian hyperstimulation and IUI increases the chance of pregnancy per cycle. Approximately one in ten to one in five cycles results in a successful pregnancy. This combination therapy is often used in unexplained fertility and mild fertility problems for 3 or 4 months (Davies et al. 2009).

Ovulation induction is the imitation of normal activity of the ovary with assistance of medication. Clomiphene is most often used as medication; alternatives are FSH injections. It is the aim to release one egg per cycle; however, 10% of pregnancies conceived with clomiphene administration will be multiple pregnancies. Treatment of women with PCOS is very successful with this method. Moreover, these women can enhance their chances by moderate weight loss (5–10% of starting weight). Weight reduction is also recommended in women with a body mass index greater than 30, before ovulation induction. Otherwise they are not likely to respond to medication (Davies et al. 2009).

In vitro fertilization (IVF) is the procedure where an egg and sperm are joined in vitro or outside the body. The technique was very experimental at the time the first *test-tube* baby was born (Louise Brown in 1978); since then, the technique has become very successful. It is particularly indicated to bypass damaged fallopian tubes, where a blockage prevents eggs and sperm for meeting. Prior to the IVF procedure, a number of medications are administered to the woman:

- Gonadotrophins or FSH in order to stimulate the ovaries to produce a large number of eggs (start during the period and given for 10–12 days).
- GnRH analogue or GnRH antagonist is given in order to block the hormone that triggers ovulation, in order to prevent for early ovulation.
- hCG is administered when the follicles have reached the desired size in order to mature the eggs.

Administration of these medications is monitored securely by vaginal ultrasounds in order to count the number and size of developing eggs. Blood analyses are performed in order to assess oestrogen levels. Egg collection is guided by vaginal ultrasound and takes about 30 min. At the same day, the male partner will supply a semen sample. Consequently, eggs of the best quality will be brought together with a prepared sample of sperm in vitro, and 2–6 days after egg collection, the best embryos will be selected for transfer into the uterus (Davies et al. 2009).

Success rates of IVF are strongly dependent on maternal age. In young women, with a large number of embryos available, in her first IVF cycles, it is advised to transfer only one embryo, in that her chances for a multiple pregnancy are high (De Sutter et al. 2002). In older women, when embryo quality is poor or after a number of IVF cycles, more embryos can be transferred in order to increase the chance on live birth. When the IVF procedure was not successful, a new treatment can start after at least 1 month. In some countries, a couple of IVF cycles are covered by insurance (see further).

Intra-cytoplasmic sperm injection (ICSI) is an advanced IVF technique where one single sperm is selected under the microscope and injected into the centre of the egg. This procedure is indicated in men with low sperm counts or sperm of poor quality. When a man is unable to produce sperm or when the number or quality of sperm is too low to achieve pregnancy, **sperm donation** may be a solution. Sperm donation may also be used when there is a risk for inherited disease in the couple or when there is no male partner in a couple or a single woman (Davies et al. 2009).

Assisted reproduction is not without risks. Ovarian hyperstimulation syndrome (OHSS) is an iatrogenic condition and only happens when women receive medication to stimulate their ovaries (gonadotrophins). Within treatment, chemical substances may make small blood vessels more porous, and fluid may leak out, making ovaries larger and tender. Sometimes fluid can build up in the abdomen and—rarely—around the lungs and heart. Women with polycystic ovaries, lean women and young women are more prone to develop OHSS. Usually, symptoms are mild and last a few days to a few weeks; sometimes hospital admission is required.

5.5.6 Expectations of ART

Since the remarkable year 1978, when the first IVF baby was born, assisted reproduction has evolved significantly. In the beginning of assisted reproduction, only a fraction of transferred embryos led to a succesfull pregnancy. As a consequence, there was an aggressive ovarian stimulation protocol in those days, and multiple embryos were transferred. This resulted in a multiple pregnancy epidemic and a high incidence of ovarian hyperstimulation syndrome (Niederberger et al. 2018). As the technique became more effective and twin-prone mothers were more easily detected (young women with a large number of high-quality embryos available at pick-up), the multiple pregnancy rate after assisted reproduction diminished (De Sutter et al. 2002). Because of less aggressive stimulation of ovaries, the incidence of ovarian hyperstimulation diminished dramatically, although it still occurs from time to time. Currently, in European countries, there is a pregnancy rate of 29.6% per aspiration in IVF and 27.8% for ICSI. In cycles where frozen embryos were used, the pregnancy rate per thawing was 27.0% (Calhaz-Jorge et al. 2017).

There are several techniques that may enhance the success of assisted reproduction. **Blastocyst transfer** is a procedure where embryos are only transferred at days

5–6 (blastocyst stage) within assisted reproduction. At this stage, embryos have the best potential for implantation. This procedure increases pregnancy rates when couples have several good-quality embryos available.

In vitro maturation is a process where immature eggs are collected from the ovaries and matured in vitro before fertilization. As such, ovarian stimulation can be avoided, and this technique is consequently of interest in women at danger for hyperstimulation and in women with newly diagnosed cancer, where time is lacking between diagnosis and treatment to start the procedure of ovary stimulation. **Embryo freezing** can be done when embryos resulting from an IVF or ICSI process that were not transferred can be used in a subsequent cycle. The embryos can be frozen in liquid nitrogen for 5 years or more. The freezing and thawing cycle may be detrimental for some embryos, and success rates of ART with thawed embryos are lower than with fresh embryos, but ovarian stimulation can be avoided this way (Davies et al. 2009).

5.5.7   Psychological Impact of Fertility Treatment

Fertility problems have a large impact on the personal life of couples. A lot of people go through a mourning process in that they 'lost' a future they have dreamt of. Different studies assessed higher rates of depression (up to 40%) and anxiety (15%) in women undergoing IVF. As such, infertility is found to be as stressful as other major medical disorders. The levels of stress vary during the IVF treatment. Higher levels are reported between embryo transfer and pregnancy diagnosis. A higher degree of stress and sexual dysfunction has been assessed in men as well (Niederberger et al. 2018).

According to Boivin (2019), patients coping and adapting strategies can be identified during the fertility process. Screening is thus important and patients at risk should be supported during treatment. It is usually necessary to point out to couples that psychological help is available in the fertility clinic and people need to be invited to make use of it (Boivin 2019). Avoidance coping seems to be correlated with poor adjustment to the condition of infertility; dispositional optimism is associated with better coping. Because women and men tend to cope differently, relational problems may occur during fertility treatment; however, some studies have shown that a considerable proportion of couples (25–50%) report a strengthened relationship during fertility treatment (Niederberger et al. 2018).

5.5.8   Current and Future Possibilities to Postpone Parenthood

Women can **freeze their eggs** without immediate fertilization. This can be done to secure fertility in case that a woman does not have a partner yet or before cancer treatment. It is recommended to freeze eggs before the age of 35 to have some success (30–40% success when there are ten eggs available). Nevertheless, egg freezing is expensive (between 1500 and 3000 € per cycle) and therefore not an option for many women across the globe.

When a woman no longer has eggs of her own or only eggs of very poor quality, **egg donation** may be a solution. Medical conditions in which donor eggs may be indicated are premature ovarian insufficiency, after chemotherapy or in Turner syndrome. Success rates are high in egg donation (30–35% per embryo transfer); however, finding a donor may be difficult. In this process, the egg receiver takes hormone supplements to prepare the womb for embryo implantation; the egg donor goes through ovarian simulation and egg collection. Cycles of both the donor and recipient need to be adjusted to synchronize with each other (Davies et al. 2009).

Recently, Yamashiro et al. (2018) found that induced pluripotent stem cells (IPSCs) may differentiate into cells similar to immature oocytes in the human foetus. These oogonia need 8 months to mature into oocytes in vivo. As women are born with their finite number of gametes, **in vitro production of human oocytes** may open new opportunities in reproductive technology (Yamashiro et al. 2018).

Some women are born without a uterus, have their uterus removed at reproductive age or have a uterus anomaly which is not compatible with pregnancy. When this is the case, it is considered absolute uterine factor infertility (AUFI). Until recently, this condition was untreatable and women with AUFI had to remain childless, to adopt or to make use of the services of a surrogate mother. In 2014, a healthy boy was born by elective caesarean section after **uterus transplantation** (UTx). A uterine allograft is a type of vascularized composite allograft transplantation, such as the face and hand. The difference with transplantation of the hand and face is that uterine allograft may use live donors. In spite of this advantage, uterine allograft is a more complicated procedure compared to other allograft transplantations, in that the blood flow of a uterine graft will be shared by both mother and foetus. Moreover, other than most transplantations, the success of UTx is not demonstrated within days but only after more than a year after transplantation (with the possible delivery of a healthy child). Once the woman has a healthy child, hysterectomy will be performed after a couple of months in order to diminish the risk of immunosuppression—associated side effects, such as nephrotoxicity, diabetes and certain malignancies. Swedish researchers started preparations on this research in 1999; in the meanwhile, more than ten UTX babies have been born (eight in Sweden, one in the United States, one in Brazil (from a deceased donor)) (Niederberger et al. 2018).

5.5.9 Economic Inequities in Fertility Treatment

Efforts have been made in some countries to provide reasonable access to assisted reproduction for everyone, including couples with limited financial resources (Boivin and Pennings 2005). As such, costs of one or more cycles are refunded in Belgium, France, the Netherlands and the United Kingdom. In other countries, fertility treatment is not refunded, and consequently, costs of $1618 per cycle (in Pakistan) to $12,146 per cycle (in the United States) are very difficult, if not impossible, to cover for couples with low resources (IVF-Worldwide n.d.). Consequently, in case of fertility problems, creating a family is the privilege for those who can afford medical treatment. Support of fertility care in resource-poor countries is often neglected because of limited resources, an emphasis on HIV/AIDS prevention and overpopulation in these countries. Nonetheless, involuntary childlessness in developing countries has often a higher societal impact when compared to Western countries, and lack of medical help means neglect of reproductive rights of women in these settings (Ombelet and Goossens 2017). Prevention of sexually transmitted infections (STIs) and education on family planning and STIs are a first step in the good direction for these countries, but low-cost fertility treatment should be available as well. A low-cost ovarian stimulation protocol (Ferraretti et al. 2015) and low-cost IVF techniques (Ombelet 2014) have been assessed in developing countries with promising results. Because of the destructive impact of childlessness on the personal life of million couples, fertility problems should not be applied as a medium to handle overpopulation. Next to prevention of STIs, education about family planning and assessment of lifestyle factors (e.g. tobacco use and obesity), access to low-cost therapy should be provided in order to meet the Human Rights, Article 16:1, which states that 'Men and women of full age, without any limitation due to race, nationality or religion have the right to marry and found a family' (WHO 2014).

5.6   Fertility Knowledge

Studies on fertility awareness and attitudes towards parenthood prove that highly educated people have a positive attitude towards parenthood; nonetheless these young people are often not sufficiently aware of the higher mentioned impact of age on fertility (Virtala et al. 2011; Peterson et al. 2012; Sørensen et al. 2016; Lampic et al. 2006; Tydén et al. 2006; Chan et al. 2015; Skoog Svanberg et al. 2006; Bretherick et al. 2010). At the question 'at what age are women most fertile?' in studies using the Swedish Fertility Awareness Questionnaire, 63% of female Swedish undergraduate students in the study of Lampic et al. (2006) reported the correct answer (age 20–24) versus 46% of male Swedish undergraduate students ($P < 0.001$). A similar study in the United States shows comparable results (Peterson et al. 2012); however, no significant difference was found between men and women.

A few studies assessed knowledge about the age where a marked decrease in women's ability to become pregnant can be expected. In the Swedish studies, a large proportion of men and women responded correctly (35–39 years); nevertheless, more than 40% undergraduate Swedish students and more than 30% postgraduate Swedish students think that a marked decrease in women's fertility can be expected at age 40 or later. In Finland and the United States, the optimistic perception about female fertility is even higher.

The success rates of assisted reproductive techniques are overestimated in students. A significant proportion (40%) of Swedish students thought that there was a 40–100% chance of getting pregnant after a first IVF attempt; in the United States, half of the students estimated a 40–100% chance of having a child with IVF.

Lampic et al. (2006) and authors of similar studies concluded that university students are planning their children at ages when female fertility is decreasing. Her results also revealed that these students were not sufficiently aware of the effect of female age on fertility. An important consequence of this lack of knowledge may be that an increasing number of couples will experience infertility in the future (Almeida-Santos et al. 2017).

5.6.1 Knowledge of Fertility Among Medical Students

Nouri and colleagues (2014) compared fertility awareness between Austrian medical students and non-medical students. Medical students had a higher awareness of age on fertility than non-medical students, particularly in identifying the correct age when a woman is most fertile (Nouri et al. 2014). The general knowledge level was however low also among medical students, which has been found also in Ukrainian and Saudi Arabian studies (Alfaraj et al. 2019; Nouri et al. 2014; Mogilevkina et al. 2016). As an example more than 60% of Ukrainian medical students think that female fertility decreases only after the age of 45 years (Mogilevkina et al. 2016). However, (Szücs et al. 2017) found that Hungarian, Serbian and Romanian female university students in health sciences had significantly more knowledge about the menstrual cycle when compared with other university students (Szűcs et al. 2017).

An American study among obstetrics and gynaecology (OB/GYN) resident physicians found that almost half of residents overestimated the age at which a marked decline in a woman's ability to get pregnant occurs (Yu et al. 2016). A majority (83%) believed an OB/GYN should initiate discussions about age-related fertility decline with patients (Yu et al. 2016), and four out of ten thought they should have discussions about oocyte cryopreservation (Peterson et al. 2018). Overestimation of age-related decline was more common among residents who were unwilling to initiate discussion about oocyte cryopreservation (Peterson et al. 2018). More international studies in medical students are needed before general conclusions can be drawn, but it is not favourable that future health-care providers par excellence, apt to help future couples with their family planning, are not sufficiently aware of fertility either. Both the general public and health professionals should be sufficiently informed about the increased reproductive risks associated with higher maternal age (Schmidt et al. 2012).

5.6.2 Knowledge of the Impact of Lifestyle Factors on Fertility and Pregnancy Outcome

In a study on fertility awareness in Flanders (Belgium), only 10–20% of adolescents and students think that age has an impact on female fertility. Alcohol, drugs and tobacco are considered as more dangerous (Table 5.1).

Table 5.1 Response of Flemish adolescents and students to the question 'Which lifestyle factors have an impact on female fertility?'

	Adolescents			Students		
	M (N = 442)	F (N = 423)	p-Value	M (N = 105)	F (N = 235)	p-Value
Factors that decrease female fertility	%	%		%	%	
Alcohol	32.5	20.1	<0.001	42.5	35.6	NS
Drugs	30.0	24.1	<0.05	27.4	14.0	<0.01
Smoking	33.4	28.9	NS	56.6	55.5	NS
Diseases, infections	18.8	23.8	NS	20.8	31.4	<0.05
Stress	2.2	4.9	<0.05	17.9	19.9	NS
Weight	8.5	4.0	<0.01	6.6	16.9	<0.05
Nutrition	13.5	9.2	<0.05	9.4	14.4	NS
Medication	3.1	2.5	NS	8.5	14.4	NS
Lifestyle	8.9	6.5	NS	15.1	21.2	NS
Psychological factors	0.3	0.7	NS	0.9	1.3	NS
Genetic factors	1.7	3.9	NS	9.4	8.5	NS
Environmental factors	1.9	5.9	NS	6.6	7.6	NS
Age	12.1	7.1	<0.05	10.4	18.2	NS

5.6.3 Knowledge of Fertility, Fertility Awareness, Reproductive Intentions and Behaviour: What Is the Link?

In summary, existing literature suggests the knowledge of fertility and fertility awareness is low, both among the general population and medical students/professionals. Still, only a handful of studies have evaluated the effect of knowledge interventions on behavioural outcomes, and none of the few studies that have had found any effect on behavioural outcomes despite increased knowledge levels among participants. The relation between knowledge of fertility, fertility awareness, reproductive intentions and behaviour is indeed complex. Several theoretical models of health behaviour can be used to explain it (a full account is too extensive for this chapter but see, e.g. the Health Belief Model and the Theory of Planned Behavior), none of which suggests a linear correlation between increased knowledge and behaviour change. However, although not the only factor, knowledge of fertility is indisputable one important factor for informed decision-making regarding reproductive health.

5.7 Interventions for Increasing Fertility Awareness

There are a growing number of studies on fertility awareness in the last decade. Online education offers interesting possibilities in this matter, in order to reach the target population in a tailored manner. The extent to which online fertility education is effective in increasing knowledge and change of behaviour requires longitudinal follow-up. However, online fertility education is accessible whenever needed and is, as such, a convenient platform for those seeking information.

Several campaigns have been launched in Western countries in the last decade, such as *Protect your fertility* (American Society for Reproductive Medicine) and *National Infertility Awareness Week* (InfertilityAwareness.org) in the United States and *Get Britain Fertile* and *Fertility Education initiative* in Great Britain. Some of these campaigns were criticized because the focus was particularly on women and because the public did not always appreciated being confronted with declining fertility with age, particularly not those couples already struggling with their fertility (Gray 2013).

5.7.1 Online Information and Education

Almeida-Santos et al. (2017) found that websites rather than doctors were the main source of information for participants (aged 15–45) to learn about fertility (Almeida-Santos et al. 2017). What information is available online regarding fertility and preconception care? Agricola and colleagues (2013) compared international guidelines for preconception health and care with information in Italian found by women of childbearing age and health professionals when googling for it. The information found through online searches by both groups were poor and inaccurate, which highlight the need for easy accessed and appealingly presented evidence-based information from trustworthy sources (Agricola et al. 2013). Several ambitious websites have since been launched in different countries, published by health-care profession associations, governmental health authorities or research groups, as standalone source of information or part of larger campaigns/efforts (Table 5.2).

5.7.2 How Effective Is Online Education?

Wantland et al. (2004) and Webb et al. (2010) found that online interventions can have a positive impact on health behaviours (Wantland et al. 2004; Webb et al. 2010). Online health information may thus be a cost-effective manner to disseminate fertility awareness. This was confirmed by the study by Wojcieszek and Thompson (2013). They exposed 137 undergraduate students online to a brief brochure on fertility, ART and delayed childbearing and found a significant increase in fertility knowledge and a decrease in intended age at first birth (Wojcieszek and Thompson 2013). Also Daniluk and Koert (2015) assessed the effectiveness of an online education in increasing knowledge of fertility and assisted reproductive technologies and in changing beliefs about the timing of parenthood in 199 childless men and women. They found that knowledge and beliefs were influenced immediately after reading ten online posts related to fertility (MyFertilityChoices.com). However, 6 months later there was no longer a significant change in knowledge and beliefs. This was particularly the case for men (Daniluk and Koert 2015).

Table 5.2 Examples of websites aimed to increase fertility awareness and promote preconception health

	Target group	Origin	Language	Publisher
YourFertility.org.au	General public and health-care professionals	AU	English	The Fertility Coalition
nhs.uk/livewell/infertility	General public	UK	English	NHS, Department of Health and Social Care
MyFertilityChoices.com	General public	CA	English	Canadian Institutes of Health Research and The University of British Columbia
ReproduktivLivsplan.se	General public	SE	Swedish English French Spanish Somali Arabic Greek	Uppsala University
BeforeAndBeyond.org	Health-care professionals	US	English	National Preconception Health and Health Care Initiative
ShowYourLoveToday	Adults of reproductive age	US	English	National Preconception Health and Health Care Initiative
OneKeyQuestion	General public and health-care professionals	US	English	Power to Decide
PensiamociPrima.net	General public and health-care professionals	IT	Italian	ICBD and the Italian Health Department
www.Zwangerwijzer.nl	General public	NL	Dutch	Erasmus MC
www.slimmerzwanger.nl	General public	NL	Dutch	Erasmus MC
GezondZwangerWorden.be	General public and health-care professionals	BE	Flemish	Flemish Minister of Welfare, Public Health and Family

5.7.3 Tools for Increasing Fertility Awareness

To enable women personalized risk assessment and guiding regarding their fertility status and to improve health seeking behaviour, Bunting and Boivin (2010) developed the Fertility Status Awareness Tool (FertiSTAT). The FertiSTAT is available online (fertistat.com) in English and Portuguese and can be used by both individuals (women) and couples.

Jack and colleagues have developed a health information technology system to promote and provide preconception care through an online conversational agent 'Gabby' (Gardiner et al. 2013). African American women who tested the system found it positive and showed more preconception risk reduction than controls (Jack et al. 2015).

5.7.4 Reproductive Life Plan

5.7.5 What Is a Reproductive Life Plan?

Reproductive life planning is a concept coined in the United States to decrease poor pregnancy outcomes and prevent unintended pregnancies (Allaire and Cefalo 1998; Johnson et al. 2006) and can also be used to increase fertility awareness (Stern et al. 2013). A reproductive life plan (RLP) refers to an individual's reproductive goals and strategies to fulfil these within the context of personal life goals and values (Moos et al. 2008). By receiving a set of non-normative questions about having or not having children, both men and women can be encouraged to reflect on and thereby formulate their own RLP and find strategies for successful family planning, i.e. to have the desired number of children and to avoid unwanted pregnancies as well as ill-health that may threaten reproduction (Moos 2003; Sanders 2009; Files et al. 2011). The main question is "Do you plan to have any (more) children at any time in your future?" followed by different questions and information depending on the answer. More recently, the One Key Question™ has become popular, 'Would you like to become pregnant in the next year'. The concept of RLP and One Key Question™ (and related questions) have been implemented in clinical settings in several forms, including personal consultations with health-care providers and written materials such as leaflets/booklets and websites.

A theoretical understanding of the RLP was presented by Liu and colleagues [2016]. Their concept analysis described RLP as preceded by reproductive potential, the need for reproductive planning and health literacy. Six aspects were attributed to the RLP: inclusive of both sexes, responsibility, lifelong plan, communication, flexibility and personalization. Given these attributes, the outcomes are family planning, contraception, preconception care and empowerment.

Criticism has been raised that the RLP concept might be challenging or less meaningful for women with ambivalent feelings towards pregnancy and thereby might alienate rather than empower women. RLPs also don't take into account the social determinants of health that may make planning for the future difficult. People with lack of access to education and economic opportunity and young adults with a low sense of agency may not have the privilege of feeling that they can plan anything in their lives. It is necessary for health-care providers to have an open-minded and patient-centred approach to be able to tailor the counselling accordingly to the caretakers' point of view to avoid causing pain and mistrust (Stern et al. 2015; Callegari et al. 2017; Morse and Moos 2018).

5.7.5.1 Experiences with Reproductive Life Plan

The RLP concept has been evaluated as a tool in counselling in various settings in the United States (Dunlop et al. 2010; Mittal et al. 2014; Bommaraju et al. 2015), Sweden (Stern et al. 2013; Bodin et al. 2018) and Iran (Fooladi et al. 2018). The consultations were provided by physicians or nurse-midwives and targeted women with chronic diseases, young women, women of reproductive age or both women and men. RLP-based counselling increased the target groups knowledge (Stern et al. 2013; Mittal et al. 2014; Fooladi et al. 2018) and fertility awareness (Bodin et al. 2018) but had no effect on effective contraceptive use (Bommaraju et al. 2015). Three studies evaluated possible effects on participants' personal reproductive life plans. In the Swedish studies, a higher proportion expressed the goal to have children in their life after the counselling (Stern et al. 2013; Bodin et al. 2018), and among young women, the expressed age for having their last child was lowered (Stern et al. 2013). However, no effect on participants' reproductive life plan was seen in the Iranian study (Fooladi et al. 2018). All studies exploring participants' experiences with the RLP found them to be predominantly positive (Stern et al. 2013; Dunlop et al. 2010; Bodin et al. 2018; Fooladi et al. 2018), more so among women than men (Dunlop et al. 2010; Bodin et al. 2018).

Two studies have explored the implementation of RLP counselling in clinical setting (Stern et al. 2015; Robbins et al. 2017). Health-care providers reported positive experiences of using the RLP, and a majority adopted the concept in their counselling (Stern et al. 2015). Among a nationally representative sample of US health centres providing family planning services, almost six out of ten had a written protocol for RLP assessments, and almost nine out of ten frequently assessed RLP during family planning counselling (Robbins et al. 2017).

5.8   Conclusion and Recommendations for Practice

There have been significant changes in relation to family planning and fertility in the last 50 years. Availability of reliable contraception in some parts of the world and longer education contributed to emancipation of women in these countries. As a consequence, it was possible for people to decide when they wanted children and how many. Among others, these changes resulted in a 50% reduction of fertility rate worldwide.

Nonetheless, reproductive decisions are not personal for everybody. Cultural, religious and professional aspects may have an impact on family planning as well. Even when contraception is available, the rate of unintended pregnancies is still very high. Although a large number of unintended pregnancies end up being wanted children, planning of pregnancy proves beneficial for the mental and physical health of both mother and child. On the other hand, millions of couples suffer from infertility worldwide. In Western countries, the choice to postpone parenthood may add to fertility problems, in that maternal age has an important impact on the chance of conceiving. Although assisted reproduction techniques (ART) evolved quickly in the last decade and chances to conceive are still increasing, not all couples will be able to accomplish their desired family with ART nor may they have the financial resources to access ART. Age is an important determinant for ART as well.

A large number of studies on fertility awareness show that there is a lack of knowledge on the correlation between age and fertility within the public. Furthermore, people have unrealistic expectations of ART. A growing number of educational tools (mostly online) on fertility awareness are available, and some of them are promising. It is of importance that these tools are developed in dialogue with the target audience, in that paternalism should be avoided. Couples dealing with infertility may be very sensitive for campaigns with an emphasis on issues these couples cannot control at that point (such as age). It should be emphasized that fertility is a couples-issue and not a woman-issue. 'The Reproductive Life Plan' has been introduced in some countries and merits further exploration in order to raise fertility awareness. Fertility awareness should receive enough attention in the education of health-care providers as well, in order to enable them to provide correct information and to discuss reproduction with their clients.

Knowledge on fertility is a first step towards informed decision-making in reproductive health. In the past, education already proved successful in empowerment of women and increasing reproductive rights. Next to education on reproductive aspects, governmental interventions are needed to improve access to cheap and effective contraception worldwide on the one hand and to fertility treatment on the other hand, because founding a family is a human right.

Acknowledgements The authors wish to thank professor Petra De Sutter (Ghent University, Belgium) for her advice on the medical topics.

References

Agricola E, Gesualdo F, Pandolfi E, Gonfiantini MV, Carloni E, Mastroiacovo P, et al. Does googling for preconception care result in information consistent with international guidelines: a comparison of information found by Italian women of childbearing age and health professionals. BMC Med Inform Decis Mak. 2013;13(1):14.

Akande VA. Tubal disease: towards a classification. Reprod Biomed Online. 2007;15(4):369–75.

Alfaraj S, Aleraij S, Morad S, Alomar N, Al Rajih H, Alhussain H, et al. Fertility awareness, intentions concerning childbearing, and attitudes toward parenthood among female health professions students in Saudi Arabia. Int J Health Sci (Qassim). 2019;13(3):34–9. [cited 2019 Jun 9]. https://www-ncbi-nlm-nih-gov.zuid.vives.ezproxy.kuleuven.be/pmc/articles/PMC6512144/pdf/IJHS-13-34.pdf

Allaire AD, Cefalo RC. Preconceptional health care model. Eur J Obstet Gynecol Reprod Biol. 1998;78:163–8.

Almeida-Santos T, Melo C, Macedo A, Moura-Ramos M. Are women and men well informed about fertility? Childbearing intentions, fertility knowledge and information-gathering sources in Portugal. Reprod Health. 2017;14:91.

Baird DT, Bajos N, Cleland J, Glasier A, La Vecchia C, Leridon H, et al. Why after 50 years of effective contraception do we still have unintended pregnancy? A European perspective. Hum Reprod. 2018;33(5):777–83. [cited 2019 Jun 7]. http://www.ncbi.nlm.nih.gov/pubmed/29659848

Barrett G, Smith SC, Wellings K. Conceptualisation, development, and evaluation of a measure of unplanned pregnancy. J Epidemiol Community Heal. 2004;58:426–33.

Bodin M, Tydén T, Käll L, Larsson M. Can Reproductive Life Plan-based counseling increase men's fertility awareness? Ups J Med Sci. 2018;123(4):255–63.

Boivin J. How does stress, depression and anxiety affect patients undergoing treatment? Curr Opin Obstet Gynecol. 2019;31(3):195–9.

Boivin J, Pennings G. Parenthood should be regarded as a right. Arch Dis Child. 2005;90:784–5.

Bommaraju A, Malat J, Mooney JL. Reproductive life plan counseling and effective contraceptive use among urban women utilizing title X services. Women's Heal Issues. 2015;25(3):209–15.

Bos HM, Van Rooij FB. The influence of social and cultural factors on infertility and new reproductive technologies. J Psychosom Obstet Gynaecol. 2007;28(2):65–8. [cited 2019 Aug 23]; https://www.tandfonline.com/action/journalInformation?journalCode=ipob20

Brahem S, Mehdi M, Elghezal H, Saad A. The effects of male aging on semen quality, sperm DNA fragmentation and chromosomal abnormalities in an infertile population. J Assist Reprod Genet. 2011;28:425–32.

Bretherick KL, Fairbrother N, Avila L, Harbord SH, Robinson WP. Fertility and aging: do reproductive-aged Canadian women know what they need to know? Fertil Steril. 2010;93(7):2162–8.

Bunting L, Boivin J. Development and preliminary validation of the fertility status awareness tool: FertiSTAT. Hum Reprod. 2010;25(7):1722–33.

Calhaz-Jorge C, De Geyter C, Kupka MS, De Mouzon J, Erb K, Mocanu E, et al. Assisted reproductive technology in Europe, 2013: results generated from European registers by ESHRE. The European IVF-monitoring Consortium (EIM), for the European Society of Human Reproduction and Embryology (ESHRE). Hum Reprod. 2017;32(10):1957–73.

Callegari LS, Aiken AR, Dehlendorf C, Cason P, Borrero S. Addressing potential pitfalls of reproductive life planning with patient-centred counseling. Am J Obstet Gynecol. 2017;216(2):129–34.

Chan CHY, Chan THY, Peterson BD, Lampic C, Tam MYJ. Intentions and attitudes towards parenthood and fertility awareness among Chinese university students in Hong Kong: a comparison with Western samples. Hum Reprod. 2015;30(2):364–72.

Channon MD, Harper S. Educational differentials in the realisation of fertility intentions: is sub-Saharan Africa different? PLoS One. 2019;14(7):e0219736. [cited 2019 Aug 23]. https://doi.org/10.1371/journal.pone.0219736.

Dain L, Auslander R, Dirnfeld M. The effect of paternal age on assisted reproduction outcome. Fertil Steril. 2011;95(1):1–8.

Daniluk JC, Koert E. Fertility awareness online: the efficacy of a fertility education website in increasing knowledge and changing fertility beliefs. Hum Reprod. 2015;30(2):353–63.

Daniluk JC, Koert E, Cheung A. Childless women's knowledge of fertility and assisted human reproduction: identifying the gaps. Fertil Steril. 2012;97(2):420–6. https://doi.org/10.1016/j.fertnstert.2011.11.046.

Davies M, Webber L, Overton C. Infertility. Oxford: Oxford University Press; 2009.

De Sutter P, Gerris J, Dhont M. A health-economic decision-analytic model comparing double with single embryo transfer in IVF/ICSI. Hum Reprod. 2002;17(11):2891–6.

Delbaere I, Verstraelen H, Goetgeluk S, Martens G, De Backer G, Temmerman M. Pregnancy outcome in primiparae of advanced maternal age. Eur J Obs Gynecol Reprod Biol. 2007;135(1):41–6.

Devlieger R, Martens E, Goemaes R, Cammu H. Perinatale activiteiten in Vlaanderen 2017. Studiecentrum voor Perinatale Edidemiologie (SPE). 2018.

Drevin J, Kristiansson P, Stern J, Rosenblad A. Measuring pregnancy planning: a psychometric evaluation and comparison of two scales. J Adv Nurs. 2017;73(11):2765–75.

Dunlop AL, Logue KM, Miranda MC, Narayan DA. Integrating reproductive planning with primary health care: an explanation among low-income, minority women and men. Sex Reprod Healthc. 2010;1(2):37–43.

Eurostat. Being young in Europe today. 2015. [cited 2018 Mar 6].

Ferraretti AP, Gianaroli L, Magli MC, Devroey P. Mild ovarian stimulation with clomiphene citrate launch is a realistic option for in vitro fertilization. Fertil Steril. 2015;104(2):333–8.

Files JA, Frey KA, David PS, Hunt KS, Noble BN, Mayer AP. Developing a reproductive life plan. J Midwifery Womens Health. 2011;56:468–74.

Finer LB, Zolna MR. Declines in unintended pregnancy in the United States, 2008–2011. N Engl J Med. 2016;374(9):843–52. [cited 2019 Aug 26]. http://www.nejm.org/doi/10.1056/NEJMsa1506575

Fooladi E, Weller C, Salehi M, Rezaee Abhari F, Stern J. Using reproductive life plan-based information in a primary health care center increased Iranian women's knowledge of fertility, but not their future fertility plan: a randomized, controlled trial. Midwifery. 2018;67:77–86.

Gardiner PM, Hempstead MB, Ring L, Bickmore T, Yinusa-Nyahkoon L, Tran H, et al. Reaching women through health information technology: the Gabby preconception care system. Am J Health Promot. 2013;27:eS11–20.

Goossens J, Van Den Branden Y, Van der Sluys L, Delbaere I, Van Hecke A, Verhaeghe S, et al. The prevalence of unplanned pregnancy ending in birth, associated factors, and health outcomes. Hum Reprod. 2016;31(12):2821–33.

Goossens J, Verhaeghe S, Van Hecke A, Barrett G, Delbaere I, Beeckman D. Psychometric properties of the Dutch version of the London measure of unplanned pregnancy in women with pregnancies ending in birth. PLoS One. 2018;13(4):e0194033.

Gray E. "Get Britain fertile": does this fertility ad campaign "sham" women? Huffpost. 2013. https://www.huffpost.com/entry/get-britain-fertile-fertility-ad-campaign-british-shame-women_n_3353160?guce_referrer=aHR0cHM6Ly93d3cuYmluZy5jb20vc2VhcmNo-P3E9Z2V0K2JyaXRhaW4rZmVydGlsZSZmb3JtPUVER0VBUiZxcz1QUiRiZjdmlkPTg4M2I1-MDg1ZGVkMTQyMzFiYjc2NWViMjk5MmMwOW

Habbema JDF, Eijkemans MJC, Leridon H, te Velde ER. Realizing a desired family size: when should couples start? Hum Reprod. 2015;30(9):2215–21.

Hamilton BE, Martin JA, Osterman MJK, Rossen LM. Vital statistics rapid release births: provisional data for 2018. 2018. [cited 2019 Aug 26]. https://www.cdc.gov/nchs/products/index.htm.

IVF-Worldwide. IVF costs in different countries. n.d. https://ivf-worldwide.com/education/introduction/ivf-costs-worldwide/the-costs-of-ivf-in-different-countries.html

Jack BW, Bickmore T, Hempstead MB, Yinusa-Nyahkoon L, Sadikova E, Suzanne M, et al. Reducing preconception risks among African American women with conversational agent technology. J Am Board Fam Med. 2015;28:441–51.

Johnson K, Posner S, Biermann J, Cordero J, Atrash H, Parker C, et al. Recommendations to improve preconception health and health care—United States. A report of the CDC/ATSDR Preconception Care Work Group and the Select Panel on Preconception Care. MMWR Recomm Rep. 2006;55(RR-6):1–23.

Lampic C, Svanberg AS, Karlström P, Tydén T. Fertility awareness, intentions concerning childbearing, and attitudes towards parenthood among female and male academics. Hum Reprod. 2006;21(2):558–64.

Leridon H. Can assisted reproduction technology compensate for the natural decline in fertility with age? A model assessment. Hum Reprod. 2004;19(7):1548–53.

Mackenzie SC, Wickins-Drazilova D, Wickins J. The ethics of fertility treatment for same-sex male couples: considerations for a modern fertility clinic. Eur J Obstet Gynecol Reprod Biol. 2019;244:71–5. https://doi.org/10.1016/j.ejogrb.2019.11.011.

Max R. Our world in data: fertility rate. 2017. https://ourworldindata.org/fertility-rate

Mercier RJ, Garrett J, Thorp J, Siega-Riz AM. Pregnancy intention and postpartum depression: secondary data analysis from a prospective cohort. BJOG. 2013;120(9):1116–22.

Mills M, Rindfuss RR, McDonald P, te Velde E. Why do people postpone parenthood? Reasons and social policy incentives. Hum Reprod Update. 2011;17(6):848–60.

Mittal P, Dandekar A, Hessler D. Use of a modified reproductive life plan to improve awareness of preconception health in women with chronic disease. Perm J. 2014;18(2):28–32.

Mogilevkina I, Stern J, Melnik D, Getsko E, Tydén T. Ukrainan medical students' attitudes to parenthood and knowledge of fertility. Eur J Contracept Reprod Heal Care. 2016;21(2):189–94.

Moos M-K. Unintended pregnancies: a call for nursing action. MCN Am J Matern Child Nurs. 2003;28(1):24–30.31.

Moos M-K, Dunlop AL, Jack BW, Nelson L, Coonrod DV, Long R, et al. Healthier women, healthier reproductive outcomes: recommendations for the routine care of all women of reproductive age. Am J Obstet Gynecol. 2008;199:S280–9.

Moreau C, Bohet A, Le Guen M, Regnier Loilier A, Bajos N. Unplanned or unwanted? A randomized study of national estimates of pregnancy intention. Fertil Steril. 2014;102:1663–70.

Morse JE, Moos M-K. Reproductive life planning: raising the questions. Matern Child Health J. 2018;22:439–44.

Niederberger C, Pellicer A, Cohen J, Gardner DK, Palermo GD, O'Neill CL, et al. Forty years of IVF. Fertil Steril. 2018;110(2):185–324.e5.

Nouri K, Huber D, Walch K, Promberger R, Buerkle B, Ott J, et al. Fertility awareness among medical and non-medical students: a case-control study. Reprod Biol Endocrinol. 2014;12:94.

Olive DL. Endometriosis in clinical practice. London and New York: Taylor & Francis; 2005.

Ombelet W. Is global access to infertility care realistic? The Walking Egg Project. Reprod Biomed Online. 2014;28(3):267–72. https://doi.org/10.1016/j.rbmo.2013.11.013.

Ombelet W, Goossens J. Global reproductive health—why do we persist in neglecting the undeniable problem of childlessness in resource-poor countries? Facts Views Vis Obgyn. 2017;9(1):1–3.

Peterson B, Gordon C, Boehm JK, Inhorn MC, Patrizio P. Initiating patient discussions about oocyte cryopreservation: attitudes of obstetrics and gynaecology resident physicians. Reprod Biomed Soc Online. 2018;6:72–9.

Peterson BD, Pirritano M, Tucker L, Lampic C. Fertility awareness and parenting attitudes among American male and female undergraduate university students. Hum Reprod. 2012;27(5):1375–82.

Robbins CL, Gavin L, Carter MW, Moskosky SB. The link between reproductive life plan assessment and provision of preconception care at publicly funded health centres. Perspect Sex Reprod Health. 2017;49(3):167–72.

Ross L. Reproductive justice: an introduction. Oakland, CA: University of California Press; 2017.

Sanders L. Reproductive life plans. MCN Am J Matern Child Nurs. 2009;34:342–7.

Schmidt L, Sobotka T, Bentzen JG, Andersen A, ESHRE Reproduction and Society Task Force. Demographic and medical consequences of the postponement of parenthood. Hum Reprod Update. 2012;18(1):29–43.

Skoog Svanberg A, Lampic C, Karlström PO, Tydén T. Attitudes toward parenthood and awareness of fertility among postgraduate students in Sweden. Gend Med. 2006;3(3):187–95.

Sobotka T, Lutz W. Misleading policy messages derived from the period TFR: should we stop using it? Comp Popul Stud—Zeitschrift für Bevölkerungswissenschaft. 2010;35(3):637–64.

Sørensen NO, Marcussen S, Grønbaek Backhausen M, Juhl M, Schmidt L, Tydén T, et al. Fertility awareness and attitudes towards parenthood among Danish university college students. Reprod Health. 2016;13:146. [cited 2019 Jun 9]. https://www-ncbi-nlm-nih-gov.zuid.vives.ezproxy.kuleuven.be/pmc/articles/PMC5154162/pdf/12978_2016_Article_258.pdf

Stern J, Bodin M, Grandahl M, Segeblad B, Axen L, Larsson M, et al. Midwives' adoption of the reproductive life plan in contraceptive counselling: a mixed methods study. Hum Reprod. 2015;30(5):1146–55.

Stern J, Larsson M, Kristiansson P, Tydén T. Introducing reproductive life plan-based information in contraceptive counselling: an RCT. Hum Reprod. 2013;28(9):2450–61.

Szűcs M, Bitó T, Csíkos C, Párducz Szöllősi A, Furau C, Blidaru I, et al. Knowledge and attitudes of female university students on menstrual cycle and contraception. J Obstet Gynaecol. 2017;37(2):210–4.

Tydén T, Svanberg AS, Karlström P-O, Lihoff L, Lampic C. Female university students' attitudes to future motherhood and their understanding about fertility. Eur J Contracept Reprod Health Care. 2006;11(3):181–9.

United Nations. The Millennium Development Goals Report. 2015. https://www.un.org/millenniumgoals/2015_MDG_Report/pdf/MDG2015rev(July 1).pdf.

Urrutia RP, Polis CB, Jensen ET, Greene ME, Kennedy E, Stanford JB. Effectiveness of fertility awareness-based methods for pregnancy prevention: a systematic review. Obstet Gynecol. 2018;132(3):591–604.

Van Bavel J. Choice of study discipline and the postponement of motherhood in Europe: the impact of expected earnings, gender composition, and family attitudes. Demography. 2010;47:439–58. [cited 2019 Jun 7]. https://www.ncbi.nlm.nih.gov/pmc/articles/PMC3000018/pdf/dem-47-0439.pdf

Virtala A, Vilska S, Huttunen T, Kunttu K. Childbearing, the desire to have children, and awareness about the impact of age on female fertility among Finnish university students. Eur J Contracept Reprod Health Care. 2011;16(2):108–15.

Waldenström U. Postponing parenthood to advanced age. Ups J Med Sci. 2016;121(4):235–43.

Wantland DJ, Portillo CJ, Holzemer WL, Slaughter R, McGhee EM. The effectiveness of Web-based vs. non-Web-based interventions: a meta-analysis of behavioral change outcomes. J Med Internet Res. 2004;6(4):e40.

Webb TL, Joseph J, Yardley L, Michie S. Using the internet to promote health behavior change: a systematic review and meta-analysis of the impact of theoretical basis, use of behavior change techniques, and mode of delivery on efficacy. J Med Internet Res. 2010;12(1):e4.

WHO. WHO laboratory manual for the examination and processing of human semen. 2010.

WHO. Reproductive health strategy to accelerate progress towards the attainment of international development goals and targets. 2014. https://apps.who.int/iris/bitstream/handle/10665/68754/WHO_RHR_04.8.pdf;jsessionid=F1280361A7D9F858A79EC094FBCBC201?sequence=1

Wojcieszek AM, Thompson R. Conceiving of change: a brief intervention increases young adults' knowledge of fertility and the effectiveness of in vitro fertilization. Fertil Steril. 2013;100(2):523–9.

Yamashiro C, Sasaki K, Yabuta Y, Kojima Y, Nakamura T, Okamoto I, et al. Generation of human oogonia from induced pluripotent stem cells in vitro. Science. 2018;362(6412):356–60.

Yu L, Peterson B, Inhorn M, Boehm J, Patrizio P. Knowledge, attitudes, and intentions toward fertility awareness and oocyte cryopreservation among obstetrics and gynecology resident physicians. Hum Reprod. 2016;32(1):403–11.

Nutrition

6

Zainab Akhter, Melissa van der Windt,
Rianne van der Kleij, Nicola Heslehurst,
and Régine Steegers-Theunissen

6.1 Introduction

This chapter will provide an overview of preconception nutrition for both women and men. Healthy nutrition is important for people's health and wellbeing across the life course. Nutrition prior to conception is important to optimize fertility, gamete function, and set a foundation for the infant's first 1000 days; from conception to 2 years of age. As there is little change in dietary patterns between preconception and pregnancy, it is important for young adults to establish healthy nutrition behaviours, meeting the daily recommended nutrient intakes (RNI) to improve overall wellbeing, reproductive health for conception, and health throughout pregnancy as well as to prevent adverse pregnancy outcomes associated with nutrient deficiencies (Table 6.1)

Z. Akhter
Institute of Health and Society, Newcastle University, Newcastle upon Tyne, UK

M. van der Windt
Department of Obstetrics and Gynaecology, Erasmus MC,
Rotterdam, The Netherlands

R. van der Kleij
Department of Public Health & Primary Care, Leiden University Medical Center,
Leiden, The Netherlands

Department of Obstetrics and Gynaecology, Erasmus MC,
Rotterdam, The Netherlands

N. Heslehurst
Institute of Health and Society, Newcastle University, Newcastle upon Tyne, UK

R. Steegers-Theunissen (✉)
Department of Conception Epidemiology, Sophia Children's Hospital, Erasmus MC,
Rotterdam, The Netherlands
e-mail: r.steegers@erasmusmc.nl

© Springer Nature Switzerland AG 2020
J. Shawe et al. (eds.), *Preconception Health and Care: A Life Course Approach*,
https://doi.org/10.1007/978-3-030-31753-9_6

Table 6.1 Summary of micronutrients function, sources, and daily recommended nutrient intakes (RNI) for women, pregnant women, and men

Nutrient	Function	Sources	Daily RNI[a]
Folate (vitamin B9)	DNA synthesis and repair, red blood cell production, brain and spinal cord development	Green leafy vegetables, meat, whole grains	Women: 400 µg Pregnancy: 600 µg Men: 400 µg
Cobalamin (vitamin B12)	DNA synthesis and repair, red blood cell production, healthy nervous system maintenance	Meat, seafood, dairy, fortified non-dairy drinks	Women: 2.4 µg Pregnancy: 2.6 µg Men: 2.4 µg
Thiamine (vitamin B1)	Neuron communication, immunity, digestion	Nuts, legumes, rice, whole grains	Women: 1.1 mg Pregnancy: 1.4 mg Men: 1.2 mg
Riboflavin (vitamin B2)	Regulates thyroid activity, adrenal function, antibody production	Dairy, dark green vegetables	Women: 1.1 mg Pregnancy: 1.4 mg Men: 1.3 mg
Vitamin A	Vision, cellular differentiation, immunity	Eggs, meat, fish, or for β-carotene red-yellow fruits and vegetables	Women: 500 µg Pregnancy (β-carotene): 4.8 mg Men: 600 µg
Vitamin C	Immunity, growth and repair of tissues	Citrus fruits, berries	Women: 45 mg Pregnancy: 55 mg Men: 45 mg
Vitamin D	Calcium absorption	Sunlight, oily fish, egg yolks	Women: 5 µg Pregnancy: 5 µg Men: 5 µg
Vitamin E	Protects cells, antioxidant	Nuts, seeds, vegetable oils	Women: 7.5 mg Pregnancy: 10 mg Men: 10 mg
Vitamin K	Blood clotting, wound healing	Green leafy vegetables	Women: 55 µg Pregnancy: 55 µg Men: 65 µg
Iron[a]	Transports oxygen around the body	Meat, lentils, green leafy vegetables	Women: 7.5–22.6 mg Pregnancy: 10–30 mg Men: 7.5–22.6 mg
Zinc[b]	DNA synthesis	Meat, shellfish, nuts	Women: 3–9.8 mg Pregnancy: 4.2–14 mg Men: 4.2–14 mg
Iodine	Produces thyroid hormones, regulates metabolism	Iodized salt, white fish, dairy products, potato skins	Women: 150 µg Pregnancy: 200 µg Men: 150 µg
Calcium	Maintains bones and teeth, regulates muscle contractions	Dairy products, fortified non-dairy milk	Women: 1000 mg Pregnancy: 1200 mg Men: 1000 mg

[a]Recommended nutrient intake (RNI) is the daily intake which meets the nutrient requirements of almost all (97.5%) apparently healthy individuals in an age- and sex-specific population according to World Health Organization recommendations

[b]RDA ranges for iron and zinc range from high bioavailability for mixed diets to low bioavailability for vegan and vegetarian diets

(Inskip et al. 2009). This chapter will cover micronutrients (vitamins and minerals) and diet quality (including macronutrients proteins, fats, and carbohydrates). Healthy sources of these nutrients, including both natural and fortified foods, will be introduced, as well as recommendations for supplements. Information is also provided for men and women following special diets including vegan and vegetarian, particularly in relation to micronutrients. Because dietary intake also affects mental wellbeing, and a growing body of evidence suggests dietary intake before and during pregnancy even affects the mental health of future children, this chapter includes information on preconception nutrition and mental health.

Micronutrients are vitamins and minerals which are essential for the healthy functioning of the human body. They are only required in miniscule amounts, but failing to meet these small quantities can result in physical and mental health complications. Micronutrient deficiencies are associated with health risks for young adults as well as high reproductive risks including subfertility, anaemia, and congenital anomalies (Berti et al. 2009). Some deficiencies also present with depressive symptoms such as low mood, but there is limited evidence for the impact of micronutrient supplementation for maternal mental health (Nguyen et al. 2017). Deficiencies in micronutrients can occur due to undernutrition, which is common in women in low- and middle-income countries, eating foods with low nutritional density (relative undernutrition), or as a consequence of medication use and/or chronic diseases. Women's undernutrition can lead to the birth of a baby starting life with nutritional deficits which are associated with impaired physical development, and also cognitive, motor, socioemotional, and behavioural development (Vohr et al. 2017).

Adequate calorie intake is not sufficient to support foetal development—the quality of a woman's diet matters too. Unfortunately, the reported dietary intakes of pregnant women in high-income countries, including Europe, the USA, and Australia, do not meet national dietary intake recommendations for folate, iron, or vitamin D (Blumfield et al. 2013). The physiological demands of growing a baby can worsen any underlying micronutrient deficiencies or increase the risk of developing one. The first few weeks after the last menstrual period, even before confirmation of pregnancy, are critical periods of embryonic, placental, and organ development; therefore it is essential to ensure vitamin and mineral intake for women is adequate to support both mother's and baby's health.

The potential effects of nutritional factors on male reproductive health are becoming increasingly apparent. In particular, certain micronutrients have been associated with sperm factors including sperm count and motility. Men's undernutrition, in particular a shortage of micronutrient intake, detrimentally affects these sperm factors as well as sperm DNA quality and its epigenetic (re)programming (Schagdarsurengin and Steger 2016). This is supported with the association between strong adherence to a preconception micronutrient rich "Mediterranean diet" by couples undergoing IVF/ICSI treatment and the increased success of achieving pregnancy (Vujkovic et al. 2010). These positive associations between micronutrient intake, adherence to specific dietary patterns, and semen parameters in men emphasize the importance of also paying attention to men's nutrition.

6.2   Micronutrients

This section describes the characteristics, function, sources, deficiency, and supplements for the following vitamins and minerals: folate; cobalamin; thiamine; riboflavin; vitamins A, C, D, E, and K; zinc; iron; iodine; and calcium. The RNI are presented in Table 6.1.

6.2.1   Vitamins

6.2.1.1 Folate (Vitamin B9/11)

Characteristics and Function
Folate is a water-soluble B vitamin naturally present in foods and human tissues. In general, the term folate refers to the vitamin in its natural form, whereas the term folic acid is used for the more stable synthetic form of this vitamin. The bioavailability of folic acid is approximately 70% higher than that of folate, although there are wide variations depending on the measurement methodology used (McNulty and Pentieva 2004). Folate is essential for healthy cell development and for the metabolism of specific biochemical reactions in the body (Steegers-Theunissen et al. 2013). Folate is part of the one-carbon (1-C) metabolism and provides essential 1-C moieties and methyl groups for various cellular processes. The reduced form of folate, tetrahydrofolate (THF), acts as a substrate in the synthesis of DNA, transfer RNA, several amino acids, and lipids. In addition, 5-methyl THF is the most active form of folate in tissues and serves as a methyl donor for methylation of DNA, histones, lipids, and proteins. Other main substrates and cofactors of 1-C metabolism for synthesis and methylation of these substances are choline, methionine, cobalamin (vitamin B12), and pyridoxine (vitamin B6) (Wagner 1995; Shane 1995).

The 1-C metabolism is important for the synthesis, repair, and epigenetic (re) programming of DNA and synthesis of proteins and lipids for cell membranes and endocrine, inflammation, signalling, and other pathways (see Chap. 2). Folate provides a critical methyl group for the creation of a high-energy methylating intermediate of the 1-C metabolism, i.e. S-adenosyl-methionine (SAM). This methylating intermediate is the most important methyl donor in the body for the methylation of lipids, proteins, and DNA. During the preconception period, gametogenesis and folliculogenesis take place, in which the requirement for folate is enhanced (Kelly et al. 2005). After fertilization, the blastocyst is demethylated, followed by the selective methylation of genes (Finnell et al. 2002). Moreover, developing embryos are rapidly producing new cells and are therefore especially sensitive to reduced levels of folates. Ectoderm and early neural epithelium tissue may be the embryonic tissues that are most heavily affected by folate deficiency.

There is some evidence that the use of multivitamin supplements, in particular of folic acid, may decrease the risk of subfertility in women and men (McNulty and Pentieva 2004). Most evidence, however, is available about the preventive effect of folic acid use in the periconception period to reduce the occurrence and recurrence of congenital anomalies, particularly neural tube defects (NTDs) (De-Regil et al. 2015). Neural tube defects (NTDs) are common complex congenital malformations resulting from failure of the neural tube closure during embryogenesis. Closure of the cranial neural tube should take place between 21 and 28 days after conception and is essential not only for continued development of the brain but also for initial formation of the skull. If neural tube closure fails, the embryo develops an NTD. Specific types include anencephaly, encephaloceles, spina bifida, and tethered cord (Botto et al. 1999).

Low-level evidence indicates that there might be a modest association between maternal folic acid supplement use and the reduction of preeclampsia and gestational hypertension risk (Bulloch et al. 2018; De Ocampo et al. 2018). The suggested underlying mechanisms of these associations with adverse maternal pregnancy and neonatal outcome are early placental impairments of cell division, angiogenesis, and other essential processes in the early establishment of pregnancy due to a primary shortage of folate and secondary hyperhomocysteinemia and DNA hypomethylation. In general, folate deficiency can be treated by a folate-rich dietary pattern and folic acid intake (Mignini et al. 2005; Williams et al. 2011). It has been shown that periconception maternal folic acid supplement use significantly increases the methylation of the imprinted IGF2 DMR gene in offspring, a gene involved in embryogenesis and atherosclerosis, which warrants further investigation with regard to health in later life (Steegers-Theunissen et al. 2009; Pauwels et al. 2017).

Men's folate deficiency as well as methionine and choline as substrates of the 1-C metabolism can also have a direct, measurable effect on sperm parameters, such as sperm concentration, morphology and motility, DNA damage, and epigenetic (re) programming (Schagdarsurengin and Steger 2016; Salas-Huetos et al. 2017). There is increasing evidence for the positive relationship between the adequacy of men's folate levels and semen quality and embryonic growth. Since there is no full understanding of the benefits and risks of paternal folic acid supplement use for embryonic growth trajectories, pregnancy outcomes, and health and disease risks of the children in later life, so far only a folate-rich diet and not the use of a folic acid supplement is recommended for men (see Chap. 2).

Sources

Humans are entirely dependent on dietary sources or supplements for their folate supply (Scholl and Johnson 2000). Folate can be derived from leafy green vegetables, such as spinach, kale, and arugula, and as well in some fruits and whole-grain products (World Health Organization and Food and Agriculture Organization of the United Nations 2004).

Deficiency

Folate is a water-soluble vitamin, meaning that it is not stored in the body for a long period of time and is excreted rapidly from the body after absorption (Mahmood 2014). Since folate is mandatory for a variety of essential molecular biological pathways, it is not surprising that folate deficiency results in DNA damage, reduced cell multiplication, and increased cell death with consequences for derangements in foetal and placental growth and development. A primary deficiency of natural folate results in an increase of the total homocysteine concentration that can be detrimental to the quality of the oocyte, subsequent fertilization, implantation, embryogenesis, and foetal outcome (Hague 2003; Steegers-Theunissen and Steegers 2003; Ebisch et al. 2007). The main cause of folate deficiency is having an unhealthy diet that does not include enough folate-rich foods. Clinically, severe folate deficiency can cause megaloblastic anaemia where the bone marrow produces large, structurally abnormal red blood cells and symptoms include fatigue and dizziness (Green and Miller 1999).

Supplements
Folic acid is the synthetic and most stable form of folate and is used in supplements and in fortified foods (McNulty and Pentieva 2010). A daily folic acid supplement of 400 µg is internationally recommended to women from ideally 3 months before conception to 12 completed weeks of pregnancy (World Health Organization and Food and Agriculture Organization of the United Nations 2004). For women with an increased risk of having a pregnancy affected by a NTD, such as women with pre-pregnancy obesity or diabetes, some countries recommend a higher dose of 4–5 mg folic acid (NICE 2008).

6.2.1.2 Cobalamin (Vitamin B12)

Characteristics and Function
Cobalamin is a water-soluble B vitamin that participates as a pivotal co-enzyme to maintain the body's homeostasis. It acts as an essential cofactor in DNA synthesis, in particular in 1-C metabolism which is a vitamin B12-dependent metabolic path-way (Steegers-Theunissen et al. 2013; Selhub 2002). In addition, cobalamin is needed for red blood cell production and synthesis of fatty acids in myelin, which plays an important role in conduction of nerve impulses (Ralapanawa et al. 2015).

A diet low in vitamin B12 preconceptionally and during pregnancy is associated with an increased risk of a child with a congenital heart disease (Verkleij-Hagoort et al. 2006). Furthermore, a marginal maternal vitamin B12 status also increases the risk of offspring with spina bifida (Groenen et al. 2004). A more prolonged defi-ciency results in subfertility by causing changes in ovulation or development of the ovum or changes leading to defective implantation (Bennett 2001). In the context of assisted reproduction, ovarian responsiveness to gonadotrophin treatment has been shown to be affected by levels of dietary folate, vitamin B12, and other 1-C sub-strates and cofactors (Twigt et al. 2011).

Vitamin B12 is important in cellular replication, especially for the synthesis of RNA and DNA, and deficiency in men has been associated with decreased sperm count and motility (Sinclair 2000). Intervention studies have shown that administer-ing vitamin B12 supplements, in different dosages, to subfertile men leads to an increase in standard sperm parameters, sperm concentration, and motility (Isoyama et al. 1986, 1984; Kumamoto et al. 1988).

Sources
Cobalamin is best derived from animal-based food products such as meats, fish, seafood, poultry, eggs, cheese, and milk (Chandra-Hioe et al. 2019). For those prac-ticing a vegetarian or vegan lifestyle, a possible vitamin B12 deficiency is one of the greatest nutritional concerns. However, several vegan cereals, plant-based milk, and soy products are fortified with vitamin B12 and are therefore an excellent artificial source of this vitamin for persons who avoid animal products.

Deficiency

In general, as B vitamins are water-soluble, they can easily dissolve in water and are excreted from the body rapidly since they are not stored for long periods of time, except for cobalamin. About 2–5 mg of cobalamin can be stored in the body, mainly in the liver up to 3–5 years' worth of vitamin B12 (Chatterjea and Shinde 2011). Therefore, due to this valuable pathway, cobalamin deficiency is extremely rare. Conditions that affect the small intestine and interfere with nutrient absorption, such as Crohn's disease, celiac disease, bacterial growth, or a parasite, might cause a cobalamin deficiency (Weisshof and Chermesh 2015).

Cobalamin deficiency is associated with hematologic, neurologic, and psychiatric problems. It is a common cause of macrocytic (megaloblastic) anaemia. Neurologic symptoms from vitamin B12 deficiency arise from both central and peripheral nerve damage. Psychiatric issues from vitamin B12 deficiency include impaired memory, irritability, depression, dementia, and, rarely, psychosis (Lee 1999; Lindenbaum et al. 1988).

6.2.1.3 Thiamine (Vitamin B1)

Characteristics and Function

Thiamine is a water-soluble B vitamin, which is known to be involved in energy metabolism and breaking down sugars and carbon skeletons. Thiamine pyrophosphate is the active form of thiamine and serves as a cofactor for several enzymes involved primarily in carbohydrate catabolism. Other functions important for women's health connected to this vitamin are neuronal communication, immune system activation, signalling and maintenance processes in cells and tissues, and cell membrane dynamics (Manzetti et al. 2014).

Adequate thiamine levels are crucial for embryonic and foetal brain development due to its involvement in the synthesis of myelin and several neurotransmitters. The deficiency also leads to neural membrane dysfunction since thiamine is the structural component of mitochondrial and synaptosomal membranes (Kloss et al. 2018). It has been suggested that thiamine deficiency is also a cause of intrauterine growth restriction (IUGR). One study found that mothers with normal pregnancy had significantly higher thiamine levels in the blood cells than mothers whose pregnancies were complicated by IUGR (Heinze and Weber 1990). There is lack of data for effects of men's thiamine intake on reproductive health.

Sources

Thiamine is found in a wide variety of foods; nuts, legumes, rice, and whole grains have among the highest contents of thiamine (NIH 2018; Ladipo 2000). Whole grain flours and brown (unrefined) rice contain thiamine within their outer shell. However, modern roller milling processes remove much of the bran and germ of the grains of these cereals, along with their naturally occurring thiamine content. Therefore, the Council on Foods and Nutrition of the American Medical Association advocated for the enrichment of thiamine and other B vitamins in white flour and white bread in 1939. Nowadays, 28% of industrially milled flour is fortified, often with thiamine and other B vitamins (Hoogendoorn et al. 2016). There is no evidence of thiamine toxicity by oral administration, and no tolerable upper intake limit has been set (World Health Organization and Food and Agriculture Organization of the United Nations 2004).

Deficiency

Deficiency of thiamine can affect the cardiovascular, nervous, and immune system. However, nutritional deficiency for thiamine is rare in people who consume a moderately varied diet that contains whole grains. However, insufficient intake of thiamine is associated with beriberi disease and Wernicke encephalopathy (Lonsdale 2018). Excessive vomiting in pregnancy, also known as hyperemesis gravidarum, can cause thiamine depletion and, in exceptional cases, might lead to maternal Wernicke's encephalopathy (Oudman et al. 2019). There is little data available on the long-term effects of thiamine deficiency on women's health or the impact on foetal development in either the short or long term.

6.2.1.4 Riboflavin (Vitamin B₂)

Characteristics and Function

Riboflavin, also known as vitamin B_2, is a water-soluble vitamin naturally found in food. Its most important biologically active forms are flavin adenine dinucleotide (FAD) and flavin mononucleotide (FMN). Multiple flavin-dependent proteins that utilize FMN or/and FAD, so-called flavoproteins, participate in a range of redox reactions in the tricarboxylic acid (TCA) cycle, fatty acid beta-oxidation, amino acid degradation, and electron transport chain (ETC) which are essential functions to produce adenosine triphosphate (ATP), the body's energy supply (Powers 2003; Lienhart et al. 2013). Riboflavin is also needed to regulate thyroid activity and adrenal function.

Associations between periconception riboflavin status and reproductive outcome have scarcely been reported. Women who are riboflavin deficient have a higher risk for developing preeclampsia compared to women with adequate riboflavin levels (odds ratio 4.7, 95% confidence interval 1.8–12.2) (Wacker et al. 2000). There is lack of data for effects of men's riboflavin intake or deficiency on reproductive health.

Sources

High concentrations of riboflavin are found in milk and other dairy products and in dark green vegetables such as spinach and broccoli. Whole grains, meats, and fatty fish are also good sources of riboflavin (World Health Organization and Food and Agriculture Organization of the United Nations 2004).

Pregnancy demands higher riboflavin intake than the recommended daily allowance as it crosses the placenta and contributes to foetal growth and development. Especially in the third trimester of pregnancy, when energy and protein needs are greater for foetal development, higher riboflavin intake is required. There is no evidence of riboflavin toxicity by oral administration, and no tolerable upper intake limit has been defined (World Health Organization and Food and Agriculture Organization of the United Nations 2004).

Deficiency

Riboflavin deficiency is relatively common when dietary intake is insufficient because it is continuously excreted in the urine of healthy individuals and often occurs alongside other B vitamin deficiencies (Brody 1998). People who adopt a vegan lifestyle are at higher risk for a riboflavin deficiency, since vegans restrain from consuming animal products. Deficiency can be avoided by consuming a diverse range of fruits and vegetables. In consideration of the major metabolic pathways that flavoproteins influence, riboflavin deficiencies impact red blood cell production and lead to anaemia. Other consequences include sore throat, hyperaemia, swelling of oral and mucous membranes, cheilosis, and glossitis, which further leads to loss of hair, inflammation of the skin, and cataract development (Thakur et al. 2017). Deficiency of riboflavin during pregnancy can result in birth defects including congenital heart defects and limb deformities (Smedts et al. 2008; Robitaille et al. 2009).

6.2.1.5 Vitamin A

Characteristics and Function

Vitamin A is a fat-soluble vitamin which is important for immune function, vision, and reproduction (Clagett-Dame and Knutson 2011). Vitamin A is a component of a protein called rhodopsin which absorbs light in the retinal receptors which makes it critical for vision (Wolf 2001). Vitamin A is also required for growth, tissue development, and cellular differentiation which are all processes that occur particularly during embryo development in pregnancy. There are two forms of vitamin A found in diets: preformed vitamin A and provitamin A carotenoids. Preformed vitamin A (retinol) comes from animal sources such as dairy and meat. Provitamin A carotenoids are plant pigments, the most important one being beta-carotene. High doses of vitamin A in the retinol form, such as prescription acne medications, for the mother can increase the risk of birth defects; therefore it is essential that any vitamin A in supplements taken are in the beta-carotene form (Rothman et al. 1995).

Vitamin A also plays an essential role in male fertility, in particular in the maintenance of spermatogenesis. However, the role of vitamin A supplement use in subfertile men is unclear.

Sources

Beta-carotene is a red-orange plant pigment and is therefore found in red and yellow fruits and vegetables such as sweet potatoes, carrots, and apricots and also green leafy vegetables. Fish liver oil supplements and liver food products such as pâté should be avoided by women who could become pregnant as they are high in the retinol form of vitamin A.

Deficiency

Vitamin A deficiency is a problem in low- and middle-income countries, and pregnant and breastfeeding mothers are at a higher risk than the general population. Since vitamin A is crucial for visual health, one of the main symptoms of vitamin A deficiency is night blindness where the ability for vision to adapt in dim lighting reduces or is lost (Katz et al. 1995).

6.2.1.6 Vitamin C

Characteristics and Function

Vitamin C, known as ascorbic acid, is a water-soluble vitamin with antioxidant function. Vitamin C is required for collagen synthesis and helps growth and repair of tissues and also immune function. The ovary is a site of high ascorbic acid accumulation and turnover which indicates it is important for reproductive health; its roles include preventing damage from free radicals and promoting follicular development and ovulation (Jeyaseelan et al. 1995). Vitamin C may also help raise levels of progesterone which is a hormone that prepares the uterus for conception (Henmi et al. 2003).

Human spermatozoa contain high concentrations of polyunsaturated fatty acids and also have a significant ability to generate reactive oxygen species, mainly superoxide anion and hydrogen peroxide. These features make spermatozoa particularly susceptible to peroxidative damage. Antioxidants such as vitamin C, vitamin E, and carotenoids can repair the appropriate pro-oxidant-antioxidant balance and maintain the genetic integrity of sperm cells by preventing damage to sperm DNA (Kodentsova et al. 1994). Clinical studies have shown that vitamin C supplementation might improve sperm count, sperm motility, and sperm morphology in infertile men, as well as in men who smoke (Akmal et al. 2006). Additional vitamin C supplement use might have a place to improve the semen quality towards conception.

Sources

Sources of vitamin C include citrus fruits, bell peppers, and berries. Vitamin C content is higher in raw produce compared to after heating or boiling. As vitamin C cannot be stored in the body, it is essential to include it in the diet every day.

Deficiency

Vitamin C deficiency is rare but can result in scurvy with symptoms such as weakness, joint pain, bleeding gums, and easy bruising. Vitamin C helps the absorption of iron in the body; therefore vitamin C deficiency might appear alongside an iron deficiency.

6.2.1.7 Vitamin D

Characteristics and Function

Vitamin D is a fat-soluble vitamin which is necessary to facilitate calcium absorption in the body but also plays a role in reproductive health. Women with higher vitamin D levels have been shown to have a higher success of embryo implantation after in vitro fertilization (IVF) (Farzadi et al. 2015). Additionally, vitamin D deficiency in pregnancy is associated with adverse short- and long-term outcomes including maternal preeclampsia, foetal bone mass, and childhood asthma (Aghajafari et al. 2013; Erkkola et al. 2009).

The role of vitamin D in the modulation of testes functions, including hormone production and spermatogenesis, has been investigated in animals and humans. Experimental studies support a beneficial effect of vitamin D on male fertility. However, clinical studies in humans have shown conflicting results (de Angelis et al. 2017).

Sources
Human bodies create vitamin D when exposed to sunlight; therefore deficiencies are common in northern countries such as the UK. Dietary sources of vitamin D include oily fish, red meat, and egg yolks. For vegetarians and vegans, foods such as breakfast cereals and milk are fortified with vitamin D.

Deficiency
Vitamin D deficiency is common, especially in people who live far from the equator, people with darker skin tones, and people who spend a lot of time indoors or cover their skin when outside. Additionally, obesity is associated with increased risk of vitamin D deficiency (Vimaleswaran et al. 2013). Symptoms of vitamin D deficiency include fatigue, bone pain, and low mood.

Supplements
As vitamin D deficiency is common, a 10 µg daily supplement is recommended during pregnancy and for high-risk groups, such as people with darker skins and obesity (NICE 2008).

6.2.1.8 Vitamin E

Characteristics and Function
Vitamin E is a fat-soluble antioxidant which protects cell membranes and interacts closely with vitamin C. Oxidative stress is associated with decreased female fertility; therefore it is important to include antioxidant vitamins C and E in the diet (Ruder et al. 2009). The combination of vitamin E and selenium might improve the motility and morphology of spermatozoa, even in men without reproductive problems (Vezina et al. 1996). However, the potential harmful effects and the optimal dose of vitamin E supplements need to be established.

Sources
Vitamin E is present in most food, and high sources include nuts, seeds, and vegetable oils.

Deficiency
Vitamin E deficiency is rarely due to lack of dietary intake but rather due to issues with dietary fat absorption or metabolism. When deficiency does occur, symptoms include the results of oxidative stress, such as muscle weakness. Neuron sheaths are composed of fats, and lack of vitamin E can result in damage to the nervous system (Traber et al. 1987).

6.2.1.9 Vitamin K

Characteristics and Function
Vitamin K is a fat-soluble vitamin essential for blood clotting and wound healing. Vitamin K is required to produce prothrombin, a protein involved in the process of blood coagulation.

Sources
The main dietary sources of vitamin K are green leafy vegetables such as broccoli and spinach.

Deficiency
Vitamin K deficiency, although rare, leads to an inability to form blood clots and therefore results in easy bruising and excessive bleeding. Having a vitamin K deficiency in pregnancy increases the risk of haemorrhage in the mother or baby which can result in brain damage or death for either (Shahrook et al. 2018).

6.2.2   Minerals

6.2.2.1 Zinc

Characteristics and Function
Zinc plays an important role in fertility, especially for ovarian function. Zinc is required for DNA synthesis and is therefore vital for oocyte development (Ebisch et al. 2006). Zinc is an antioxidant and seems to have a positive effect on sperm quality when administered together with folic acid (Wong et al. 2002). Total normal sperm count increases after combined zinc sulphate and folic acid treatment in both subfertile and fertile men. Despite this beneficial effect on male fertility, the potential harmful effects and the optimal remain to be established before wide-scale implementation of combined zinc and folic acid administration.

Sources
Sources of zinc include meat, shellfish, beans, and nuts.

Deficiency
Symptoms of zinc deficiency include slower than expected growth and poor immune system function. Zinc deficiency in the preconception period impairs oocyte maturation and can block ovulation (Tian and Diaz 2012). The preconception deficiency can result in developmental delay post-implantation even if zinc is included in the diet after conception (Anthony et al. 2014).

6.2.2.2 Iron

Characteristics and Function
Iron is an important component of haemoglobin, which carries oxygen in red blood cells to transport around the body. It also plays an important role in improving

immunity and muscle strength. Women have an increased need for iron due to blood loss during menstruation. During pregnancy, the body increases its blood volume by up to 50% to supply the growing foetus and placenta; therefore iron demands also increase (Soma-Pillay et al. 2016). There is lack of data for the effect of paternal iron intake on reproductive health.

Sources
Iron-rich foods include lean meat, lentils, and green leafy vegetables. Additionally, some breakfast cereals are fortified with iron.

Deficiency
The most common symptoms of iron deficiency are lack of energy and shortness of breath. Iron deficiency anaemia is the most common deficiency in women worldwide and can block ovulation therefore decreasing chances of conception (Chavarro et al. 2006). However, when pregnancy does occur, iron deficiency can result in adverse outcomes such as preterm delivery and small for gestational age babies (Allen 2000). There is also evidence that iron deficiency anaemia increases the risk of postpartum haemorrhage, which is the leading cause of maternal mortality worldwide, and 99% of cases occur in low- and middle-income countries (Kavle et al. 2008).

6.2.2.3 Iodine

Characteristics and Function
Iodine is essential to produce thyroid hormones and regulate metabolism. Maternal iodine intake during the preconception period and pregnancy is crucial for foetal brain development (Melse-Boonstra and Jaiswal 2010). The impact of iodine intake on the male reproductive function is not entirely known. One study suggests that an increase in semen iodine levels is associated with different variables related to male infertility (Partal-Lorente et al. 2017). Moreover, there are implications that the global decline in sperm concentrations may be caused by a higher iodine intake, which has mainly been caused by iodine supplements (Sakamoto et al. 2004).

Sources
If iodized salt is not available, then other sources to include in the diet are white fish such as cod, dairy, and eggs. Those following vegan and vegetarian diets should be aware they are at higher risk of iodine deficiency but can find iodine in potato skins, prunes, and seaweed.

Deficiency
The highest prevalence of iodine deficiency in the world is in Europe where nearly 60% of the general population is deficient (de Benoist et al. 2003). Iodine deficiency is the main preventable cause of cognitive impairment. Symptoms include unexpected weight gain from slowed metabolism and slowed heart rate leading to feelings of weakness.

6.2.2.4 Calcium

Characteristics and Function
Calcium is most known for maintaining healthy bones and teeth but is also involved in regulating muscle contractions, including the heartbeat, and blood clotting. Sufficient calcium intake is important in childhood and early adulthood while bone mass is still building up in preparation for the rapid bone loss experienced after menopause to reduce the risk of osteoporosis. During pregnancy, foetal bone development requires calcium and will absorb some of this from the maternal skeleton; therefore it is important to ensure adequate calcium intake from preconception to reduce the risk of bone disorders in later life (Kovacs 2001). There is lack of data for effects of paternal calcium intake on reproductive health.

Sources
Dietary sources of calcium include dairy products (milk, cheese, and yoghurt), and vegan sources include non-dairy fortified drinks, beans, and nuts.

Deficiency
Symptoms of calcium deficiency include muscle aches, fatigue, and weak bones.

6.2.3   Diet Quality

Diet quality refers to dietary balance of food groups and composition of macronutrients, which are nutrients required in larger quantities to provide energy. Better maternal diet quality during pregnancy has been shown to be postively associated with child neurodevelopment and cognition (Borge et al. 2017). The three macronutrient groups are proteins, carbohydrates, and fats. Macronutrient intakes of women from high-income countries do not match recommendations, due to overconsumption of saturated fat and underconsumption of fibre and polyunsaturated fat (Blumfield et al. 2012). In low- and middle-income countries, the daily caloric intake is insufficient, and cereals contribute to over half of the daily intake (Lee et al. 2013).

Protein builds up every cell in the body and is essential for growth and healthy body maintenance as hormones, antibodies, and enzymes are all made of protein. Women's protein intake before conception and throughout pregnancy is strongly associated with birth weight (Moore et al. 2004; Cucó et al. 2006). Good sources of proteins include meat, fish, and eggs. Plant sources of proteins include legumes and nuts.

Carbohydrates are the body's energy source and should make up the majority of the diet. Whole grains and fibre-rich fruits and vegetables are the best source of healthy carbohydrates unlike refined grains and foods with added sugar.

Fats are also essential for healthy functioning of the body and for increased vitamin and mineral absorption. Trans- and saturated fat, found in butter and red meat, should be limited, and unsaturated fats such as omega-3 and omega-6 fatty acids should be taken instead. These essential fatty acids are required for the structure of cell membranes and the formation of new tissues, but cannot be synthesized by the human body (Hornstra 2000). Omega-3 fatty acids, found in nuts and fatty fish such as salmon, are important for foetal neurodevelopment. Docosahexaenoic acid (DHA) in particular is a major structural fat that makes up the human brain and eyes and therefore is required during pregnancy for brain development (Greenberg et al. 2008).

However, men's dietary patterns are as well of importance to reproductive health. Those with strong adherence to a healthy dietary pattern (featuring high consumption of fruits, vegetables, whole grain, legumes, seafood, low-fat dairy, and poultry) had a significantly higher level of sperm concentration compared with those following an unhealthy dietary pattern (characterized by high consumption of red or processed meat, refined grain, high-fat dairy, and potatoes) (Arab et al. 2018).

6.2.4 Preconception Nutrition and Mental Health

In the last 20 years, the relationship between nutrition and mental health across the life span has become more apparent (Sarris et al. 2015). Dietary intake affects mental wellbeing, and a growing body of evidence suggests dietary intake before and during pregnancy affects the mental health of future children (Baskin et al. 2015).

One specific area of interest is the relationship between the dietary pattern of both men and women, and mental health. Recent studies suggest nutrition might be a potent predictor of maternal mental health status and the mental health of their offspring (Farr and Bish 2013; Stephenson et al. 2018). This relationship between diet and maternal mental health is suggested to be reciprocal and invigorating. Excessive distress is associated with an unhealthy diet, and an unhealthy dietary pattern is also associated with distress and other adverse mental health outcomes (Farr and Bish 2013; Stephenson et al. 2018). Moreover, the prevalence of psychological disorders and (excessive) mental distress might mediate the relation between poor women's nutritional habits and adverse health outcomes. For instance, if the woman is feeling depressed or is exposed to high levels of work-related stress, this might impact nutritional habits, leading to poorer food choices and subsequently worse maternal and neonatal health outcomes (Farr and Bish 2013). Whether women's preconception nutrition is related to the future mental health of the offspring is less clear. Multiple reviews revealed pre-pregnancy obesity of the mother was related to cognitive and psychiatric problems in the offspring. Specifically, they found that these children suffered an increased risk of reduction in IQ scores, attention deficit hyperactivity disorder (ADHD), psychotic disorders, and eating disorders in later life (Van Lieshout et al. 2011; Contu and Hawkes 2017). Although it is highly likely these women also had unhealthier dietary patterns, this association should be explored. Another recent study found that women's fasting plasma total homocysteine increased the risk of adverse neurodevelopmental outcome in their offspring (Roige-Castellvi et al. 2019).

The association between preconception nutrition and mental health is not only suggested for women, but also for men. Although the subject of paternal preconception care is gaining more attention, evidence for the association in men, especially in comparison to women, is relatively small (Kotelchuck and Lu 2017). Animal studies have demonstrated that the nutritional habits of men, in specific folate intake, are associated with the methylation of certain genes that influence the development of several mental diseases (Lambrot et al. 2013). More research is needed to determine how, and to what degree, maternal and paternal preconception nutrition are related to the mental health of women, men, and their (future) children.

6.2.5   Summary

Preconception nutrition is important for both women and men; for their own wellbeing, optimal fertility, and early stages of foetal development and to prevent adverse outcomes of pregnancy that can have lifelong implications for the health and wellbeing of children. The majority of nutritional requirements can be met through dietary intake, with the exception of folic acid and vitamin D which require supplementation. Some populations and high-risk groups may require further supplementation or specific alterations to their diet to achieve the nutritional requirements for healthy living and for healthy pregnancy, such as women following vegan or vegetarian diets. There is strong evidence on the importance of certain nutrients, such as folate and folic acid. However, there is limited data on other nutrients especially for male reproductive health or on the role of preconception nutrition and maternal mental health. While some evidence exists specifically in the context of preconception nutrition and global health such as higher prevalence of vitamin A deficiency, further research is also needed in low- and middle-income countries. There are inequalities in opportunity to follow a healthy diet preconceptionally that need to be addressed both between low-, middle-, and high-income countries but also within them.

6.3   Recommendations for Practice

- Men and women should be advised on the importance of preconception nutrition and to follow a varied diet to meet the nutritional requirements.
- Men and women should be provided with information on daily recommended nutrient intake requirements and sources of nutrients.
- All women should be advised to take a daily folic acid supplement of 400 µg from 3 months before conception to 12 weeks of pregnancy; some countries may have guidelines for higher doses for certain high-risk populations, such as women with diabetes or obesity.
- All women should take a 10 µg supplement of vitamin D.
- Women should be advised if they require preconception vitamin A supplementation, or if they choose to take multivitamin supplementation, then it is essential that any vitamin A supplements are in the beta-carotene form.

- Vegan and vegetarian women may require additional amendments to the diets and/or supplementation to meet the recommended daily nutrient intake requirements.
- Some sub-populations, such as women with fertility problems, obesity, or diabetes, may require additional nutritional support in the preconception period.
- Policies are needed to address the lack of access to high-nutritional-quality food in communities to improve health and wellbeing preconceptionally and throughout the life course.

References

Aghajafari F, Nagulesapillai T, Ronksley PE, Tough SC, O'Beirne M, Rabi DM. Association between maternal serum 25-hydroxyvitamin D level and pregnancy and neonatal outcomes: systematic review and meta-analysis of observational studies. BMJ. 2013;346:f1169.

Akmal M, Qadri JQ, Al-Waili NS, Thangal S, Haq A, Saloom KY. Improvement in human semen quality after oral supplementation of vitamin C. J Med Food. 2006;9(3):440–2.

Allen LH. Anemia and iron deficiency: effects on pregnancy outcome. Am J Clin Nutr. 2000;71(5):1280S–4S.

Anthony K, Tian X, Diaz FJ, Neuberger T. Preconception zinc deficiency disrupts postimplantation fetal and placental development in mice. Biol Reprod. 2014;90(4):83.

Arab A, Rafie N, Mansourian M, Miraghajani M, Hajianfar H. Dietary patterns and semen quality: a systematic review and meta-analysis of observational studies. Andrology. 2018;6(1):20–8.

Baskin R, Hill B, Jacka FN, O'Neil A, Skouteris H. The association between diet quality and mental health during the perinatal period. A systematic review. Appetite. 2015;91:41–7.

Bennett M. Vitamin B12 deficiency, infertility and recurrent fetal loss. J Reprod Med. 2001;46(3):209–12.

Berti C, Calabrese S, Cetin I. Role of micronutrients in the periconceptional period. Hum Reprod Update. 2009;16(1):80–95.

Blumfield ML, Hure AJ, Macdonald-Wicks L, Smith R, Collins CE. Systematic review and meta-analysis of energy and macronutrient intakes during pregnancy in developed countries. Nutr Rev. 2012;70(6):322–36.

Blumfield ML, Hure AJ, Macdonald-Wicks L, Smith R, Collins CE. Micronutrient intakes during pregnancy in developed countries: systematic review and meta-analysis. Nutr Rev. 2013;71(2):118–32.

Borge TC, Aase H, Brantsæter AL, Biele G. The importance of maternal diet quality during pregnancy on cognitive and behavioural outcomes in children: a systematic review and meta-analysis. BMJ Open. 2017;7(9):e016777.

Botto LD, Moore CA, Khoury MJ, Erickson JD. Neural-tube defects. N Engl J Med. 1999;341(20):1509–19.

Brody T. Nutritional Biochemistry. 2nd ed. Berkeley, CA: University of California; 1998. 1006 p

Bulloch RE, Lovell AL, Jordan VMB, McCowan LME, Thompson JMD, Wall CR. Maternal folic acid supplementation for the prevention of preeclampsia: a systematic review and meta-analysis. Paediatr Perinat Epidemiol. 2018;32(4):346–57.

Chandra-Hioe MV, Lee C, Arcot J. What is the cobalamin status among vegetarians and vegans in Australia? Int J Food Sci Nutr. 2019;70:1–12.

Chatterjea MN, Shinde R. Textbook of Medical Biochemistry. 8th ed. London: JP Medical Ltd; 2011. p. 163–96.

Chavarro JE, Rich-Edwards JW, Rosner BA, Willett WC. Iron intake and risk of ovulatory infertility. Obstet Gynecol. 2006;108(5):1145–52.

Clagett-Dame M, Knutson D. Vitamin A in reproduction and development. Nutrients. 2011;3(4):385–428.

Contu L, Hawkes CA. A review of the impact of maternal obesity on the cognitive function and mental health of the offspring. Int J Mol Sci. 2017;18(5):E1093.

Cucó G, Arija V, Iranzo R, Vilà J, Prieto MT, Fernández-Ballart J. Association of maternal protein intake before conception and throughout pregnancy with birth weight. Acta Obstet Gynecol Scand. 2006;85(4):413–21.

de Angelis C, Galdiero M, Pivonello C, Garifalos F, Menafra D, Cariati F, et al. The role of vitamin D in male fertility: a focus on the testis. Rev Endocr Metab Disord. 2017;18(3):285–305.

de Benoist B, Andersson M, Takkouche B, Egli I. Prevalence of iodine deficiency worldwide. Lancet. 2003;362(9398):1859–60.

De Ocampo MPG, Araneta MRG, Macera CA, Alcaraz JE, Moore TR, Chambers CD. Folic acid supplement use and the risk of gestational hypertension and preeclampsia. Women Birth. 2018;31(2):e77–83.

De-Regil LM, Pena-Rosas JP, Fernandez-Gaxiola AC, Rayco-Solon P. Effects and safety of periconceptional oral folate supplementation for preventing birth defects. Cochrane Database Syst Rev. 2015;12:CD007950.

Ebisch IM, Thomas CM, Peters WH, Braat DD, Steegers-Theunissen RP. The importance of folate, zinc and antioxidants in the pathogenesis and prevention of subfertility. Hum Reprod Update. 2007;13(2):163–74.

Ebisch IMW, Thomas CMG, Peters WHM, Braat DDM, Steegers-Theunissen RPM. The importance of folate, zinc and antioxidants in the pathogenesis and prevention of subfertility. Hum Reprod Update. 2006;13(2):163–74.

Erkkola M, Kaila M, Nwaru BI, Kronberg-Kippilä C, Ahonen S, Nevalainen J, et al. Maternal vitamin D intake during pregnancy is inversely associated with asthma and allergic rhinitis in 5-year-old children. Clin Exp Allergy. 2009;39(6):875–82.

Farr SL, Bish CL. Preconception health among women with frequent mental distress: a population-based study. J Women Health. 2013;22(2):153–8.

Farzadi L, Khayatzadeh Bidgoli H, Ghojazadeh M, Bahrami Z, Fattahi A, Latifi Z, et al. Correlation between follicular fluid 25-OH vitamin D and assisted reproductive outcomes. Iranian J Reprod Med. 2015;13(6):361–6.

Finnell RH, Spiegelstein O, Wlodarczyk B, Triplett A, Pogribny IP, Melnyk S, et al. DNA methylation in Folbp1 knockout mice supplemented with folic acid during gestation. J Nutr. 2002;132(8 Suppl):2457S–61S.

Green R, Miller JW. Folate deficiency beyond megaloblastic anemia: hyperhomocysteinemia and other manifestations of dysfunctional folate status. Semin Hematol. 1999;36(1):47–64.

Greenberg JA, Bell SJ, Ausdal WV. Omega-3 fatty acid supplementation during pregnancy. Rev Obstet Gynecol. 2008;1(4):162–9.

Groenen PM, van Rooij IA, Peer PG, Gooskens RH, Zielhuis GA, Steegers-Theunissen RP. Marginal maternal vitamin B12 status increases the risk of offspring with spina bifida. Am J Obstet Gynecol. 2004;191(1):11–7.

Hague WM. Homocysteine and pregnancy. Best Pract Res Clin Obstet Gynaecol. 2003;17(3):459–69.

Heinze T, Weber W. Determination of thiamine (vitamin B1) in maternal blood during normal pregnancies and pregnancies with intrauterine growth retardation. Z Ernahrungswiss. 1990;29(1):39–46.

Henmi H, Endo T, Kitajima Y, Manase K, Hata H, Kudo R. Effects of ascorbic acid supplementation on serum progesterone levels in patients with a luteal phase defect. Fertil Steril. 2003;80(2):459–61.

Hoogendoorn A LC, Parvanta I, Garrett GS. Food Fortification Global Mapping Study 2016. European Commission; 2016

Hornstra G. Essential fatty acids in mothers and their neonates. Am J Clin Nutr. 2000;71(5 Suppl):1262s–9s.

Inskip HM, Crozier SR, Godfrey KM, Borland SE, Cooper C, Robinson SM. Women's compliance with nutrition and lifestyle recommendations before pregnancy: general population cohort study. BMJ. 2009;338:b481.

Isoyama R, Baba Y, Harada H, Kawai S, Shimizu Y, Fujii M, et al. Clinical experience of methylcobalamin (CH3-B12)/clomiphene citrate combined treatment in male infertility. Hinyokika Kiyo. 1986;32(8):1177–83.

Isoyama R, Kawai S, Shimizu Y, Harada H, Takihara H, Baba Y, et al. Clinical experience with methylcobalamin (CH3-B12) for male infertility. Hinyokika Kiyo. 1984;30(4):581–6.

Jeyaseelan I, Luck MR, Scholes RA. Ascorbic acid and fertility. Biol Reprod. 1995;52(2):262–6.

Katz J, Khatry SK, West KP, Humphrey JH, Leclerq SC, Pradhan EK, et al. Night blindness is prevalent during pregnancy and lactation in rural Nepal. J Nutr. 1995;125(8):2122–7.

Kavle JA, Stoltzfus RJ, Witter F, Tielsch JM, Khalfan SS, Caulfield LE. Association between anaemia during pregnancy and blood loss at and after delivery among women with vaginal births in Pemba Island, Zanzibar, Tanzania. J Health Popul Nutr. 2008;26(2):232–40.

Kelly TL, Neaga OR, Schwahn BC, Rozen R, Trasler JM. Infertility in 5,10-methylenetetrahydrofolate reductase (MTHFR)-deficient male mice is partially alleviated by lifetime dietary betaine supplementation. Biol Reprod. 2005;72(3):667–77.

Kloss O, Eskin NAM, Suh M. Thiamin deficiency on fetal brain development with and without prenatal alcohol exposure. Biochem Cell Biol. 2018;96(2):169–77.

Kodentsova VM, Vrzesinskaya OA, Spirichev VB. Male fertility: a possible role of vitamins. Ukr Biokhim Zh (1978). 1994;66(5):17–22.

Kotelchuck M, Lu M. Father's role in preconception health. Matern Child Health J. 2017;21(11):2025–39.

Kovacs CS. Calcium and bone metabolism in pregnancy and lactation. J Clin Endocrinol Metabol. 2001;86(6):2344–8.

Kumamoto Y, Maruta H, Ishigami J, Kamidono S, Orikasa S, Kimura M, et al. Clinical efficacy of mecobalamin in the treatment of oligozoospermia—results of double-blind comparative clinical study. Hinyokika Kiyo. 1988;34(6):1109–32.

Ladipo OA. Nutrition in pregnancy: mineral and vitamin supplements. Am J Clin Nutr. 2000;72(1 Suppl):280S–90S.

Lambrot R, Xu C, Saint-Phar S, Chountalos G, Cohen T, Paquet M, et al. Low paternal dietary folate alters the mouse sperm epigenome and is associated with negative pregnancy outcomes. Nat Commun. 2013;4:2889.

Lee GR. Pernicious anemia and other causes of vitamin B12 (cobalamin) deficiency. In: Lee GR, et al., editors. Wintrobe's Clinical Hematology. Baltimore: Williams & Wilkins; 1999. p. 941–64.

Lee SE, Talegawkar SA, Merialdi M, Caulfield LE. Dietary intakes of women during pregnancy in low- and middle-income countries. Public Health Nutr. 2013;16(8):1340–53.

Lienhart WD, Gudipati V, Macheroux P. The human flavoproteome. Arch Biochem Biophys. 2013;535(2):150–62.

Lindenbaum J, Healton EB, Savage DG, Brust JC, Garrett TJ, Podell ER, et al. Neuropsychiatric disorders caused by cobalamin deficiency in the absence of anemia or macrocytosis. N Engl J Med. 1988;318(26):1720–8.

Lonsdale D. Thiamin. Adv Food Nutr Res. 2018;83:1–56.

Mahmood L. The metabolic processes of folic acid and Vitamin B12 deficiency. J Health Res Rev. 2014;1(1):5–9.

Manzetti S, Zhang J, van der Spoel D. Thiamin function, metabolism, uptake, and transport. Biochemistry. 2014;53(5):821–35.

McNulty H, Pentieva K. Folate bioavailability. Proc Nutr Soc. 2004;63(4):529–36.

McNulty H, Pentieva K. Folate bioavailability. In: Bailey LB, editor. Folate in health and disease. 2nd ed. Boca Raton: CRC Press, Taylor and Francis Group; 2010. p. 25–47.

Melse-Boonstra A, Jaiswal N. Iodine deficiency in pregnancy, infancy and childhood and its consequences for brain development. Best Pract Res Clin Endocrinol Metab. 2010;24(1):29–38.

Mignini LE, Latthe PM, Villar J, Kilby MD, Carroli G, Khan KS. Mapping the theories of pre-eclampsia: the role of homocysteine. Obstet Gynecol. 2005;105(2):411–25.

Moore VM, Davies MJ, Willson KJ, Worsley A, Robinson JS. Dietary composition of pregnant women is related to size of the baby at birth. J Nutr. 2004;134(7):1820–6.

Nguyen PH, DiGirolamo AM, Gonzalez-Casanova I, Pham H, Hao W, Nguyen H, et al. Impact of preconceptional micronutrient supplementation on maternal mental health during pregnancy and postpartum: results from a randomized controlled trial in Vietnam. BMC Womens Health. 2017;17(1):44.

NICE. Maternal and child nutrition—Public health guideline [PH11]: National Institute for Health and Care Excellence; 2008 [updated November 2014]. https://www.nice.org.uk/guidance/PH11/chapter/4-Recommendations.

NIH. Office of Dietary Supplements. Thiamin: National Institutes of Health; 2018 [updated 2018]. https://ods.od.nih.gov/factsheets/Thiamin-HealthProfessional/#h3.

Oudman E, Wijnia JW, Oey M, van Dam M, Painter RC, Postma A. Wernicke's encephalopathy in hyperemesis gravidarum: a systematic review. Eur J Obstet Gynecol Reprod Biol. 2019;236:84–93.

Partal-Lorente AB, Maldonado-Ezequiel V, Martinez-Navarro L, Herrera-Contreras I, Gutierrez-Repiso C, Garcia-Fuentes E, et al. Iodine is associated to semen quality in men who undergo consultations for infertility. Reprod Toxicol. 2017;73:1–7.

Pauwels S, Ghosh M, Duca RC, Bekaert B, Freson K, Huybrechts I, et al. Maternal intake of methyl-group donors affects DNA methylation of metabolic genes in infants. Clin Epigenetics. 2017;9:16.

Powers HJ. Riboflavin (vitamin B-2) and health. Am J Clin Nutr. 2003;77(6):1352–60.

Ralapanawa DM, Jayawickreme KP, Ekanayake EM, Jayalath WA. B12 deficiency with neurological manifestations in the absence of anaemia. BMC Res Notes. 2015;8:458.

Robitaille J, Carmichael SL, Shaw GM, Olney RS. National Birth Defects Prevention S. Maternal nutrient intake and risks for transverse and longitudinal limb deficiencies: data from the National Birth Defects Prevention Study, 1997–2003. Birth Defects Res A Clin Mol Teratol. 2009;85(9):773–9.

Roige-Castellvi J, Murphy M, Fernandez-Ballart J, Canals J. Moderately elevated preconception fasting plasma total homocysteine is a risk factor for psychological problems in childhood. Public Health Nutr. 2019;22(9):1615–23.

Rothman KJ, Moore LL, Singer MR, Nguyen U-SDT, Mannino S, Milunsky A. Teratogenicity of high vitamin A intake. N Engl J Med. 1995;333(21):1369–73.

Ruder EH, Hartman TJ, Goldman MB. Impact of oxidative stress on female fertility. Curr Opin Obstet Gynecol. 2009;21(3):219–22.

Sakamoto KQ, Ishizuka M, Kazusaka A, Fujita S. Iodine intake as a possible cause of discontinuous decline in sperm counts: a re-evaluation of historical and geographic variation in semen quality. Jpn J Vet Res. 2004;52(2):85–94.

Salas-Huetos A, Bullo M, Salas-Salvado J. Dietary patterns, foods and nutrients in male fertility parameters and fecundability: a systematic review of observational studies. Hum Reprod Update. 2017;23(4):371–89.

Sarris J, Logan AC, Akbaraly TN, Amminger GP, Balanzá-Martínez V, Freeman MP, et al. Nutritional medicine as mainstream in psychiatry. Lancet Psychiatry. 2015;2(3):271–4.

Schagdarsurengin U, Steger K. Epigenetics in male reproduction: effect of paternal diet on sperm quality and offspring health. Nat Rev Urol. 2016;13(10):584–95.

Scholl TO, Johnson WG. Folic acid: influence on the outcome of pregnancy. Am J Clin Nutr. 2000;71(5 Suppl):1295S–303S.

Selhub J. Folate, vitamin B12 and vitamin B6 and one carbon metabolism. J Nutr Health Aging. 2002;6(1):39–42.

Shahrook S, Ota E, Hanada N, Sawada K, Mori R. Vitamin K supplementation during pregnancy for improving outcomes: a systematic review and meta-analysis. Scientific Rep. 2018;8(1):11459.

Shane B. Folate chemistry and metabolism. In: Bailey LP, editor. Folate in health and disease. New York: Marcel Dekker; 1995. p. 1–22.

Sinclair S. Male infertility: nutritional and environmental considerations. Altern Med Rev. 2000;5(1):28–38.

Smedts HP, Rakhshandehroo M, Verkleij-Hagoort AC, de Vries JH, Ottenkamp J, Steegers EA, et al. Maternal intake of fat, riboflavin and nicotinamide and the risk of having offspring with congenital heart defects. Eur J Nutr. 2008;47(7):357–65.

Soma-Pillay P, Nelson-Piercy C, Tolppanen H, Mebazaa A. Physiological changes in pregnancy. Cardiovasc J Afr. 2016;27(2):89–94.

Steegers-Theunissen RP, Obermann-Borst SA, Kremer D, Lindemans J, Siebel C, Steegers EA, et al. Periconceptional maternal folic acid use of 400 microg per day is related to increased methylation of the IGF2 gene in the very young child. PLoS One. 2009;4(11):e7845.

Steegers-Theunissen RP, Steegers EA. Nutrient-gene interactions in early pregnancy: a vascular hypothesis. Eur J Obstet Gynecol Reprod Biol. 2003;106(2):115–7.

Steegers-Theunissen RP, Twigt J, Pestinger V, Sinclair KD. The periconceptional period, reproduction and long-term health of offspring: the importance of one-carbon metabolism. Hum Reprod Update. 2013;19(6):640–55.

Stephenson J, Heslehurst N, Hall J, Schoenaker D, Hutchinson J, Cade JE, et al. Before the beginning: nutrition and lifestyle in the preconception period and its importance for future health. Lancet. 2018;391(10132):1830–41.

Thakur K, Tomar SK, Singh AK, Mandal S, Arora S. Riboflavin and health: a review of recent human research. Crit Rev Food Sci Nutr. 2017;57(17):3650–60.

Tian X, Diaz FJ. Zinc depletion causes multiple defects in ovarian function during the periovulatory period in mice. Endocrinology. 2012;153(2):873–86.

Traber MG, Sokol RJ, Ringel SP, Neville HE, Thellman CA, Kayden HJ. Lack of Tocopherol in peripheral nerves of vitamin E-deficient patients with peripheral neuropathy. N Engl J Med. 1987;317(5):262–5.

Twigt JM, Hammiche F, Sinclair KD, Beckers NG, Visser JA, Lindemans J, et al. Preconception folic acid use modulates estradiol and follicular responses to ovarian stimulation. J Clin Endocrinol Metab. 2011;96(2):E322–9.

Van Lieshout RJ, Taylor VH, Boyle MH. Pre-pregnancy and pregnancy obesity and neurodevelopmental outcomes in offspring: a systematic review. Obes Rev. 2011;12(5):e548–59.

Verkleij-Hagoort AC, de Vries JH, Ursem NT, de Jonge R, Hop WC, Steegers-Theunissen RP. Dietary intake of B-vitamins in mothers born a child with a congenital heart defect. Eur J Nutr. 2006;45(8):478–86.

Vezina D, Mauffette F, Roberts KD, Bleau G. Selenium-vitamin E supplementation in infertile men. Effects on semen parameters and micronutrient levels and distribution. Biol Trace Elem Res. 1996;53(1–3):65–83.

Vimaleswaran KS, Berry DJ, Lu C, Tikkanen E, Pilz S, Hiraki LT, et al. Causal relationship between obesity and vitamin D status: bi-directional Mendelian randomization analysis of multiple cohorts. PLoS Med. 2013;10(2):e1001383.

Vohr BR, Poggi Davis E, Wanke CA, Krebs NF. Neurodevelopment: the impact of nutrition and inflammation during preconception and pregnancy in low-resource settings. Pediatrics. 2017;139(Supplement 1):S38–49.

Vujkovic M, de Vries JH, Lindemans J, Macklon NS, van der Spek PJ, Steegers EA, et al. The preconception Mediterranean dietary pattern in couples undergoing in vitro fertilization/intracytoplasmic sperm injection treatment increases the chance of pregnancy. Fertil Steril. 2010;94(6):2096–101.

Wacker J, Fruhauf J, Schulz M, Chiwora FM, Volz J, Becker K. Riboflavin deficiency and preeclampsia. Obstet Gynecol. 2000;96(1):38–44.

Wagner C. Biochemical role of folate in cellular metabolism. In: Bailey LP, editor. Folate in health and disease. New York: Marcel Dekker; 1995. p. 23–42.

Weisshof R, Chermesh I. Micronutrient deficiencies in inflammatory bowel disease. Curr Opin Clin Nutr Metab Care. 2015;18(6):576–81.

Williams PJ, Bulmer JN, Innes BA, Broughton PF. Possible roles for folic acid in the regulation of trophoblast invasion and placental development in normal early human pregnancy. Biol Reprod. 2011;84(6):1148–53.

Wolf G. The discovery of the visual function of vitamin A. J Nutr. 2001;131(6):1647–50.

Wong WY, Merkus HM, Thomas CM, Menkveld R, Zielhuis GA, Steegers-Theunissen RP. Effects of folic acid and zinc sulfate on male factor subfertility: a double-blind, randomized, placebo-controlled trial. Fertil Steril. 2002;77(3):491–8.

World Health Organization and Food and Agriculture Organization of the United Nations. Vitamin and mineral requirements in human nutrition. 2004.

Lifestyle: Weight

Annick Bogaerts, Amanda Bye, Margriet Bijlholt,
Kate Maslin, and Roland Devlieger

7.1 Introduction

Strong links between women and men's health *before* pregnancy and maternal and child health outcomes have been demonstrated to have consequences across generations. Poor nutritional status among women and men of reproductive age, including underweight, overweight, and obesity, is becoming more common. This chapter describes the epidemiology of weight disorders, makes connections between weight and health outcomes for women and children, and describes strategies for addressing this critical issue.

Many men, women, and adolescent girls have inadequate or imbalanced daily diets, leading to underweight, overweight, and obesity, often alongside micronutrient deficiencies. Undernutrition among women and children is the underlying cause of 3.5 million deaths annually worldwide, as well as accounting for 35% of the disease burden in children younger than 5 years and of 11% of total global disability-adjusted life years. Women's underweight (BMI < 18.5 kg/m^2) (Table 7.1) ranges from 10% to 19% in most countries and can result in poor fetal development (Black et al. 2013). It is associated with poor obstetric outcomes such as increased risk for

A. Bogaerts (✉) · M. Bijlholt
Department of Development and Regeneration,
KU Leuven University, Leuven, Belgium
e-mail: annick.bogaerts@kuleuven.be

A. Bye
UCL Great Ormond Street Institute of Child Health, London, UK

King's College London, London, UK

K. Maslin
Faculty of Health, University of Plymouth, Plymouth, Devon, UK

R. Devlieger
Department of Development and Regeneration, KU Leuven University,
Leuven, Belgium

© Springer Nature Switzerland AG 2020
J. Shawe et al. (eds.), *Preconception Health and Care: A Life Course Approach*,
https://doi.org/10.1007/978-3-030-31753-9_7

Table 7.1 Definition and categorization of body mass index (weight in kg/squared height in meters)

Underweight	$<18.5\ kg/m^2$
Healthy weight	$18.5–24.9\ kg/m^2$
Overweight	$25.0–29.9\ kg/m^2$
Obesity	$\geq30\ kg/m^2$

preterm birth and low birth weight and can lead to lifelong problems for women themselves. Differences between high- and low-income countries have become less distinct. Globally it is estimated that 35% of adult women are overweight or obese, putting them at greater risk for preexisting health risks before conception and at increased risks for developing pregnancy and childbirth complications. Weight retained from a previous pregnancy may also predict subsequent obesity and cardio-metabolic problems. Infants born to women who are overweight or obese tend to be larger and may be at risk of developing obesity, type 2 diabetes and neurocognitive disorders in later life (Godfrey et al. 2017).

Because lifestyle interventions during pregnancy have limited impact on maternal and child health outcomes, intervening prior to conception is essential. An increased focus on developing and testing interventions to help young adults achieve a healthy weight is needed to improve health in current and future generations and to reduce the increasing burden of chronic diseases. The international *EarlyNutrition* research project (http://www.project-earlynutrition.eu) developed recommendations for dietary practice for women before pregnancy, taking long-term health consequences into account. Healthcare providers should be encouraged and trained to support and provide advice on nutrition, including optimizing adolescent nutrition and health. In fact, adherence to good dietary and lifestyle habits should start in childhood and adolescence. Particular attention should be paid to the intake and status of specific micronutrients, especially folate, in women of reproductive age. Dietary supplementation with iron, vitamin D, vitamin B12, iodine, and others may be indicated in women at risk of poor intake and insufficiency of these micronutrients (Koletzko et al. 2019). This is further discussed in Chap. 5. Healthcare systems and communities should provide the services and support needed to ensure access to affordable healthy foods, nutrition counselors, and safe places to exercise.

Healthcare providers should pay particular attention to the weight status of women and men of reproductive age. Where appropriate they should provide advice for modifying weight by improving lifestyle including diet and physical activity. Weight management may be a sensitive and difficult issue for healthcare professionals to approach, particularly in women of reproductive age (Knight-Agarwal et al. 2014; Atkinson and McNamara 2017). Discussing weight management with men may be challenging for different reasons, as men are less likely to perceive their weight as a problem and less likely to engage with weight loss services (Robertson et al. 2014). Although many women may successfully lose excess weight, weight regain is common and related to underlying psychological factors such as self-efficacy as well as to the many competing priorities that women face (Annesi 2018). Research has also shown that women may be disproportionately affected by food insecurity, particularly in resource-poor settings, making preparation and access to healthy food more difficult (Ivers and Cullen 2011).

Underweight must not be neglected, as underweight women are more likely to be deficient in important nutrients and their diets should be supplemented if required. Concurrently, the number of women of reproductive age with eating disorders is increasingly recognized, as are the increasing number of women having bariatric surgery. Both groups require specific attention to their nutrition and will be discussed further later in this chapter. In delivering preventive, wellness care, professionals must use existing evidence-based practices as well as innovative mechanisms, trying to integrate preconception care into ongoing healthcare programs. Currently, preconception care is usually *not* an integrated part of existing care paths. Healthcare providers should take advantage of every opportunity they have with people of reproductive age to provide health information and interventions to improve their well-being and that of any children they may wish to have in the future.

7.2   Measuring Weight Status

Overweight and obesity are defined as abnormal or excessive fat accumulation in adipose tissue that poses a risk for health (World Health Organization 2000). Overweight and obesity are assessed by using different anthropometric measurements and techniques. BMI is most commonly used, which is calculated as weight in kilograms divided by the square of height in meters (kg/m^2). Waist circumference is a useful proxy for abdominal fat but is subject to measurement error (Verweij et al. 2013). Skinfold thicknesses can be measured by using a caliper and provide information on the percentage of body fat. More direct measures of body fat and body fat distribution can be assessed by using instruments such bioelectrical impedance analysis, magnetic resonance imaging, dual energy X-ray absorptiometry, and air displacement plethysmography.

Although BMI is highly correlated with the degree of fat mass, it does not directly measure the percentage of body fat or fat distribution. A higher amount of fat-free tissue, such as muscle, is associated with health benefits, whereas excess fat is harmful. The ability of measured BMI to detect people with excess body fat percentage (BF%) is highly specific, but measured BMI has a poor sensitivity as it fails to identify nearly half of the adults (Okorodudu et al. 2010) and a quarter of children (Javed et al. 2015) with excess BF%. Ideally BF% should also be calculated. In a recent study including a thousand 25-year-old adults, nearly 40% of those who were not obese according to BMI had excess body adiposity according to BF% cutoffs ($\geq 25\%$ for men, $\geq 35\%$ for women), and 2% who were obese by BMI were not obese according to BF% (Kumpulainen et al. 2016). This is important as measuring individuals who have BMI within the normal range, but who have high BF% may have an increased risk for cardio-metabolic diseases (Gomez-Ambrosi et al. 2012). Nevertheless, BMI offers a more accurate assessment of adiposity than weight alone and is a well-reproducible indicator of metabolic risk. Due to its simplicity, most epidemiological and clinical studies consider BMI as a useful and easy method to measure this surrogate marker for increased health risks relating to excess body fat (Fattah et al. 2009).

It is recommended that body weight should be measured, instead of relying on self-report. When using self-reported weight to calculate BMI, approximately one in six to seven individuals with obesity will be misclassified due to underestimation of BMI (Onubi et al. 2016). Fortunately, no time trends were found in the accuracy of self-report BMI categories, so at least increases in obesity rates based on self-reported height and weight are likely to reflect increases and are not inflated by changes in reporting accuracy (Hattori and Sturm 2013). It is argued that under-recognition of overweight and obesity, which is common in both lay people and medical practitioners, is due to recalibration of visual body weight norms. Because larger body sizes are now common, this has caused a recalibration to the range of body sizes that are perceived as being "normal" and increased the visual threshold for what constitutes "overweight," which ultimately may be a hindrance to weight management or intervention efforts (Robinson 2017). This misperception of weight category has important implications, given that risk of adverse pregnancy outcomes increases in a dose-relationship pattern with increasing maternal BMI (Aune et al. 2014), which will be discussed further later in this chapter.

Data on measured and self-reported BMI, derived from a recent Food Consumption Survey (FCS, $N = 1213$) 2014 were used to assess possible misreporting. Correction factors (measured BMI/self-reported BMI) were calculated as a function of a combination of background variables such as region, gender, educational level, and age group. When compared with the measured BMI, the self-reported BMI in the FCS was underestimated by a mean of 0.97 kg/m^2 (corresponding with approximately 2.5–3 kg), and 28% of people with obesity (18–64 years) underestimated their BMI. After applying the correction factors on self-reported BMI data in the Health Interview Survey 2013 (HIS, $N = 6545$), the prevalence of obesity increased from 13% based on original self-reported BMI to 17% based on the corrected HIS data, which approximated the measured prevalence derived from FCS data. This implies that the problem of obesity is probably 4% points higher in this cohort than initially thought based on self-reported HIS data. Applying the correction factor on the self-reported BMI of National Health Interview Surveys probably leads to a more accurate estimation of the obesity prevalence, which is important for policy and decision-making (Drieskens et al. 2018). This needs to be taken into account if we compare the rates of maternal BMI categories between different countries.

7.3   Prevalence of Underweight, Overweight, and Obesity

The prevalence of obesity in women of reproductive age varies across countries with increased prevalence in non-white ethnic groups, especially non-Hispanic black women (55.8%) (Poston et al. 2016; Ogden et al. 2014). Figure 7.1 indicates the estimated overweight and obesity prevalence worldwide with the red areas showing those regions with highest overweight and obesity rates. In low- and

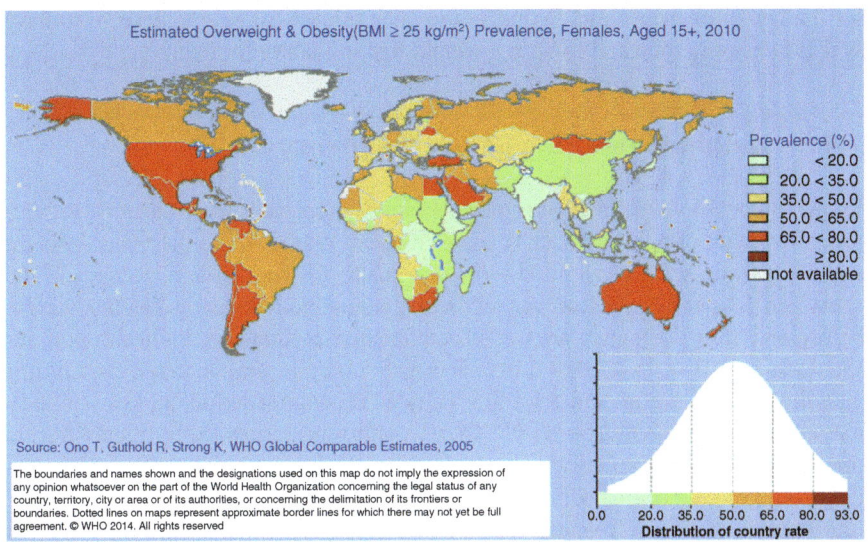

Estimated Overweight & Obesity(BMI ≥ 25 kg/m²) Prevalence, Females, Aged 15+, 2010

Fig. 7.1 Estimated overweight and obesity prevalence worldwide

middle-income countries, a shift to more energy-dense food and more sedentary lifestyle resulted in a global transition from undernutrition to more over-nutrition and micronutrient deficits. Excess weight is now becoming more common than underweight in women of reproductive age in many developing countries in Asia and Africa (Mendez et al. 2005; Ng et al. 2014; Onubi et al. 2016). This may be due to, increased urbanization, leading to increased access to energy-dense foods and motorized transportation. Traditionally considered a problem of high-income countries, obesity has received greater attention in low-income and middle-income countries (LMICs) in recent years.

In 2008, there were almost three overweight or obese women of childbearing age for each underweight woman in LMICs (Black et al. 2013), which raises the question of whether maternal overweight is now more important than maternal underweight in influencing the long-term chronic disease burden in these countries. An analysis of adult body mass index (BMI) in 200 countries from 1975 to 2014 with over 19 million participants found that the age-standardized global proportion of underweight women (BMI <18.5 kg/m²) decreased from 15% to 10%; South Asia had the highest proportion of underweight women with an estimated 24% in 2014. Although the proportion of women who are underweight has decreased, the proportion of obese women globally has risen from 6% to 15% from 1975 to 2014.

In many low-, middle-, and high-income countries, up to 50% of women are overweight or obese when they become pregnant (Collaboration NCDRF 2016). On the other hand, in South Asia 24% of women are underweight. Discussions about using different cutoffs for the classification in BMI categories of these Asian population are ongoing. In the meantime, the health implications of underweight in women need to be addressed too, not only for the benefit of the individual but also for the health of their children and future generations. All people deserve to have access to healthy food and to be at a weight that is healthy for them.

7.4   Weight Monitoring Before Pregnancy

Being at a healthy weight is an important part of a person's life trajectory, regardless of whether or not they want to have children. Women's pre-pregnancy weight and postpartum weight retention influence health for women and children in the short and longer term. However, clinical guidelines addressing healthy weight before and after pregnancy are not systematically implemented in health policies (Scott et al. 2014). In a 2014 cross-sectional survey in 66 countries, the clinical guidelines regarding maternal weight included recommendations to assess maternal weight at first prenatal visit (90%), to monitor gestational weight gain during pregnancy (81%) and to provide recommendations to women about healthy gestational weight gain (62%). Guidelines related to preconception (42%) and postpartum weight (13%) were less common. Recommendations regarding maternal weight management are not widely known in many countries. Moreover, there are many inconsistencies and variance in practices related to establishing a healthy weight before and after pregnancy. There is a lack of international consensus on guidelines around healthy weight before, during, and after pregnancy. Recommendations and evidence-based interventions in this arena are urgently needed (Skouteris et al. 2019).

Most countries across the world do not report data on pre-gestational body mass index (BMI) systematically. Data for pre-pregnancy BMI are mainly based on data from women of reproductive age in National Health and Nutrition Examination Surveys (Poston et al. 2016). Moreover, information about pre-gestational weight and height is often based on recalled self-reported data, which, as previously discussed, can be biased. Alternatively, it is based on a measurement at the first antenatal visit, when the woman is already several weeks pregnant. Because of a rising incidence of obesity among women, Euro-Peristat has recently added the monitoring of mother's pre-pregnancy BMI, categorized as a *recommended*—i.e., considered desirable for a more complete picture of perinatal health across the member states—perinatal health indicator (www.europeristat.com) (Zeitlin et al. 2009). They recommend recording pre-pregnancy BMI or if unavailable measurements at first prenatal assessment. Preferably all women of reproductive age should be routinely screened for BMI to monitor the success of public health programs aimed at reducing weight.

7.5   Weight Monitoring During Pregnancy

There are, many controversies around the value of repeated weighing during pregnancy. Measuring weight during pregnancy is problematic as it is a proxy for not only fat accumulation but also for intra- and extravascular fluid retention, fetal growth, amniotic fluid, and growth of breast tissue. The National Institute for Health Care and Excellence (NICE) guidelines on weight management before, during, and after pregnancy (2010) clearly indicate that health professionals should advise, encourage, and help women with a BMI of 30 kg/m² or more to reduce weight before becoming pregnant. Losing 5–10% of their weight would have significant health benefits and could increase their chances of becoming pregnant. They suggest that evidence-based behavioral change techniques including motivational support techniques are used and that women are encouraged to check their weight periodically. In the meantime, routine weighing during pregnancy was phased out on recommendations of the National Institute for Health Care and Excellence (NICE); the rationale for this was a potential increased perceived maternal stress without proven benefit. In contrast, researchers from an Australian group concluded that women were satisfied with being weighed antenatally and they accepted the reintroduction of weighing in the antenatal clinic (Brownfoot et al. 2016). More information about monitoring weight and related health indicators during regular well women care is needed.

Weighing during routine appointments ro has potential advantages: the recorded weight can initiate discussions on appropriate weight and about lifestyle modifications in order to achieve healthy weight. In women, weight gain can induce anxiety and stress, even when related to a "physiologic condition" like pregnancy or postnatal periods. Appropriate measurements and counseling in these situations can have a possible anxiety-reducing effect (Bogaerts et al. 2013a). Reassurance and stress reduction are crucial components of good perinatal care and impact on weight trajectories. Indeed, the authors showed that anxiety in early pregnancy is strongly associated with gestational weight gain and postnatal weight retention (Bogaerts et al. 2013b, c). At the same time, research has demonstrated a strong positive dose-response association between pre-pregnancy BMI and the likelihood of major depressive disorders. Compared with a BMI of 18, the adjusted odds ratios for women with BMIs of 23, 28, and 33 were 1.4, 1.9, and 2.6, respectively. This risk was aggravated by gestational weight gain outside the Institute of Medicine (IOM) recommendations (inadequate and excessive gestational weight gain) (Bodnar et al. 2009). Overall the relationship between psychosocial factors and weight gain in pregnancy is complex, with depression, body dissatisfaction, and social support appearing to have a direct relationship with excessive gestational weight gain (Hartley et al. 2015). A systematic review has identified protective psychological factors for excess gestational weight gain, namely, internal locus of control for weight gain, lower than recommended target weight gain and higher self-efficacy for healthy eating (Kapadia et al. 2015). This indicates that maternal weight monitoring and management have an underlying psychological component which cannot be neglected during periconception counseling.

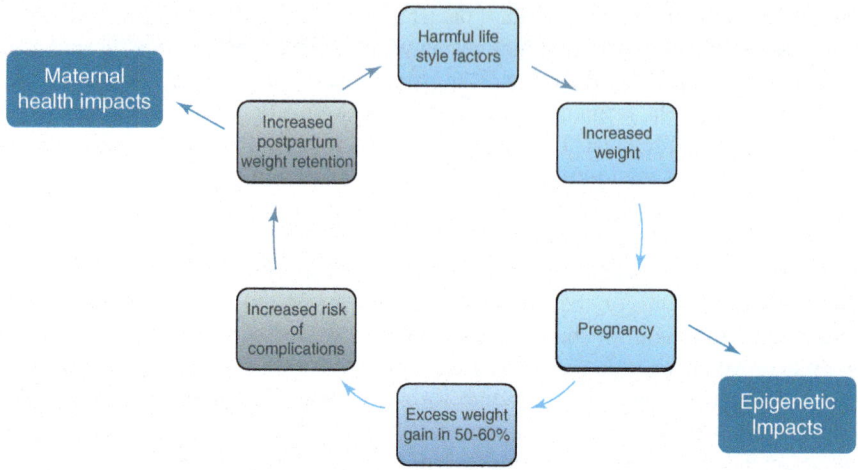

Fig. 7.2 Cycle of weight gain in women across the reproductive years

7.6   Associations Between Maternal Weight and Reproductive Outcomes

An unhealthy weight in women of reproductive age affects the woman's health but also places her offspring at risk, particularly of developing childhood obesity and its later metabolic, cardiovascular, and neurocognitive consequences. This cycle can therefore repeat in subsequent generations (Fig. 7.2).

7.7   Impact on Women and Men

Pre-pregnancy BMI is associated with many important pregnancy outcomes, for both women and their offspring. These are listed in Table 7.2. Compared to women with a healthy weight before pregnancy, those who are overweight or obese, as well as those women who are underweight, are at increased risk of adverse pregnancy and birth outcomes (Bogaerts et al. 2012). A dose-response relationship between increasing maternal BMI and adverse childbirth outcomes has been reported in a systematic review and meta-analyses of 44 studies. This review highlighted that even modest increases in maternal BMI were associated with increased risk of fetal death, stillbirth, neonatal, and perinatal death. Although the greatest risk was for those with a BMI of >40 kg/m², a threshold of increased risk existed at between 24 and 27 kg/m² for most outcomes (Aune et al. 2014). Typically, other research studies and systematic reviews haven't always discriminated between the risks of maternal overweight versus obesity. However, this oversight should be considered against the backdrop of underestimation of overweight and obesity by both lay people and health professionals and the increased visual threshold for what constitutes "overweight" (Robinson 2017). There is a sense among midwives that encountering

Table 7.2 Maternal obesity and short- and long-term outcomes

Preconception	Pregnancy	Postpartum	
Maternal outcomes	Maternal outcomes	Maternal outcomes	Offspring outcomes
	Early pregnancy loss	Postpartum hemorrhage	Increased risk childhood obesity
Fertility treatment less successful	Congenital fetal malformations	Increased weight retention	Asthma, wheezing
Comorbidities: T2 diabetes, chronic hypertension	Decreased detection of fetal abnormalities	Decreased intention and continuation of breastfeeding	Poorer neurocognitive development
	Large-for-gestational-age baby, small-for-gestational-age baby	Increased risk for wound infection	Autism spectrum disorder
	Shoulder dystocia	Increased risk T2 diabetes	Cognitive abnormality
	Spontaneous and medically indicated premature birth	Increased risk of postpartum depression	
	Stillbirth	Increased risk of metabolic syndrome[a]	
	Gestational diabetes		
	Preeclampsia		
	Labor difficulties: prolonged onset, increased risk of induction, anesthetic complications, birth trauma, intrapartum monitoring difficulties		
	Instrumental and caesarean birth		
	Increased risk of depression		

[a]For both mother and child
Sources: Godfrey et al. (2017), Poston et al. (2016), Bogaerts et al. (2012, 2013d, 2015), Bodnar et al. (2015), Guelinckx et al. (2008), Leonard (2017), Yang et al. (2017)

pregnant women with a BMI > 30 kg/m² is considered normal and that the "cutoff" scores for referral for services for pregnant women based on BMI has increased (Schmied et al. 2011).

Undernutrition must not be neglected, as underweight women are more likely to be deficient in important nutrients, and their diets should be carefully assessed and supplemented as required. A systematic review and meta-analysis of population-based cohort studies in LMICs revealed a double burden: maternal underweight is associated with higher risk of preterm, low birth weight, and small-for-gestational-age (SGA) birth, and by contrast, maternal obesity increases the risk of gestational diabetes, pregnancy-induced hypertension, preeclampsia, caesarean delivery, and postpartum hemorrhage (Rahman et al. 2015; Marchi et al. 2015). Particular attention should be paid to the intake and status of some micronutrients, especially folate, in women of reproductive age (Koletzko et al. 2019). This is discussed further in Chap. 5.

The rise in obesity prevalence in women of reproductive age is considered to be the major determinant of the striking increase in preexisting type 2 diabetes among pregnant women. Pregnant women with preexisting diabetes are at increased risk of poor maternal, fetal, and neonatal outcomes, including pregnancy loss, perinatal mortality, fetal macrosomia, and congenital malformations. Chronic hypertension is also an increasing problem in obese women of reproductive age. Studies indicate that pregnant women with preexisting chronic hypertension show an increased risk of superimposed preeclampsia, caesarean delivery, preterm delivery, low birth weight, neonatal unit admission, and perinatal death (Bramham et al. 2014). This reinforces the need for an early pregnancy screening for comorbidities in women with preconception obesity and a greater emphasis on a multifaceted approach to achieve an optimal weight before conception in women of reproductive age.

Women with obesity who are intending to become pregnant take longer on average to conceive, and time to pregnancy increases with the degree of obesity. Ovulatory dysfunction, the most common infertility diagnosis among women with obesity, appears to be independent of age and parity and is likely to result from suboptimal glycemic control and insulin resistance associated with obesity. Assisted reproductive technology is more often required in women who are obese but is less successful than in lean women: women with obesity experience a 68% reduction in livebirths from an assisted reproductive technology cycle compared with women of normal weight (Poston et al. 2016).

In the meantime, the global increase in obesity among men (3–11% between 1975 and 2014) is of relevance; paternal obesity has been linked to impaired fertility by affecting sperm quality and quantity and is associated with increased chronic disease risk in offspring (Collaboration NCDRF 2016). The cumulative contribution of both maternal and paternal obesity on the risk of obesity in future generations has been suggested by several studies and causal pathways involving interaction between genetic, epigenetic, and environmental factors are emerging (Godfrey et al. 2017).

7.8   Postpartum Weight Retention

Maternal obesity and postpartum weight retention, which are often mentioned together as inter-pregnancy weight change, are all related to poorer maternal physical and mental health. Inter-pregnancy weight change, which is the net result of weight gain (particularly fat gain) during pregnancy, weight loss after pregnancy, and weight change after the postpartum period until the start of the next pregnancy, is linked to increased risk for gestational hypertension, diabetes, stillbirth, and infant mortality (Bogaerts et al. 2013b; Cnattingius and Villamor 2016; Villamor and Cnattingius 2006). Even women who were initially healthy weight before the start of their first pregnancy and who had an increase in BMI at the start of a next pregnancy were at increased risk for developing gestational diabetes and hypertension, compared to those who kept their BMI stable (−1 to +1 units BMI) between pregnancies (Bogaerts et al. 2013b). Therefore, stabilizing maternal weight between pregnancies and turning the inter-pregnancy period into an optimal time frame for action is worthwhile. Concurrently, failure to lose pregnancy-related weight in an appreciable time of 6 months after delivery is an important indicator of obesity in midlife and, alongside other factors, may contribute to an intergenerational cycle of obesity (Fig. 7.2). Increased attention to and investment in the inter-pregnancy period is needed, including better, practical, and evidence-based strategies.

Childbearing is associated with long-term maternal weight gain. Within a 7- to 10-year period, childbearing women gain on average 2–3 kg more than non-childbearing women, and nearly one in four gains more than 5 kg (Kirkegaard et al. 2015). The additional fat mass tends to accumulate in the abdomen (Gunderson et al. 2004), which is physiologically the most harmful location for excess fat storage. Maternal weight gain increases the risk of obesity, obesity-related diseases later in life (Rooney and Mathiason 2005), and complications in subsequent pregnancies (Bogaerts et al. 2013b; Villamor and Cnattingius 2006). Complications in subsequent pregnancies were also noted in women who had a healthy pre-pregnancy BMI for both pregnancies (Yang et al. 2017). Weight retention during the postpartum period has been identified as a strong risk factor for long-term maternal weight gain. Smoking cessation, reduced breastfeeding, less physical activity, more sedentary activity, high calorie intake and specifically high intake of junk or fried foods intake postpartum are maternal behaviors which have been associated with postpartum weight retention within the first 2 years after delivery. These factors are inextricably linked to the underlying additional time commitment and responsibilities of caring for a baby and family. Psychological factors including stress and anxiety can also influence maternal weight. Women with elevated levels of stress and anxiety consume more fats, oils, sweets, and snacks and have decreased intakes of vitamins and are therefore described as "emotional eaters." Obese women are more likely to suffer from higher levels of anxiety and depression compared to normal-weight women (Devlieger et al. 2016). Screening for psychological and behavioral characteristics within families needs to be part of the lifestyle intervention to prevent weight retention (Kirkegaard et al. 2015).

7.9 Impact on the Child

Although underlying mechanisms are only beginning to emerge, epidemiological studies and observational cohorts show significant associations between women's weight and offspring outcomes in the short as well as in the longer term (Table 7.1). Pre-pregnancy obesity has been hypothesized to exert long-term health effects on the developing child through "early life programming." Long-term adverse health outcomes in the offspring include lifelong risk of obesity and metabolic dysregulation with increased insulin resistance, type 2 diabetes, hypertension, and dyslipidemia, as well as behavioral problems and risk of asthma (O'Reilly and Reynolds 2013). Recent studies confirm that high maternal BMI across the child-bearing period increases the risk of obesity in the offspring during childhood, but a high pre-pregnancy BMI has a stronger influence than either gestational weight gain or postpartum weight retention (Leonard 2017). The additional effect of gestational weight gain in women who are overweight or obese before pregnancy is small. Given the large population impact, future interventions aiming to reduce the preva-lence of childhood overweight and obesity should focus on maternal weight status before pregnancy, in addition to weight gain during pregnancy (O'Reilly and Reynolds 2013; Adane et al. 2018; Patton et al. 2018; Voerman et al. 2019).

Emerging evidence suggests that maternal obesity could be associated with poorer cognition in offspring and an increased risk of neurodevelopmental disor-ders, including cerebral palsy. Moreover, maternal and childhood obesity is more and more found to be associated with a child's cognitive and mental health prob-lems (Godfrey et al. 2017). The impact of an unhealthy and obese preconception and intrauterine environment, on cognitive function, is gaining support from scien-tific evidence. Maternal pre-pregnancy BMI trajectories have significant impact on offspring's early childhood physical and cognitive development up to the average age of 5 years. Children born to chronically obese women are more likely to be clas-sified as developmentally vulnerable/at risk on gross and fine motor skills, commu-nication skills, and general knowledge. They also had an elevated risk of suspected gross motor delay compared with children born to women with a normative BMI trajectory (Adane et al. 2018).

7.10   Maternal Weight and Mental Well-Being

Around one in four mothers experience symptoms of anxiety and depression in the perinatal period. More commonly, perinatal maternal depression seems to be a con-tinuation of pre-pregnancy mental health problems into pregnancy and the postpar-tum period. Mental health should therefore be part of preconception care as maternal mental health problems are associated with adverse obstetric, neonatal, and child-hood physical and mental health outcomes that will continue to affect families throughout generations (Patton et al. 2018; Attoe et al. 2018). Persistence of precon-ception mental health risks into the postpartum period affects mother-infant bond-ing with a greater likelihood of maternal over-intrusiveness, emotional withdrawal, and failure to sensitively engage. Mental health problems might be important medi-ators of the relation between preconception factors such as poor nutrition and smok-ing and some of the associated adverse outcomes in the offspring (See also Sect. 7.5). There is a need for interdisciplinary research to bring together scientists with expertise in nutrition, exercise, mental health, public health, and preventive care to identify practical, evidence-based strategies for supporting women's health. The chapter on mental health includes a more extensive discussion on this topic.

7.11 Eating Disorders

Eating disorders are a group of serious mental illnesses characterized by severe disturbances of eating behaviors that can significantly impair health and psychosocial functioning (for example Micali et al. 2015; Keshaviah et al. 2014). The three main types of eating disorders are anorexia nervosa, bulimia nervosa, and binge eating disorder (American Psychiatric Association, 2013). Anorexia nervosa is defined as a persistent restriction of energy leading to significantly low body weight, which is accompanied by an intense fear of gaining weight despite significantly low body weight or engaging in behaviours that interfere with weight gain. Bulimia nervosa is characterized by recurrent episodes of binge eating (eating an unusually large amount of food in a defined period of time) with the feeling of a lack of control over eating, followed by engagement in compensatory behaviors which attempt to counteract the effects of the binge eating (e.g., self-induced vomiting, misuse of laxatives, or excessive exercise). Similarly, binge eating disorder involves recurrent episodes of binge eating with a loss of control, but unlike bulimia nervosa, binge eating episodes are not followed by compensatory behaviors. There is also an additional category intended to capture those individuals with eating disorder symptoms that cause significant distress or impairment, but who do not meet all the criteria for a full threshold eating disorder, referred to as other specified feeding or eating disorders (OSFED).

There is currently insufficient research to accurately determine how many women are affected by eating disorders in the period before and during pregnancy with prevalence estimates ranging between 2 and 5% of women (Bye et al. 2020; Watson et al. 2013) in early pregnancy. Women with eating disorders can be at an increased risk of adverse maternal and infant outcomes, with variation between the types of eating disorders, including infertility, unplanned pregnancies, miscarriage, prematurity, low and high birth weight babies, and difficulties with infant feeding (Watson et al. 2017; Solmi et al. 2014; Micali et al. 2007a; Easter et al. 2011). There is evidence to suggest some adverse outcomes associated with perinatal eating disorders may be mediated by pre-pregnancy BMI and gestational weight gain (Watson et al. 2017; Micali and De Stavola 2012). The majority of women with eating disorders tend to experience a decrease in eating disorder symptoms during pregnancy but remain at risk of postnatal relapse of symptoms and often continue to experience high levels of depression and anxiety symptoms throughout the perinatal period (Easter et al. 2015; Micali et al. 2007b). Furthermore, the experience of being pregnant can be emotionally challenging for some women with eating disorders, including those who are considered in remission, as they adjust to changes in their body shape and weight, appetite, and sense of identity (Taborelli et al. 2016; Claydon et al. 2018).

Considering the adverse risks associated with eating disorders, it is imperative that women with a current or prior history of eating disorders are identified and offered support before, during and following pregnancy (National Institute for Health and Care Excellence 2014, 2017). To enhance identification of women affected by eating disorders, all women at their first contact with health services to discuss preconception care should be asked about any current or past mental illness (National Institute for Health and Care Excellence 2014). Health professionals need to understand that some women may find it difficult or upsetting to have these discussions about their mental health as they may feel shameful and fear negative perceptions of them as a future mother (Bye et al. 2018). Active and supportive listening can help women to begin to discuss their illness and identify what support is needed in a safe environment. Women who are identified as having current or past eating disorders should be referred to a mental health service, preferably a specialist perinatal mental health service or eating disorder service, for preconception counseling and a comprehensive assessment of current mental health needs (National Institute for Health and Care Excellence 2017). Treatment options available to women with eating disorders include a range of psychological or cognitive behavioral approaches (National Institute for Health and Care Excellence 2017). Health professionals should discuss a woman's diet and eating habits with her and respond to any concerns she may have. Advice and education should include the importance of healthy eating, achieving a healthy body weight and ceasing behaviours such as binge eating, self-induced vomiting, misuse of laxatives, and excessive exercise. Health professionals should advise women that good nutrition is very important to give them the best chance of a healthy pregnancy and a healthy baby. It may also be appropriate to begin sensitive discussions with a woman about her future plans for infant feeding, which may include brief education about the benefits of breastfeeding, and these discussions can then be followed up in pregnancy and postnatally.

7.12   Adolescents and Young Adults

Puberty marks a transition to adolescence and a life phase during which girls and boys acquire resources that are essential for becoming parents of the next generation. It also marks the beginning of the reproductive life with a transition to functional gamete production. The preconception phase, that is, adolescence, varies markedly in length. This has implications for the acquisition of the social, financial, and educational assets and nutritional, health, and interpersonal risks that underlie intergenerational processes. The 3 months before conception, when male and female gamete maturation is achieved, represents a crucial period during which parental exposures, including nutrition, obesity, substance use, stress, endocrine disruptors, and physical activity, may influence gamete structure and function. Until we have strong evidence from early lifestyle interventions on the impact of crucial development periods and long-term health outcomes in the offspring, we can, as healthcare providers, at least stimulate an early healthy lifestyle from puberty throughout pregnancy and thereafter. The rationale is based on life course epidemiology, developmental (embryo) programming around the time of conception, women's motivation, and disappointing results from interventions starting in pregnancy.

The preconception phase presents a period of special opportunity for intervention. It is important to inform adolescents about the impact of early lifestyle on crucial periods during development and that these exposures have long-term effects.

Identification of people contemplating pregnancy provides a window of opportunity to improve health before conception, such as optimizing maternal weight, and is essential to improve outcomes (Stephenson et al. 2018). Adolescence is an important time frame to address poor nutrition related to healthy weight. Unfortunately, a link to a healthy preconception weight is not being made by this group. With their increased autonomy over eating, at least in high-income countries, and their tendency to focus on education, employment, and partner choice, it is unlikely that adolescents and young adults will consider conception in the future as a motivator for healthy eating. They might be more amenable to an argument that improved nutrition will lead to better muscle mass, improved cognition, and healthier skin complexion. Interventions must emphasize the importance of healthy food that is cheap, easy to reach, and part of the social norm (The 2018), alongside promoting physical activity in the school and community environments.

Adolescents and young adults are usually assumed to be generally healthy, and this group seldom accesses healthcare services, as they might not believe that they behave unhealthily. Young adulthood is a period when lifelong health behaviors and habits can be established and modified. Those of low socioeconomic status or low educational attainment, migrants, and displaced groups are hard-to-access members of the young population and need attention too. New approaches are needed to work with young adults on nutrition, exercise, and mental wellness. This includes information sharing with the aim of engaging their interest, encouraging them to join in a new initiative, political will to provide capacity, and the development of opportunities for change. Very little is known about what adolescents eat and why. A co-creation design in developing new strategies is important as they know best what they need and how to reach their peers with messages that lead to change and action. All societies owe their adolescents the chance to make their future healthier. Additionally, the political leaders must give adolescent health priority in national health strategies, plans, and budgets. Only these actions will enable and support the transformation required (Hanson et al. 2016).

7.13 Effects of Lifestyle Interventions During the Preconception Period

Detailed information is needed about the interconnections among nutrition, physical activity, smoking, other environmental stressors, and metabolic exposures that influence perinatal outcomes. A sharper focus on intervention before conception is needed to improve maternal and child health and reduce the growing burden of non-communicable diseases. Alongside continued efforts to reduce smoking, alcohol consumption, and obesity in the population, heightened awareness of preconception health, particularly regarding nutrition, is needed. Importantly, health professionals should be alerted to ways of identifying women who are planning a pregnancy (Stephenson et al. 2018).

Prevention of unhealthy weight among women of reproductive age should be viewed as a global public health priority. Effective interventions, tailored to ethnicity and culture are important to improve the health of women, children, and families in the context of the global obesity epidemic. Promoting a healthy weight before pregnancy is imperative to improve maternal and newborn health as well as to support the overall health of populations across the globe. While adverse pregnancy and childbirth outcomes related to alcohol, smoking, certain medications, caffeine, and poor nutritional status during pregnancy are widely accepted, the effect of malnutrition in all its forms, i.e., underweight, overweight and obesity, undernutrition, and nutrient deficiency before conception, is less well understood (The 2018). In the postnatal period, breastfeeding and support for resuming activity are important modifiable factors influencing women's ability to return to their pre-pregnancy weight (Gaillard et al. 2018).

Being underweight before the start of a pregnancy is associated with a range of adverse maternal and infant outcomes too, yet those women are relatively neglected by many healthcare providers and in clinical pathways, where the focus is mainly on women with a high BMI (Bye et al. 2016). Provision of preconception care, including healthy lifestyle advice, could provide opportunity to advise women across the whole weight spectrum of the importance of adopting a healthy lifestyle as early as possible, including women who are underweight. Concurrently, health professionals need to consider anorexia or disordered eating behaviors in women as part of the discussion around healthy eating—not just what but how women are eating. Disordered eating needs to be considered when discussing healthy eating and weight. Screening, discussion, and treatment of eating disorders should be started in early adulthood. In the meantime, society must contribute to realistic expectations with regard to the body and the self-image. The potential clinical benefit of routine provision of preconception care, particularly for women who have a high risk of a poorer pregnancy outcome due to weight status, eating behavior, or other medical complications, needs to be explored (Bye et al. 2016).

7.14   State-of-the-Art Preconception Lifestyle Interventions

Preconception lifestyle interventions mainly focus on a healthy diet, weight management, dietary supplementation, substance use, adequate physical activity, and mental well-being of the participants. A recent follow-up study of a healthy lifestyle intervention among women with obesity and infertility showed a reduction in calorie consumption 5 years after the intervention. Additionally, women allocated to the intervention group who successfully lost weight during the intervention reported a lower energy intake and a reduced BMI in the long term, compared to women allocated to the intervention group who did not successfully lose weight and to women in the control group. Although a highly motivated population, these results show the potential sustainable effect of a preconception lifestyle intervention in this population (van Elten et al. 2019; van Dijk et al. 2017a).

Although the results from the few existing studies show promising results of intervening during the preconception period, reaching the most vulnerable women with a tailored intervention and sustained behavioral change is important. For those who have already had a child, interventions in the postpartum period and continuing until the next pregnancy offer promise, as detailed in the next section. Such inter-pregnancy interventions could potentially be a unique strategy to acquire a healthy lifestyle before a subsequent pregnancy starts. Effective lifestyle interventions for weight management among postpartum women are usually based on a combination of diet and physical activity (Lim et al. 2015). Ideally, such lifestyle interventions should go beyond education or advice alone and integrate behavioral change tech-niques such as goal setting, self-monitoring, and feedback. Mobile applications are promising tools to incorporate such behavioral change techniques for intervention efforts promoting a healthy lifestyle (Mertens et al. 2019; Van Dijk et al. 2017b, 2016). However, more research is needed to examine the effectiveness, the usability, and the critical features of the integration of eHealth into a lifestyle intervention program. Interventions must consider the social and economic context of the woman and her family. This includes access to affordable healthy food choices, knowledge about nutrition and food preparation and storage, and access to safe places for phys-ical activity. The impact of the partner is also important, and therefore a family-based approach is preferred (Choi et al. 2013; Evenson et al. 2009). Further, the impact of lack of sleep (common during the postpartum period) and daily stress on weight gain and retention should be considered and incorporated into weight man-agement programs.

7.15   Ongoing Preconception Lifestyle Intervention Studies

The interpregnAncy Coaching for a healthy future (INTER-ACT) intervention is such an eHealth-driven and face-to-face combined coaching program. This intervention is implemented between two pregnancies and during the subsequent pregnancy of women with an excessive gestational weight gain in the previous pregnancy. As half of the women with excessive gestational weight gain do not return to their pre-pregnancy weight after delivery, this is an important high-risk group to focus on, which includes women who were initially a healthy weight. INTER-ACT, which is an ongoing multicenter RCT, aims to assess the effective-ness of an eHealth inter-pregnancy lifestyle intervention on the composite out-comes score (gestational diabetes, pregnancy-induced-hypertension, caesarean delivery, large-for-gestational-age baby) in the next pregnancy. The intervention consists of two intervention phases. The first intervention phase starts at 6 weeks postpartum and lasts until 6 months postpartum. The second intervention phase starts before the 15th week of the next pregnancy and lasts until the 35th week of the pregnancy. Both intervention phases comprise face-to-face coaching and use of a mobile application. Between the two intervention phases, participants in the intervention group receive motivational reminders by e-mail every 3 months.

Coaches are trained in motivational interviewing and behavioral change tech-niques. The mobile app runs throughout the intervention periods and consists of four domains: nutrition, physical activity, weight, and mental well-being. In the nutrition domain, the participant sets nutrition goals based on the national "active food triangle" including nutrition as well as physical activity recommendations. A

Bluetooth-connected activity tracker registers the participant's activity and allows the app to assess whether the physical activity goal is reached. Weight is recorded by a Bluetooth-connected weighing scale. In the mental well-being domain, the participant can indicate her mood and her stress level. Additionally, based on the participant's progress and mood state, the app sends positive coaching messages in order to further motivate the participant. Results from this unique inter-pregnancy lifestyle interventional design are expected by the end of 2020 (Bogaerts et al. 2017).

Recently, TOP-mums for a Healthy Start was registered at the clinicaltrials.gov website (U.S. National Library of Medicine n.d.). This study evaluates the effect of a lifestyle intervention for women with a pregnancy wish who have a high risk of perinatal morbidity due to overweight or obesity. It is hypothesized that an effective lifestyle intervention directed toward healthy living, including reduction of over-weight or obesity and, if applicable, smoking reduction, can prevent health prob-lems in mothers and their offspring. The primary outcome here is reduction in body weight from baseline to 6 weeks postpartum, secondary outcomes are among other things weight retention between 6 weeks of gestation to 6 months after delivery, smoking cessation, dietary habits, physical activity habits, and relevant biomarkers. Results are anticipated by the end of 2020.

Insights provided by studies such as the INTER-ACT (Bogaerts et al. 2017) and TOP-mums studies as well as Smarter Pregnancy platform (Van Dijk et al. 2016) will facilitate the development of effective intervention strategies to counter the negative impact of an unhealthy preconception weight on the development of child-hood obesity from a broad physical, psychological, and social perspective.

An integrated approach for the management of obesity in women of reproductive age who are planning a pregnancy is crucial. Weight management should begin before conception and continue through pregnancy and the postpartum period within a multidisciplinary team focusing on mental well-being, healthy eating, and physical activity including weight management techniques. Reducing maternal obe-sity is not only a personal responsibility but also a social, environmental, political, and economic responsibility. Cost-effectiveness of regulatory frameworks increas-ing the accessibility and availability of healthy food and drinks must be balanced against the burden of reduced quality of maternal health and related costs regarding all the comorbidities in the mother as well as in the offspring (Devlieger et al. 2016).

Clear preconception health promotion targets, related to healthy diet, weight management, dietary supplementation, physical activity, and psychological well-being, are an important public health concern, for women and partners who want to become pregnant, given the intergenerational effects of suboptimal lifestyle behav-iors from conception. An agenda for timely and accurate research questions related to weight management before and after pregnancy is important to catch the attention of policy-makers and funders which can ultimately lead to the development of worldwide evidence-based guidelines for clinicians (Devlieger et al. 2016).

7.16 Limitations Regarding Preconception Lifestyle Interventions

Randomized controlled preconception trials focusing on the influence of lifestyle interventions in these critical time windows on relevant short- and long-term maternal and offspring health outcomes are scarce. They have major limitations and don't demonstrate strong effects on maternal and offspring outcomes. Many trials were performed among selected high-risk populations such as infertile women, (morbidly) obese women, or women with a previous complicated pregnancy. They usually don't focus on an integrated lifestyle advice approach targeting multiple lifestyle factors. Many trials are rather small and do not include long-term follow-up (Gaillard et al. 2018); they suffer from low adherence to the lifestyle intervention as there is most often no previous public and patient involvement during the development phase of the intervention. The latter is an important issue to take into account in future lifestyle intervention developments as this is a prerequisite to support the implementation of results from the trial world into the real world. Interventions also need to consider access to healthy and affordable food. Some communities may only have access mainly to fast food and calorie dense nutrient poor food. Fresh fruits and vegetables can be expensive, particularly in low-income neighborhoods where the price might be elevated. People must have access to safe places to exercise and healthy food in order to follow recommendations for weight management. New well-designed randomized controlled intervention trials are needed. They need to focus on interventions on a population level, targeting lifestyle in identified critical periods, with rigorous short-term and long-term maternal and offspring outcome assessments, and adequate statistical power.

7.17 Bariatric Surgery

In order to achieve a healthy weight in the preconception period, an increasing number of women of reproductive age are turning to bariatric (weight loss) surgery. Bariatric surgery in combination with lifestyle modifications is considered to be the most effective treatment to achieve successful weight loss in the long term in individuals with a BMI $\geq$ 35 kg/m^2 with comorbidities or a BMI $\geq$ 40 kg/m^2 (Jans et al. 2016). Although bariatric surgery can be very effective in weight reduction, many women are diagnosed with macro- and micronutrient deficiencies after the surgery. If women conceive while being deficient for relevant nutrients such as folic acid, B1 and B12 vitamins, and the fat-soluble (ADEK) vitamins, this can have a negative impact on the development of the fetus and neonate. The combination of physiologic changes related to pregnancy and iatrogenic postoperative alterations in the absorption and metabolism of crucial nutrients makes these women even more vulnerable, including a negative impact on the growing fetus (Johansson et al. 2015; Adams et al. 2015). Preterm birth, small-for-gestational-age and growth-restricted babies, and congenital abnormalities are more common in post-bariatric pregnant women. Additionally, nutritional deficiencies and surgical complications are frequent in these patients and require specific attention. However, research is limited, and data from large prospective cohort studies, starting before surgery and continuing until a subsequent pregnancy, have been initiated to obtain insight on reproductive issues following bariatric surgery and to optimize the healthcare of this specific population (Shawe et al. 2019).

The main knowledge gaps are related to (1) effective contraceptive counseling; (2) the optimal screening and supplementation strategy for micronutrient deficiencies after surgery before and during a subsequent pregnancy; (3) the best diagnostic method for the diagnosis of gestational diabetes mellitus; and (4) the nutritional needs of lactating women and influence on the composition of their breast milk which is needed before breastfeeding can be safely advised in this sub-population of lactating women. The AURORA database (bAriatric sUrgery Registration in wOmen of Reproductive Age) has been developed to systematically follow women of reproductive age (18–45 years) who will undergo bariatric surgery or who already underwent bariatric surgery until 6 months after a subsequent pregnancy. The findings from the AURORA study are believed to generate a significant public health impact (Jans et al. 2016). Recently, an international collaboration led to the development of evidence-based guidelines for these women, including recommendations for preconception care (Shawe et al. 2019). Finally, people without health insurance and in resource constrained environments are likely to have less access to this intervention.

7.18 Conclusion

Prevention of underweight, overweight and obesity among women of reproductive age will enhance the health and well-being of the next generation, and this should be viewed as a global public health priority. Women and their partners who have good nutrition and a healthy weight have a better life course trajectory for themselves. It can be challenging for people to remain at a healthy weight for many reasons. Resources are needed overall to help people maintain a healthy diet, including policies that assure access to healthy food. Supporting families in their journey toward motherhood/fatherhood with evidence-based treatment and programs is of high priority. Effective interventions, tailored to ethnicity and culture, are needed at each of these stages to improve the health of women, partners, and their children in the context of the global obesity epidemic.

7.19 Practical Recommendations

To tackle the developmental origins of health and chronic disease, preconception health of both the women and her partner needs sufficient and early attention, with support from their wider families, networks, and communities. The postpartum period represents an important opportunity to optimize women's health and recovery from pregnancy. As many of the physiological changes of pregnancy associated with maternal obesity are present from early pregnancy onward, providing support to women and families to optimize their weight before conception is probably the best strategy to decrease the health burden associated with maternal and childhood obesity.

In summary and based on the state of the art so far, we suggest recommendations for clinical management and policy making:

(a) **Clinical**
- Measure BMI in preconception women and advise about a healthy BMI, lifestyle, and appropriate gestational weight gain.
- Support couples to improve their lifestyle in preparation for pregnancy.
- Screen and monitor for nutritional deficiencies.
- Supplement folic acid.
- Identify vulnerable groups (e.g., those with socioeconomic problems, mental health problems, a history of bariatric surgery or eating disorders) for early screening and follow-up.
- Manage overweight, obesity, and diabetes including counseling families.
- Promote physical activity.
- Assess psychosocial problems.
- Provide educational and psychosocial counseling before and during pregnancy.
- Counsel, treat, and manage depression in women planning pregnancy and other women of childbearing age.
- Strengthen community networks and promote women's empowerment.
- Improve access to education for women of childbearing age.
- Reduce economic insecurity of women of childbearing age.

(b) **Policy**
- Standardize registration of pre-pregnancy BMI and maternal weight trajectories in perinatal databases all over the world and its associated conditions to improve estimation of health and economic burden and allow political prioritization.
- Support early prevention of unhealthy eating behavior (in schools) from a governmental prevention strategy.

References

Adams TD, Hammoud AO, Davidson LE, Laferrere B, Fraser A, Stanford JB, et al. Maternal and neonatal outcomes for pregnancies before and after gastric bypass surgery. Int J Obes. 2015;39(4):686–94.

Adane AA, Mishra GD, Tooth LR. Maternal preconception weight trajectories, pregnancy complications and offspring's childhood physical and cognitive development. J Dev Orig Health Dis. 2018;9(6):653–60.

American Psychiatric Association. Diagnostic and statistical manual of mental disorders. 5th ed. Arlington, VA: American Psychiatric Association; 2013.

Annesi JJ. Effects of self-regulatory skill usage on weight management behaviours: mediating effects of induced self-efficacy changes in non-obese through morbidly obese women. Br J Health Psychol. 2018;23(4):1066–83.

Atkinson S, McNamara PM. Unconscious collusion: an interpretative phenomenological analysis of the maternity care experiences of women with obesity (BMI≥30 kg/m^2). Midwifery. 2017;49:54–64.

Attoe C, Lillywhite K, Hinchliffe E, Bazley A, Cross S. Integrating mental and physical health care: the mind and body approach. Lancet Psychiatry. 2018;5(5):387–9.

Aune D, Saugstad OD, Henriksen T, Tonstad S. Maternal body mass index and the risk of fetal death, stillbirth, and infant death: a systematic review and meta-analysis. JAMA. 2014;311(15):1536–46.

Black RE, Victora CG, Walker SP, Bhutta ZA, Christian P, de Onis M, et al. Maternal and child undernutrition and overweight in low-income and middle-income countries. Lancet. 2013;382(9890):427–51.

Bodnar LM, Parks WT, Perkins K, Pugh SJ, Platt RW, Feghali M, et al. Maternal prepregnancy obesity and cause-specific stillbirth. Am J Clin Nutr. 2015;102(4):858–64.

Bodnar LM, Wisner KL, Moses-Kolko E, Sit DK, Hanusa BH. Prepregnancy body mass index, gestational weight gain, and the likelihood of major depressive disorder during pregnancy. J Clin Psychiatry. 2009;70(9):1290–6.

Bogaerts A, Ameye L, Bijlholt M, Amuli K, Heynickx D, Devlieger R. INTER-ACT: prevention of pregnancy complications through an e-health driven interpregnancy lifestyle intervention—study protocol of a multicentre randomised controlled trial. BMC Pregnancy Childbirth. 2017;17(1):154.

Bogaerts A, Ameye L, Martens E, Devlieger R. Weight loss in obese pregnant women and risk for adverse perinatal outcomes. Obstet Gynecol. 2015;125(3):566–75.

Bogaerts A, Van den Bergh B, Nuyts E, Martens E, Witters I, Devlieger R. Socio-demographic and obstetrical correlates of pre-pregnancy body mass index and gestational weight gain. Clin Obes. 2012;2(5–6):150–9.

Bogaerts A, Van den Bergh BR, Ameye L, Witters I, Martens E, Timmerman D, et al. Interpregnancy weight change and risk for adverse perinatal outcome. Obstet Gynecol. 2013b;122(5):999–1009.

Bogaerts A, Witters I, Van den Bergh BR, Jans G, Devlieger R. Obesity in pregnancy: altered onset and progression of labour. Midwifery. 2013d;29(12):1303–13.

Bogaerts AF, Devlieger R, Nuyts E, Witters I, Gyselaers W, Van den Bergh BR. Effects of lifestyle intervention in obese pregnant women on gestational weight gain and mental health: a randomized controlled trial. Int J Obes. 2013a;37(6):814–21.

Bogaerts AF, Van den Bergh BR, Witters I, Devlieger R. Anxiety during early pregnancy predicts postpartum weight retention in obese mothers. Obesity (Silver Spring). 2013c;21(9):1942–9.

Bramham K, Parnell B, Nelson-Piercy C, Seed PT, Poston L, Chappell LC. Chronic hypertension and pregnancy outcomes: systematic review and meta-analysis. BMJ. 2014;348:g2301.

Brownfoot FC, Davey MA, Kornman L. Women's opinions on being weighed at routine antenatal visits. BJOG Int J Obstet Gynaecol. 2016;123(2):263–70.

Bye A, Nath S, Ryan EG, Bick D, Easter A, Howard LM, et al. Prevalence and clinical characterisation of pregnant women with eating disorders. European Eating Disorders Review. 2020;28:141–5.

Bye A, Shawe J, Bick D, Easter A, Kash-Macdonald M, Micali N. Barriers to identifying eating disorders in pregnancy and in the postnatal period: a qualitative approach. BMC Pregnancy Childbirth. 2018;18(1):114.

Bye A, Shawe J, Stephenson J, Bick D, Brima N, Micali N. Differences in pre-conception and pregnancy healthy lifestyle advice by maternal BMI: findings from a cross sectional survey. Midwifery. 2016;42:38–45.

Choi J, Fukuoka Y, Lee JH. The effects of physical activity and physical activity plus diet interventions on body weight in overweight or obese women who are pregnant or in postpartum: a systematic review and meta-analysis of randomized controlled trials. Prev Med. 2013;56(6):351–64.

Claydon EA, Davidov DM, Zullig KJ, Lilly CL, Cottrell L, Zerwas SC. Waking up every day in a body that is not yours: a qualitative research inquiry into the intersection between eating disorders and pregnancy. BMC Pregnancy Childbirth. 2018;18(1):463.

Cnattingius S, Villamor E. Weight change between successive pregnancies and risks of stillbirth and infant mortality: a nationwide cohort study. Lancet. 2016;387(10018):558–65.

Collaboration NCDRF. Worldwide trends in diabetes since 1980: a pooled analysis of 751 population-based studies with 4.4 million participants. Lancet. 2016;387(10027):1513–30.

Devlieger R, Benhalima K, Damm P, Van Assche A, Mathieu C, Mahmood T, et al. Maternal obesity in Europe: where do we stand and how to move forward? A scientific paper commissioned by the European Board and College of Obstetrics and Gynaecology (EBCOG). Eur J Obstet Gynecol Reprod Biol. 2016;201:203–8.

Drieskens S, Demarest S, Bel S, De Ridder K, Tafforeau J. Correction of self-reported BMI based on objective measurements: a Belgian experience. Arch Public Health. 2018;76:10.

Easter A, Solmi F, Bye A, Taborelli E, Corfield F, Schmidt U, et al. Antenatal and postnatal psychopathology among women with current and past eating disorders: longitudinal patterns. Eur Eat Disord Rev. 2015;23(1):19–27.

Easter A, Treasure J, Micali N. Fertility and prenatal attitudes towards pregnancy in women with eating disorders: results from the Avon Longitudinal Study of Parents and Children. BJOG. 2011;118(12):1491–8.

Evenson KR, Moos MK, Carrier K, Siega-Riz AM. Perceived barriers to physical activity among pregnant women. Matern Child Health J. 2009;13(3):364–75.

Fattah C, Farah N, Barry S, O'Connor N, Stuart B, Turner MJ. The measurement of maternal adiposity. J Obstet Gynaecol. 2009;29(8):686–9.

Gaillard R, Wright J, Jaddoe VWV. Lifestyle intervention strategies in early life to improve pregnancy outcomes and long-term health of offspring: a narrative review. J Dev Orig Health Dis. 2018;10:1–8.

Godfrey KM, Reynolds RM, Prescott SL, Nyirenda M, Jaddoe VW, Eriksson JG, et al. Influence of maternal obesity on the long-term health of offspring. Lancet Diabetes Endocrinol. 2017;5(1):53–64.

Gomez-Ambrosi J, Silva C, Galofre JC, Escalada J, Santos S, Millan D, et al. Body mass index classification misses subjects with increased cardiometabolic risk factors related to elevated adiposity. Int J Obes. 2012;36(2):286–94.

Guelinckx I, Devlieger R, Beckers K, Vansant G. Maternal obesity: pregnancy complications, gestational weight gain and nutrition. Obes Rev. 2008;9(2):140–50.

Gunderson EP, Murtaugh MA, Lewis CE, Quesenberry CP, West DS, Sidney S. Excess gains in weight and waist circumference associated with childbearing: The Coronary Artery Risk Development in Young Adults Study (CARDIA). Int J Obes Relat Metab Disord. 2004;28(4):525–35.

Hanson M, Gluckman P, Bustreo F. Obesity and the health of future generations. Lancet Diabetes Endocrinol. 2016;4(12):966–7.

Hartley E, McPhie S, Skouteris H, Fuller-Tyszkiewicz M, Hill B. Psychosocial risk factors for excessive gestational weight gain: a systematic review. Women Birth. 2015;28(4):e99–e109.

Hattori A, Sturm R. The obesity epidemic and changes in self-report biases in BMI. Obesity (Silver Spring). 2013;21(4):856–60.

Ivers LC, Cullen KA. Food insecurity: special considerations for women. Am J Clin Nutr. 2011;94(6):1740S–4S.

Jans G, Matthys C, Bel S, Ameye L, Lannoo M, Van der Schueren B, et al. AURORA: bariatric surgery registration in women of reproductive age - a multicenter prospective cohort study. BMC Pregnancy Childbirth. 2016;16(1):195.

Javed A, Jumean M, Murad MH, Okorodudu D, Kumar S, Somers VK, et al. Diagnostic performance of body mass index to identify obesity as defined by body adiposity in children and adolescents: a systematic review and meta-analysis. Pediatr Obes. 2015;10(3):234–44.

Johansson K, Cnattingius S, Naslund I, Roos N, Trolle Lagerros Y, Granath F, et al. Outcomes of pregnancy after bariatric surgery. N Engl J Med. 2015;372(9):814–24.

Kapadia MZ, Gaston A, Van Blyderveen S, Schmidt L, Beyene J, McDonald H, et al. Psychological antecedents of excess gestational weight gain: a systematic review. BMC Pregnancy Childbirth. 2015;15:107.

Keshaviah A, Edkins K, Hastings ER, Krishna M, Franko DL, Herzog DB, et al. Re-examining premature mortality in anorexia nervosa: a meta-analysis redux. Compr Psychiatry. 2014;55(8):1773–84.

Kirkegaard H, Stovring H, Rasmussen KM, Abrams B, Sorensen TI, Nohr EA. Maternal weight change from prepregnancy to 7 years postpartum—the influence of behavioral factors. Obesity (Silver Spring). 2015;23(4):870–8.

Knight-Agarwal CR, Kaur M, Williams LT, Davey R, Davis D. The views and attitudes of health professionals providing antenatal care to women with a high BMI: a qualitative research study. Women Birth. 2014;27(2):138–44.

Koletzko B, Godfrey KM, Poston L, Szajewska H, van Goudoever JB, de Waard M, et al. Nutrition during pregnancy, lactation and early childhood and its implications for maternal and long-term child health: the early nutrition project recommendations. Ann Nutr Metab. 2019;74(2):93–106.

Kumpulainen SM, Heinonen K, Salonen MK, Andersson S, Wolke D, Kajantie E, et al. Childhood cognitive ability and body composition in adulthood. Nutr Diabetes. 2016;6(8):e223.

Leonard SA, Rasmussen KM, King JC, Abrams B. Trajectories of maternal weight from before pregnancy through postpartum and associations with childhood obesity. Am J Clin Nutr. 2017;106(5):1295–301.

Lim S, O'Reilly S, Behrens H, Skinner T, Ellis I, Dunbar JA. Effective strategies for weight loss in post-partum women: a systematic review and meta-analysis. Obes Rev. 2015;16(11):972–87.

Marchi J, Berg M, Dencker A, Olander EK, Begley C. Risks associated with obesity in pregnancy, for the mother and baby: a systematic review of reviews. Obes Rev. 2015;16(8):621–38.

Mendez MA, Monteiro CA, Popkin BM. Overweight exceeds underweight among women in most developing countries. Am J Clin Nutr. 2005;81(3):714–21.

Mertens L, Braeken M, Bogaerts A. Effect of lifestyle coaching including telemonitoring and tele-coaching on gestational weight gain and postnatal weight loss: a systematic review. Telemed J E Health. 2019;25(10):889–901.

Micali N, De Stavola B, dos- Santos-Silva I, Steenweg-de Graaff J, Jansen PW, Jaddoe VW, et al. Perinatal outcomes and gestational weight gain in women with eating disorders: a population-based cohort study. BJOG. 2012;119(12):1493–502.

Micali N, Simonoff E, Treasure J. Risk of major adverse perinatal outcomes in women with eating disorders. Br J Psychiatry. 2007a;190:255–9.

Micali N, Solmi F, Horton NJ, Crosby RD, Eddy KT, Calzo JP, et al. Adolescent eating disorders predict psychiatric, high-risk behaviors and weight outcomes in young adulthood. J Am Acad Child Adolesc Psychiatry. 2015;54(8):652–9.e1.

Micali N, Treasure J, Simonoff E. Eating disorders symptoms in pregnancy: a longitudinal study of women with recent and past eating disorders and obesity. J Psychosom Res. 2007b;63(3):297–303.

National Institute for Health and Care Excellence. Antenatal and postnatal mental health: clinical management and service guidance (CG192). 2014.

National Institute for Health and Care Excellence. Eating disorders: recognition and treatment (NG69). 2017.

Ng M, Fleming T, Robinson M, Thomson B, Graetz N, Margono C, et al. Global, regional, and national prevalence of overweight and obesity in children and adults during 1980–2013: a systematic analysis for the Global Burden of Disease Study 2013. Lancet. 2014;384(9945):766–81.

O'Reilly JR, Reynolds RM. The risk of maternal obesity to the long-term health of the offspring. Clin Endocrinol. 2013;78(1):9–16.

Ogden CL, Carroll MD, Kit BK, Flegal KM. Prevalence of childhood and adult obesity in the United States, 2011–2012. JAMA. 2014;311(8):806–14.

Okorodudu DO, Jumean MF, Montori VM, Romero-Corral A, Somers VK, Erwin PJ, et al. Diagnostic performance of body mass index to identify obesity as defined by body adiposity: a systematic review and meta-analysis. Int J Obes. 2010;34(5):791–9.

Onubi OJ, Marais D, Aucott L, Okonofua F, Poobalan AS. Maternal obesity in Africa: a systematic review and meta-analysis. J Public Health (Oxf). 2016;38(3):e218–e31.

Patton GC, Olsson CA, Skirbekk V, Saffery R, Wlodek ME, Azzopardi PS, et al. Adolescence and the next generation. Nature. 2018;554(7693):458–66.

Poston L, Caleyachetty R, Cnattingius S, Corvalan C, Uauy R, Herring S, et al. Preconceptional and maternal obesity: epidemiology and health consequences. Lancet Diabetes Endocrinol. 2016;4(12):1025–36.

Rahman MM, Abe SK, Kanda M, Narita S, Rahman MS, Bilano V, et al. Maternal body mass index and risk of birth and maternal health outcomes in low- and middle-income countries: a systematic review and meta-analysis. Obes Rev. 2015;16(2):758–70.

Robertson C, Archibald D, Avenell A, Douglas F, Hoddinott P, van Teijlingen E, et al. Systematic reviews of and integrated report on the quantitative, qualitative and economic evidence base for the management of obesity in men. Health Technol Assess. 2014;18(35).:v–vi, xxiii–xxix, 1–424

Robinson E. Overweight but unseen: a review of the underestimation of weight status and a visual normalization theory. Obes Rev. 2017;18(10):1200–9.

Rooney BL, Schauberger CW, Mathiason MA. Impact of perinatal weight change on long-term obesity and obesity-related illnesses. Obstet Gynecol. 2005;106:1349–56.

Schmied VA, Duff M, Dahlen HG, Mills AE, Kolt GS. 'Not waving but drowning': a study of the experiences and concerns of midwives and other health professionals caring for obese childbearing women. Midwifery. 2011;27(4):424–30.

Scott C, Andersen CT, Valdez N, Mardones F, Nohr EA, Poston L, et al. No global consensus: a cross-sectional survey of maternal weight policies. BMC Pregnancy Childbirth. 2014;14:167.

Shawe J, Ceulemans D, Akhter Z, Neff K, Hart K, Heslehurst N, et al. Pregnancy after bariatric surgery: consensus recommendations for periconception, antenatal and postnatal care. Obes Rev. 2019;20(11):1507–22.

Skouteris H, Teede HJ, Thangaratinam S, Bailey C, Baxter JA, Bergmeier HJ, et al. Commentary: obesity and weight gain in pregnancy and postpartum: an evidence review of lifestyle interventions to inform maternal and child health policies. Front Endocrinol (Lausanne). 2019;10:163.

Solmi F, Sallis H, Stahl D, Treasure J, Micali N. Low birth weight in the offspring of women with anorexia nervosa. Epidemiol Rev. 2014;36:49–56.

Stephenson J, Heslehurst N, Hall J, Schoenaker D, Hutchinson J, Cade JE, et al. Before the beginning: nutrition and lifestyle in the preconception period and its importance for future health. Lancet. 2018;391(10132):1830–41.

Taborelli E, Easter A, Keefe R, Schmidt U, Treasure J, Micali N. Transition to motherhood in women with eating disorders: a qualitative study. Psychol Psychother. 2016;89(3):308–23.

The L. Campaigning for preconception health. Lancet. 2018;391(10132):1749.

U.S. National Library of Medicine. TOP-mums, for a Healthy Start. n.d. https://clinicaltrials.gov/ct2/show/NCT02703753.

Van Dijk MR, Huijgen NA, Willemsen SP, Laven JS, Steegers EA, Steegers-Theunissen RP. Impact of an mHealth platform for pregnancy on nutrition and lifestyle of the reproductive population: a survey. JMIR Mhealth Uhealth. 2016;4(2):e53.

Van Dijk MR, Koster MP, Rosman AN, Steegers-Theunissen RP. Opportunities of mHealth in preconception care: preferences and experiences of patients and health care providers and other involved professionals. JMIR Mhealth Uhealth. 2017b;5(8):e123.

van Dijk MR, Koster MPH, Willemsen SP, Huijgen NA, Laven JSE, Steegers-Theunissen RPM. Healthy preconception nutrition and lifestyle using personalized mobile health coaching is associated with enhanced pregnancy chance. Reprod Biomed Online. 2017a;35(4):453–60.

van Elten TM, Karsten MDA, Geelen A, Gemke R, Groen H, Hoek A, et al. Preconception lifestyle intervention reduces long term energy intake in women with obesity and infertility: a randomised controlled trial. Int J Behav Nutr Phys Act. 2019;16(1):3.

Verweij LM, Terwee CB, Proper KI, Hulshof CT, van Mechelen W. Measurement error of waist circumference: gaps in knowledge. Public Health Nutr. 2013;16(2):281–8.

Villamor E, Cnattingius S. Interpregnancy weight change and risk of adverse pregnancy outcomes: a population-based study. Lancet. 2006;368(9542):1164–70.

Voerman E, Santos S, Patro Golab B, Amiano P, Ballester F, Barros H, et al. Maternal body mass index, gestational weight gain, and the risk of overweight and obesity across childhood: an individual participant data meta-analysis. PLoS Med. 2019;16(2):e1002744.

Watson HJ, Von Holle A, Hamer RM, Knoph Berg C, Torgersen L, Magnus P, et al. Remission, continuation and incidence of eating disorders during early pregnancy: a validation study in a population-based birth cohort. Psychol Med. 2013;43(8):1723–34.

Watson HJ, Zerwas S, Torgersen L, Gustavson K, Diemer EW, Knudsen GP, et al. Maternal eating disorders and perinatal outcomes: a three-generation study in the Norwegian Mother and Child Cohort Study. J Abnorm Psychol. 2017;126(5):552–64.

Yang Y, Ma CW, Yang Y, Wang X, Lin X, Fu L, et al. Effects of integrated health management intervention on overweight and obesity. Evid Based Complement Alternat Med. 2017;2017:1239404.

Zeitlin J, Mohangoo A, Cuttini M, Committee ERW, Alexander S, Barros H, et al. The European Perinatal Health Report: comparing the health and care of pregnant women and newborn babies in Europe. J Epidemiol Community Health. 2009;63(9):681–2.

Lifestyle: Substance Use—Nicotine, Alcohol and Drugs

8

Jill Shawe, Kathryn Hart, and Ann Robinson

8.1   Introduction

Use of substances including alcohol, tobacco and drugs is common in people of reproductive age, can lead to dependence and is a major global health concern. Despite targeted public health policies and campaigns, population surveys (National Institute on Drug Abuse (NIH) 2020; European Drug Report 2019) continue to highlight widespread use of substances, often in combination, which have substantial negative implications for health in general and the potential to harm future generations (Stephenson et al. 2018). Healthcare professionals need to be aware of the complex psychological, physiological and social factors that may be linked to substance use and be prepared to offer counselling and referral for specialist services. Pregnancy, however, can be a 'window of opportunity' and a motivating factor for women and their partners to change their behaviour and minimise risk with help to quit or cut down on substance use (Solomon and Quinn 2004). Preconception care offers the opportunity to further reduce risk by helping to modify consumption prior to pregnancy.

This chapter reviews the prevalence and individual effect of nicotine, alcohol, illicit drugs, new psychoactive substances and misuse of prescription drugs on reproductive health. It explores the opportunity for screening, intervention and treatment to optimise preconception health. Nicotine use through cigarette smoking, through heated tobacco products (HTPs) or via electronic nicotine delivery systems (ENDS)

J. Shawe (✉)
Faculty of Health, School of Nursing and Midwifery,
University of Plymouth, Plymouth, UK
e-mail: jill.shawe@plymouth.ac.uk

K. Hart · A. Robinson
Faculty of Health and Medical Sciences, University of Surrey, Guildford, UK

© Springer Nature Switzerland AG 2020
J. Shawe et al. (eds.), *Preconception Health and Care: A Life Course Approach*,
https://doi.org/10.1007/978-3-030-31753-9_8

is discussed. The World Health Organization (WHO 2019) estimates that 1.1 billion adults smoke tobacco worldwide and there has been an increase in use of smokeless tobacco with over 367 million users (WHO 2018a). Nicotine in tobacco and ENDS and inhalation of second-hand smoke all have a significant effect on health across the life course including fetal development, pregnancy outcomes, childhood disease (McDonnell and Regan 2019), fertility (American Society for Reproductive Medicine 2018) and health in adulthood (Wiklund et al. 2019). Although many countries have implemented anti-smoking policies, smoking is more prevalent in low- to medium-income countries where people may lack awareness of the associated health issues (WHO 2018a).

Concerns regarding drinking alcohol in relation to reproductive health are included with recommendations for preconception screening and intervention. Alcohol is readily available, and drinking is seen as a socially acceptable behaviour in many countries. However, alcohol misuse and the rise of 'binge drinking culture' can cause significant social and economic burden within populations (WHO 2018b). There is a causal association between alcohol use and more than 200 conditions of disease and injury, including mental and behavioural disorders, and even moderate use can affect the health of men and women and their offspring (WHO 2018b).

Use of Illicit drugs and new psychoactive substances (NPS) and misuse of prescription medicines is increasing globally (National Institute on Drug Abuse (NIH) 2020; European Drug Report 2019). This chapter discusses prevalence and specific concerns for reproductive health such as the rise in use of highly addictive opioids and of marijuana. Screening, assessment and interventions to optimise preconception health and prevent lifelong negative consequences are included.

8.2   Nicotine

Nicotine is a highly addictive recreational drug found naturally in the leaves of the tobacco plant. It can also be made synthetically. It has pharmacological active properties which bind to receptors in the brain increasing the flow of epinephrine and acting as a stimulant. It triggers the release of dopamine which contributes to feelings of pleasure and reward and is used for many reasons including self-medication to help with weight loss and conditions such as attention deficit hyperactivity disorder (ADHD) (Levin et al. 1996). However tobacco products and smoke also contain harmful and potentially harmful constituents (HPHCs) as listed by the FDA (2019), and it is these toxins and carcinogens that cause most harm when smoking tobacco found in cigarettes and in heated tobacco products (HTPs), which come in the form of heat sticks, pods or plugs (Tobacco Advisory Group of the Royal College of Physicians 2007). Although the health implications of electronic nicotine delivery systems (ENDS) such as e-cigarettes, which heat and vaporise a solution containing nicotine, are still unclear, with animal studies suggesting concern regarding lung disease (Siu AL, for the U.S. Preventive Services Task Force 2015), they have been seen as a safer option in containing less harmful constituents than tobacco, and their use is rising globally (WHO 2019). There is further concern that regulation of alternative nicotine delivery systems is less rigorous and that some products are flavoured (chocolate, strawberry and cherry) to attract a younger generation of user (WHO 2019).

8.2.1 Prevalence of Smoking

Smoking tobacco is a preventable cause of morbidity and mortality worldwide, responsible for the deaths of 8 million globally including 1.2 million through exposure to second-hand smoke (WHO 2019). Disease attributed to smoking confers a significant economic burden on society accounting for 1.8% of global gross domestic product (Goodchild et al. 2018).

In men and women of reproductive age, smoking is of particular concern as, in addition to detrimental effects on their own health and fertility, there is potential for direct effects on the fetus during pregnancy and on infants and children via inhalation of second-hand smoke (Mund et al. 2013). Despite tobacco control legislation, public health campaigns and general knowledge that smoking causes harm and complications, many women and their partners continue to smoke. Women of childbearing age make up the largest percentage of female smokers in the developed world and in a US survey of working women aged 18–49 years, 17.3% currently smoked cigarettes, with 75.5% of those smoking daily (Mazurek and England 2016). This sign of nicotine dependence is important as globally it is estimated that 53% of women who smoked daily continued to smoke in pregnancy causing adverse outcomes for mother and baby (Lange et al. 2018).

Nicotine is extremely addictive, and people struggle to quit smoking. In a Global Adult Tobacco Survey (WHO 2019), over 60% indicated they intended to quit smoking with 30% having tried to quit in the previous 12 months. Smoking cessation programmes are available in many countries and promoted by the WHO in order to help achieve the global target of a 30% reduction in prevalence of tobacco use by people over 15 years by 2025 (WHO 2018a).

8.2.2 The Impact on Health of Smoking and Nicotine

The health consequences of smoking for an individual and for those affected by second-hand smoke are multifarious and include cancer, cardiovascular and respiratory disease as well as morbidity associated with optical degeneration, diabetes, rheumatoid arthritis, osteoporosis, poor fertility and poor pregnancy outcomes (WHO 2019).

8.2.2.1 Nicotine and Fertility

Human and animal research has identified how smoking tobacco can negatively affect fertility and pregnancy outcomes. Smoking has a negative effect from both a female and male perspective, due to the mutagenic substances inhaled. In men, spermatogenesis, sperm quality, volume and motility are reduced, and smoking is a risk factor for erectile dysfunction [ED] with a dose-dependent effect (Cao et al. 2014;

Fullston et al. 2017). Over half of men over 40 years of age have been found to have some degree of ED (Kovac et al. 2015). Positive outcomes are seen in men choosing to stop smoking, and in a prospective cohort, participants ($n = 118$ ex-smokers) had a 25% improvement in erectile function 1 year post stopping smoking, whilst function in men who continued to smoke ($n = 163$ current smokers) remained unchanged (Pourmand et al. 2004).

Smoking by females is associated with lower fecundity and increased risk of spontaneous abortion and ectopic pregnancy (American Society for Reproductive Medicine 2018). Any dependency on nicotine appears to increase the risk of infertility (Sarokhani et al. 2017) and mechanisms for this include decreased ovarian function (Schoenaker et al. 2014) and poor quality of endometrium affecting implantation (Soares et al. 2007). Women who smoke are likely to have an earlier menopause which may affect the quality of the ova and particularly disadvantage those women leaving childbearing to later in life (Schoenaker et al. 2014). In addition, fertility may be negatively affected by treatment morbidity from cervical cancer which is increased in women who smoke (Fonseca-Moutinho 2011). This may be due to a range of mechanisms including nicotine exposure in cervical mucus and poor immune function to clear the human papilloma virus (Fonseca-Moutinho 2011).

The importance of quitting before pregnancy is paramount as smoking tobacco has been found to confer increased risk for transgenerational effects, potentially via epigenetic modification, for childhood and adult obesity, type 2 diabetes, hypertension (Rogers 2019), attention deficit hyperactivity disorder [ADHD] (Huang et al. 2018) and substance use (Cecil et al. 2016). In men, smoking prior to conception appears to alter DNA methylation in sperm (Jenkins et al. 2017). An elevated risk of leukaemia, birth defects and heart disease have been found in the children of men who smoke (Jenkins et al. 2017).

Smoking also leads to pregnancy-specific morbidity, with poor fetal and neonatal outcomes including increase in the likelihood of miscarriage, haemorrhage and pre-eclampsia, as well as premature birth and low birth weight (Lee and Lupo 2013; Pineles et al. 2014). Birth defects such as congenital heart defects, fetal septal defects (Lee and Lupo 2013) and neural tube defects (anencephaly, spina bifida and encephalocele) are all positively associated with smoking tobacco (Wang et al. 2014) and are all noted to be more severe in heavy smokers (Fullston et al. 2017). Smoking has a profound effect on placental function leading to calcification, necrosis and fibrosis, responsible for diminished utero-placental perfusion and resulting in intrauterine growth retardation, prematurity and sometimes stillbirth due to high carboxyhaemoglobin levels from carbon monoxide (Raisanen et al. 2014).

8.2.3 Interventions to Reduce Nicotine Use in Women and Men Prior to Pregnancy

Smoking cessation prior to conception is a one of the most crucial lifestyle changes people can make to avoid long-term complications for themselves and for any future children (Stephenson et al. 2018; Mund et al. 2013). The impact of stopping smoking is significant with immediate health and economic benefits (Ekpu and Brown 2015) including lowering the risks of smoking induced pathology and increased lifespan (Jayes et al. 2016). Quitting is however difficult due to the addictive nature of nicotine, and support has been found to double the chance of quitting successfully (WHO 2019). The WHO Framework Convention on Tobacco Control established policy and commitment to curbing the tobacco epidemic and supports public health programmes (WHO 2019). Two thirds of countries now have access to programmes that support cessation (WHO 2019).

Two main interventions have been found to help people quit: behavioural interventions and pharmacotherapy used individually or in combination. It is also important to consider the support for any partners and family members to quit as this has been found to increase success and prevents harm from second-hand smoke within households (World Health Organization 2013).

8.2.3.1   Behavioural Interventions

Behavioural intervention such as brief advice from health professionals or cognitive behaviour therapy involves individual and/or group meetings and is usually the first line of support for cessation (NICE 2018). Some countries have specialist 'stop smoking' counsellors to provide these services, but any health professional can give advice to motivate people to seek support and make referrals as necessary. It is important that any advice and counselling is given in a non-judgemental way and that information is clearly communicated to allow people to make informed decisions (NICE 2018). Other behavioural interventions include the use of telephone quit lines and text message support via mobile phone which have been found to increase success (Naughton et al. 2017).

For those who have tried and failed with behavioural therapy alone, then pharmacotherapy interventions are the next step but are often used in conjunction with behavioural interventions for optimal effect.

8.2.3.2   Pharmacological Interventions

Pharmacological interventions include nicotine replacement therapy (NRT) and the use of prescribed medications that alleviate the symptoms of nicotine withdrawal.

NRT aims to promote smoking cessation by helping with the physical dependence of nicotine. NRT provides the user with low levels of nicotine without the tar, carbon monoxide or chemicals from smoking tobacco. There is a range of nicotine replacement interventions such as transdermal patches, gum, inhalation cartridges, sublingual tablets and nasal spray. A Cochrane review of 150 randomised controlled trials explored the effect of different NRTs (gum, transdermal patch, nasal spray, inhalers, sublingual tablets/lozenges) compared to placebos. All forms of NRT were found effective with no overall difference in smoking cessation success by NRT type and an overall success rate suggesting that any NRT increases likelihood of quitting by 50–60% (Hartmann-Boyce et al. 2018).

Although there is no evidence that any type of NRT is more effective individually, there is however evidence to show that using a combination of NRT such as combining a nicotine patch with a faster acting form of NRT like gum achieves greater success (Hartmann-Boyce et al. 2018). Treatment should be individualised and based on preference once contraindications, cautions, possible interactions and risk of adverse effects have been considered as discussed later.

Prescribed medication is also available to support smoking cessation. Varenicline (EU Champix, US Chantix) works by reducing craving and blocking rewarding effects of nicotine, and Bupropion (Zyban) has been found to help users quit although the mechanism is unclear (NICE 2020a). Both are prescription-only medicines often used in conjunction with NRT under the guidance of a medical practitioner. It is important for prescribers to ask about pregnancy intention as neither medication is safe for use in pregnancy or if breastfeeding and if prescribed effective contraception use should be discussed to avoid unintended pregnancy.

ENDS may be of help to people wanting to quit smoking, but current evidence is limited. A large UK randomised trial found that ENDS were more effective than NRT when both products were accompanied by behavioural support (Hajek et al. 2019). In a US health survey, current cigarette smokers who had tried to quit in the last year were more likely to use ENDS than those who had not tried to quit (Schoenborn and Gindi 2014); however, the FDA has not approved ENDS for smoking cessation (Surgeon General 2020).

8.2.4 Conclusions and Recommendations for Clinical Practice

Smoking cessation guidelines and initiatives are used worldwide to intensify support for smokers to protect and save lives. The WHO report on the global tobacco epidemic (WHO 2019) presents comprehensive messages that tobacco control measures are required on global, national, local and individual levels. Smoking legislation and anti-tobacco policies such as advertising bans and plain packaging are promoted, but also clear guidance is given for health professionals on provision of cessation services. Women and men of childbearing age need clear information about the risks of smoking and support to quit for their own health and that of any children and wider family members.

8.2.4.1   Recommendations for Clinical Practice
- Identify smokers and offer both verbal and written information about the importance of quitting and the methods available to help smoking cessation.
- Ensure information is presented in a non-judgemental manner recognising that there are complex reasons for smoking and that quitting is difficult.
- Explain that stop smoking services offer evidence-based interventions that include behavioural support and advice about smoking cessation treatments and interventions.
- Explain how to access local specialist stop smoking services if available.
- Ensure all smokers and their family members, especially the vulnerable or those finding smoking cessation difficult, receive the right support and guidance to succeed.
- Advise if continuing to smoke, not to do so in the house or car.

8.3 Alcohol Use

8.3.1 Prevalence

Drinking amongst women of reproductive age is extremely common and is not automatically reduced in those who could become pregnant or even those in whom a pregnancy is recognised. Anecdotal evidence would suggest that alcohol consumption around the time of conception and into early pregnancy remains more socially acceptable than other detrimental behaviours, such as smoking, and is commonplace in developed countries. However, this is a heterogeneous behaviour; whilst binge drinking is a known reproductive risk, low but frequent consumers also represent a large but potentially under recognised at risk population.

Surveys from a range of developed countries suggest that between 50% and 80% of women of reproductive age consume alcohol, and of these 18–32% could be classified as binge drinkers dependent on the criteria used (Tough et al. 2006; Mullally et al. 2011; Mallard et al. 2013; Stephenson et al. 2014).

Active preparation for pregnancy may be associated with reduced drinking, often as part of a wider lifestyle 'overhaul', for example, Poels et al. (2017) reported that 'gathering preconception information, either by women themselves or by means of a PCC consult, is associated with women positively changing lifestyles during the preconception period' and that women who prepared for pregnancy were five times more likely to quit drinking than those who did not. However, in reality this preparatory stage cannot be assumed to bring alcohol consumption within recommended levels (see Sect. 8.3.2) due to variability in what constitutes 'planning' and a lack of awareness amongst women, their partners and the healthcare profession of the definition and importance of the preconception period. The lower priority or risk afforded to alcohol is again evidenced, with studies suggesting women are more likely to commence folic acid supplementation (Chuang et al. 2011) and to reduce caffeine (Lum et al. 2011) than to reduce alcohol.

Stephenson et al., in their 2014 survey of women attending UK maternity services (Stephenson et al. 2014), found that less than half of smokers and drinkers reduced or stopped before pregnancy, whilst in a Russian population, with high background population alcohol consumption levels (Balachova et al. 2012), substantial and positive reductions in drinking *after* pregnancy recognition were offset against the finding that there were no reductions prior to pregnancy recognition, even amongst those actively trying to conceive. This failure to stimulate behaviour change until the point of pregnancy confirmation, and the underlying lack of awareness of the vulnerable peri-conceptual period, therefore remains a key target for education and awareness raising activities. Indeed, even a proportion of women seeking fertility treatment, who clearly have a strong intention to become pregnant, report regular alcohol consumption (Joelsson et al. 2016) confirming that abstaining from alcohol is seen as a relatively low priority.

Few studies have specifically aimed to characterise male partner drinking in the peri-conception period despite its potential twofold impact on reproductive health both via changes in male fertility and via the facilitation of maternal drinking

(McBride et al. 2012; Bakhireva et al. 2011). In a retrospective survey of male partners, Bodin et al. (2017) reported only 17% had made a lifestyle adjustment before pregnancy to improve health and fertility, most commonly reducing or quitting alcohol, cigarettes or snuff or exercising more.

Once pregnancy is recognised rates of alcohol consumption further reduce, often significantly from the preconception period (Tough et al. 2006), but total abstinence is not guaranteed. Comparisons across studies and particularly between countries are difficult due to inconsistent definitions of a 'drink' or of drinking frequencies, alongside the increased potential for social desirability bias with retrospective reporting. However, in a New Zealand cohort one third of women reported drinking alcohol at some point during their pregnancy with 12% classified as being at risk of heavy alcohol exposure in early gestation (Mallard et al. 2013). UK papers published the following year suggested over half of women were consuming more than 2 units of alcohol per week in their first trimester and one quarter drank alcohol after confirmation of their pregnancy (Nykjaer et al. 2014; Smith et al. 2014).

Binge drinking specifically has been reported by 20% of pregnant women in a New Zealand cohort (>4 New Zealand standard drinks per occasion (Mallard et al. 2013)), but only 2–3% of a UK cohort (≥6 units on a single occasion (Smith et al. 2014)) and by no women in a Canadian cohort (Tough et al. 2006).

The majority of women do therefore reduce alcohol consumption once pregnancy is recognised, and in most populations abstinence becomes the predominant behaviour. However, a lack of impetus to change behaviours prior to formal pregnancy recognition, which itself may not occur until the 6th week of pregnancy, and a low relative risk attributed to alcohol consumption in comparison to other behaviours, means that many pregnancies are alcohol exposed peri-conceptually, during the first trimester and beyond.

8.3.1.1 Who Are the Drinkers?

Commonly held beliefs about the characteristics of peri-conceptual drinkers may no longer hold true. High-risk drinking behaviour and specifically binge drinking are consistently associated with a 'risk phenotype' that may include co-occurring illicit drug use, smoking, low income and/or education, low age, previous stressful life events and being unmarried (Mullally et al. 2011; Naimi et al. 2003; Witt et al. 2015; Iversen et al. 2015). However, focusing exclusively on this accepted risk population is at the expense of recognising a different but equally important sub-group of pregnancy drinkers. McCormack et al. (2017) reported that drinkers were more likely to be of high rather than low SES compared with abstainers (OR = 3.30, $p < 0.001$), and Symon et al. (2016) confirmed that, after pregnancy recognition, women from lower deprivation areas were more likely to display low but frequent drinking patterns than their more deprived counterparts, highlighting the need to target screening, interventions and support across the social spectrum.

The impact of parity and ethnicity on alcohol consumption behaviours around conception remains unclear, with studies suggesting conflicting results (Denny et al. 2012), although a tendency for greater drinking in multiparous women and those from socially disadvantaged ethnic groups, which may be country specific rather than generalisable across populations, has been identified.

8.3.2 The Impact of Alcohol

The more evidence emerges, the more negative the picture becomes regarding alcohol and reproductive health—affecting both sexes and many different stages, from early oocyte and sperm development through to pregnancy viability and duration, fetal growth and infant and future child health. These effects are not limited to the exposed generation, since alcohol's effect on gene expression allows for intergenerational transfer of negative effects (Chastain and Sarkar 2017; Mahnke et al. 2017). Similarly, detrimental outcomes are seen across the exposure range, with the consensus being that, despite the known issues associated with binge drinking in humans and animals (VandeVoort et al. 2015), there is insufficient evidence to set a safe lower level for alcohol consumption, and instead abstinence is the only truly safe option as discussed. However, this is rarely reflected in general population advice for non-pregnant women or for those men or women not actively planning a pregnancy. Whilst there have been some changes in the general population recommendations in recent years, such as the reduction in the recommended intake for men in the UK to match the level previously set for women (14 units per week), these levels are still universally at odds with the 'abstinence is best' message for pre- and perinatal health (DOH 2016).

However, it should be noted that, in addition to the issue of reporting bias already mentioned, definitive conclusions and, as such recommendations, are limited by further methodological issues inherent in this area of research. In particular the studies that do exist often have inadequate or no reporting of other known mediators and confounders of alcohol effect including, but not limited to, effects of food intake, nutritional status and supplement use, personal characteristics of the drinker such as body size and composition, maternal age and genetic influences on alcohol metabolism (Morley et al. 2007; Chiodo et al. 2010). Many studies fail to monitor all intakes across all relevant time points and are often reliant on retrospective reporting of a behaviour that we know is associated with social stigma.

Nevertheless it is widely accepted that alcohol consumption in pregnancy can cause fetal harm—a standpoint supported by a range of national professional bodies (see, e.g. the Guidelines published in 2010 by the Expert Workgroup of the Society of Obstetricians and Gynaecologists of Canada, Carson et al. 2010), who classified this statement as being supported by II-2 level evidence.

Specifically, alcohol exposure is associated with detrimental impacts on male fertility via both hormonal and tissue-specific impairments (La Vignera et al. 2013), and in women proposed mechanisms include disruptions to the menstrual cycle, hormonal derangements, direct negative effects of alcohol on ovum maturation, release and implantation or even co-occurring toxin ingestion. Whilst research remains inconclusive, a systematic review and meta-analysis by Fan et al. (2017) suggested that each alcoholic drink (12.5 g of ethanol) consumed by women of reproductive age was associated with a 2% reduction in fecundity. Both sperm and oocyte development have been reported to be affected by alcohol, likely mediated by an increase in oxidative stress (McBride and Johnson 2016; Opuwari and Henkel 2016).

Post-fertilization effects are also seen, most commonly reduced pregnancy viability due to an increased risk of spontaneous abortion (2–3 times adjusted risk in those exposed versus no exposure (Henriksen et al. 2004)). Interestingly in this study, male drinking had a greater effect on risk of spontaneous abortion, highlighting once again the potential 'hangover' effect of preconceptual behaviours on subsequent reproductive outcomes and therefore the importance of early intervention. However, these effects were only significant when consumption exceeded 10 drinks per week, and it should be noted that other studies have not found an association (Tolstrup et al. 2003). An increased risk of congenital malformations, reflecting disturbance of early fetal development (e.g. d-transposition of the great arteries, NTDs and multiple cleft lip and palate), has also been reported (Grewal et al. 2008) and again the paternal, and therefore the preconception, effect is postulated, with Zuccolo et al. (2016) suggesting a greater risk for microcephaly at birth associated with paternal rather than maternal pre-pregnancy drinking. Reducing alcohol exposure preconceptually has been estimated to reduce the live birth prevalence of specific congenital disorders by 53% (Shannon et al. 2013).

However, perhaps the most striking effect of alcohol is as a risk factor for mental retardation, specifically fetal alcohol spectrum disorders (FASD). Whilst these are primarily associated with alcohol exposure *during* pregnancy, rather than preconceptually, animal studies have uncovered an effect of chronic paternal alcohol consumption on the physical and mental development of offspring even in the absence of in utero alcohol exposure (Ouko et al. 2009). Furthermore, the artificially extended 'preconception' period created by a delayed recognition of pregnancy in many women until late in the first trimester means that pregnancies are remaining alcohol exposed at least until this point during which significant damage may occur. A recent meta-analysis of global FASD prevalence (Lange et al. 2017) estimated that 1 of every 13 pregnant women who consumed alcohol during pregnancy delivered a child with fetal alcohol spectrum disorder and that the prevalence in the general child and youth population was greater than 1% in 76 countries worldwide. Substantially increased rates in 'special' populations including children in care, those in correctional facilities and those receiving psychiatric care were found. FASD are completely preventable if a woman does not drink whilst pregnant or whilst she may become pregnant, yet there is reduced perception of prevalence, or risk, and of associated morbidity amongst both the public and health professionals (Landgraf et al. 2018) which, combined with ineffective management strategies and barriers to uptake (Poole et al. 2016), are hampering efforts to reduce their prevalence.

Later effects associated with preconceptual alcohol exposure may include reduced birth weight and increased risk of preterm birth (Nykjaer et al. 2014). Mullally et al. (2011) reported an association between high alcohol consumption reported at the booking appointment and very preterm birth (<32 weeks gestation) even after controlling for socio-demographic factors (adjusted OR 3.15 (95% CI 1.26–7.88)).

8.3.2.1 Alcohol as a Marker of Diet Quality and Other Lifestyle Behaviours

In addition to the direct physiological and biochemical effects of ethanol exposure discussed above, the role of alcohol consumption as a marker for other lifestyle behaviours and phenotypes is important to recognise.

In the general population and at extremes of intake, heavy alcohol consumption is associated with malnutrition, Wernicke-Korsakoff syndrome, folate deficiency, vitamin A depletion and pellagra (NHMRC 2009). Heavy drinking is also more consistently related to weight gain and adiposity and increases in waist circumference than light-to-moderate consumption. However several factors, in addition to frequency and intensity of alcohol consumption, appear to mediate this relationship including age, gender, type of alcohol consumed, physical activity level, sleep duration and level of eating disinhibition (Traversy and Chaput 2015). Whilst there is little if any data relating alcohol intake to other nutrient intakes or status in a preconception or inter-conception population, the theoretical risk is clear given the essentiality of these specific nutrients for reproductive health. Where the dietary intakes and/or nutritional status of alcohol-exposed pregnancies (AEP) have been investigated findings suggest a 'double jeopardy' of neurodevelopmental risk due to the co-occurrence of high-risk drinking and long-chain PUFA deficiencies (Stark et al. 2005). In men specifically it has been postulated that the effects of heavy drinking on fertility may be mediated via both an increase in seminal oxidative stress and a reduced antioxidant capacity due to an associated poor-quality diet (Opuwari and Henkel 2016). However, once again it is important not to ignore the sub-group of affluent, higher social status drinkers for whom improved diet quality and greater adherence to supplementation could be hypothesised to mediate risk from alcohol exposure yet for whom we currently have little or no data.

8.3.2.2 Current Recommendations for Alcohol Use during Preconception

Historically there has been significant disparity between countries, as to what they deem a safe alcohol intake for the population as a whole, for specific population groups, e.g. males and females, and for specific activities, e.g. driving (Furtwängler and de Visser 2012). However, despite this cross-country variability for the non-pregnant population, further complicated by methodological issues with the comparison of different alcohol measurement systems, the consensus across all major professional bodies is that abstinence is safest option for those women planning a pregnancy or who are already pregnant. Whilst this represents a significant policy shift from earlier recommendations, which tended to specify perceived vulnerable periods of pregnancy and attempted to set limits for 'safe' drinking, this 'zero tolerance' stance is now widely supported (DOH 2016; Carson et al. 2010; Australian Guidelines to Reduce Health Risks from Drinking Alcohol 2009; Danish Health and Medicines Authority 2007). However, whilst this is a positive step, few if any attempt to define the preconception period or set guidelines for the male partners of women of reproductive age.

Steegers-Theunissen et al. (2013) define the peri-conception period as a 5–6 month window in women that embraces 'oocyte growth, fertilization, conceptus formation and development to Week 10 of gestation (coinciding with the closure of the secondary palate)' suggesting that alcohol avoidance and other healthful behaviours should be adopted at least 3 months prior to conception. However, data is lacking to confirm this timeframe, and there remains a lack of robust evidence as to the latent period after alcohol exposure during which sperm defects may still be seen.

8.3.3 Interventions to Reduce Alcohol Intake in Women and Men of Reproductive Age

8.3.3.1 Screening/Identification

Given the rate of unplanned pregnancies and the need to commence behaviour change early it is widely accepted that universal screening for alcohol use is required for all women of reproductive age (Floyd et al. 2008) if we are to effectively target all those at risk of an alcohol exposed pregnancy (AEP). This is theoretically appropriate, methodologically possible (due to a range of available screening tools, see Table 8.1) and acceptable to many women (Smith et al. 2014), yet issues arise with assigning responsibility and allocating resources to this task usually assumed to be taken on within primary care. A lack of culturally sensitive instruments for minority cultures (Krulewitch 2005) has also been identified as a potential barrier.

8.3.3.2 Intervention: State of the Art

Assuming screening can be undertaken, then robust interventions are essential to refer women on to, yet there is a dearth of good-quality studies from which to conceptualise the state of the art in this field. It should be noted that if the aim is to reduce alcohol exposed pregnancies (AEP), then interventions that improve contraception behaviour and/or pregnancy planning and reduce alcohol exposure will be of benefit, individually or in combination.

As with many health interventions, improvements in knowledge are relatively easy to evidence (Elsinga et al. 2008) but whether these are translated into measurable reductions in risky behaviours and improvement in clinical endpoints (for maternal and child health) is often untested and unproven. In their 2009 systematic review, Stade et al. (2009) found only four randomised controlled trials, including 715 women, testing educational or psychological interventions to reduce alcohol consumption in women who were pregnant or planning a pregnancy. All studies were undertaken in the United States and meta-analysis was not possible due to the heterogeneity in design and outcomes, with weaknesses reported across the studies. Between group differences in rates of abstinence or absolute alcohol consumption were largely insignificant providing limited evidence for the impact of the interventions. Several studies were excluded from this review on the basis that their target population were not explicitly planning a pregnancy although, given the issue of unplanned pregnancies and delays in enacting behaviour change, their responses to

Table 8.1 Alcohol use screening tools

Tool	Source/author	Description	Available at
AUDIT Alcohol use disorders identification test	WHO Saunders et al. (1993)	10 items question, scoring 0–40 Aims to identify hazardous or harmful alcohol consumption. Developed from 6 country collaborative project Positive score: ≥8	https://www.who.int/ substance_abuse/publications/ audit/en/
AUDIT-C[a] Alcohol use disorders identification test— Consumption	Bush et al. (1998)	3 consumption questions taken from the full AUDIT tool. Score 0–12 Positive score: ≥5	https://assets.publishing. service.gov.uk/government/ uploads/system/uploads/ attachment_data/file/684826/ Alcohol_use_disorders_ identification_test_for_ consumption__AUDIT_C_.pdf
CAGE Cut down, annoyed, guilty, eye-opener	NIH National Institute on Alcohol Abuse and Alcoholism (2020)	4 item tool. Score 0–4 Aims to identify alcohol problems over the lifetime Positive score: ≥2	https://pubs.niaaa.nih.gov/ publications/arh28-2/78-79.htm
T-ACE Tolerance, annoyance, cut down and eye-opener	Sokol et al. (1989)	4 item questionnaire, score 0–5 Developed specifically for pregnant women. Can be used to identify lifetime use and prenatal use, based on the DSM–III–R criteria Positive score: ≥2[b]	https://pubs.niaaa.nih.gov/ publications/arh28-2/78-79.htm

[a]This is just one of a number of abbreviated versions of the AUDIT which have been proposed and tested (Meneses-Gaya et al. 2010)
[b]Chiodo et al. (2010) suggest raising the T-ACE total score cut-point from 2 to 3 to improve specificity with minimal loss of sensitivity in the prediction of neurobehavioral outcome in children
Biomarkers for detection of alcohol are being developed and can give an objective test for alcohol exposure where this testing is warranted. Currently they are not advised routinely for preconception care due to ethical concerns and healthcare provider/client relationship issues as discussed later in relation to substance misuse (Floyd et al. 2008)

alcohol-control intervention are still of relevance to this current review. For example, Floyd et al. (2007) targeted their RCT at risky drinking in 830 women capable of (but not planning) a pregnancy comparing the impact of four counselling sessions with personalised feedback and goals against written information. Nine months after the intervention, the group receiving counselling were twice as likely to have a reduced risk of AEP.

Lessons learnt from other health behaviour change interventions have been implemented in the AEP field and would appear to confer the expected benefits, for example, the use of tailored interventions (Hammiche et al. 2011) and motivational interviewing (Ingersoll et al. 2013), but again robust trials with longer-term clinical endpoints are lacking. It may be possible to employ more cost-effective remote strategies to increase access to interventions (Farrell-Carnahan et al. 2013), and there has been increased interest in the use of M-health technology to deliver preconception education and screening (van Dijk et al. 2017). However Velasquez et al. (2017) confirmed that outcomes may be 'dose'-dependent with participants receiving the CHOICES Plus intervention, comprising two 40 min sessions delivered by behaviour health specialists using motivational interviewing techniques to reduce risky behaviours and encourage uptake of contraceptive review, more likely than those in the Brief Advice group to reduce their risk of AEP. This would caution against excessive streamlining of services.

8.3.3.3 Recommendations for Improving Uptake and Content of Interventions in Clinical Practice

1. Increased Access and Reduction in Missed Opportunities to Act

   This means more women AND men, earlier and more regularly. (Luton et al. 2014) reported that of the 80.2% of women in their French sample who had visited a doctor within the 6 months before conception, only 13.8% discussed their planned pregnancy at this visit, whilst a scoping study of preconception health research (Toivonen et al. 2017) revealed only 11% of all studies included male participants, reflecting the female focus in the applied field too. Partner-based interventions have specifically been highlighted as a potential strategy for tackling FASD (Bakhireva et al. 2011), and moving out of the medical domain into areas such as schools and community organisations (Goossens et al. 2018) will be required if we are to reach a larger and more diverse preconception population.

2. Greater Resources and Responsibility for PCC

   Health professionals concur that a lack of contact with women but also a lack of resources and post-registration training impact on their ability to deliver PCC (Heyes et al. 2004). Agreeing who within a locality or service will take ownership of PCC, making this everybody's issue and ensuring sufficient time, education and financial resource is allocated will be essential for creating an effective and sustainable approach.

3. Communication of a Clear and Consistent Message

   This means reiterating to *all* women and men capable of conceiving and ALL professionals that deliver their healthcare and education that the only safe option regarding alcohol is total abstinence from before conception and throughout pregnancy. Messages should acknowledge that, whilst binge drinkers and those with alcohol dependency are specific at risk groups, any alcohol consumption in the peri-conception period can affect fertility and will pose a risk to the health of any subsequent fetus or baby, and it is therefore counter-productive and misleading to 'downgrade' some drinking behaviours relative to others (Mallard et al. 2013). Explanation of the specific reasons for the recommendations should be communicated to support uptake and adherence (Skagerström et al. 2015), and activities which aim to change social norms around alcohol consumption should be implemented alongside more focused preconception care.

8.4   Illicit, New Psychoactive Drug Use and Misuse of Prescription Medication

8.4.1   Introduction

Use of recreational, illicit drugs and misuse of prescription or over-the-counter medication is now common in men and in women of childbearing age, with many becoming dependent (Wong et al. 2011; Wilson and Thorp Jr 2008; Wright 2017). The use of such drugs in the peri-conception period is detrimental to women's and men's health and that of their children. It has the potential to affect not only fertility, pregnancy outcomes and fetal wellbeing but also to increase risk for future and transgenerational disease through epigenetic effects (Fleming et al. 2018) (see Chap. 2). In addition, illicit drug use is associated with lifelong negative socioeconomic consequences (Wong et al. 2011) and social vulnerability (Amaro et al. 2005; Porto et al. 2018). Risks are compounded as drug use often co-exists with alcohol, smoking and poor nutrition (Passey et al. 2014).

This section will present definitions (Table 8.2), global prevalence, effects of drugs, assessment and possible interventions for preconception management.

8.4.2   Prevalence of Psychoactive Illicit Drug Use

The number of people who use illicit drugs worldwide is unknown as use is often illegal and stigmatised which leads to difficulty in accurate estimation of prevalence. Under-reporting is likely as many surveys are self-reported and exclude those with high levels of substance use such as prisoners and people experiencing homelessness (Substance Abuse and Mental Health Services Administration (SAMHSA) 2018). Quality and availability of data also varies globally with the most reliable data coming from developed countries in Europe, North America and Australia. Data is recorded in most developed countries for four main classes of drugs: opioids, amphetamines, cocaine and cannabis (Degenhardt and Hall 2012).

Global trends show that use of drugs is increasingly common. The US National Survey of Drug Use and Health (Substance Abuse and Mental Health Services Administration (SAMHSA) 2018) found 1 in 9 (30.5 million) American people over the age of 12 had used an illicit drug in the past month, and this increased to 1 in 4 of 18–25-year-olds. In the age group 26–34 years, 28.7% had used illicit drugs in the past year.

In Europe, the European Drug Report (2019) details trends and developments in 30 European countries through the European Monitoring Centre for Drugs and Drug Addiction. Trends appear mainly consistent across countries with increasing use of illicit drugs and growth in the number of new psychoactive substances (NPS) notified. Increase in use is influenced by new markets, high availability, new psychoactive substances, internet sales and misused medicines. In 2018–2019, around 1 in 25 adults in England had used an illegal drug in the last year (Statistics on Drug Misuse England 2019).

Table 8.2 Definitions

Illicit drugs	Illicit drugs are substances classified by their ability to either stimulate (cocaine, amphetamines) or inhibit (heroin and opioids) the central nervous system, to sedate (benzodiazepine) or cause hallucinations (marijuana or LSD)
New psychoactive substances (legal highs)	New psychoactive substances formally known as legal highs are drugs which contain one or more chemical substances that produce similar effects to cocaine, cannabis and ecstasy. Examples include synthetic cannabinoids—Spice, black mamba; stimulants such as mephedrone M-CAT; sedatives GHB; and hallucinogens (N-bomb)
Controlled substances	Illicit drugs considered to be addictive are controlled substances regulated globally by international law. Drugs are categorised into 'schedules' and classes based on the balance between therapeutic use and public health risk. Country variations are seen in the regulation of new psychoactive substances
Dependence syndrome	This includes behavioural, cognitive and physiological phenomena that develop after repeated substance use. It includes a strong desire to take the substance, a high priority being given to taking the substance rather than to other activities, difficulty in controlling its use and continuing despite harmful consequences, the body adapting and becoming tolerant to the substance therefore requiring greater or more frequent use
Substance misuse or abuse	Substance misuse refers to regular use of recreational drugs, misuse of over the counter medications, misuse of prescription medications, misuse of alcohol or misuse of volatile substances, i.e. solvents or inhalants, to an extent where there is physical dependence or harm
Substance use disorder	Substance use disorder includes dependence syndrome and harmful use of alcohol and all illicit drugs including opioids, cocaine, amphetamine and cannabis but not tobacco which is treated separately
Harm reduction	Harm reduction activities are designed to reduce drug-related harm without requiring cessation of drug use
Neonatal abstinence syndrome—NAS	NAS occurs where the neonate shows signs of withdrawal from psychotropic substance exposure in utero

Adapted from United Nations Terminology and Information on Drugs (2016) https://www.unodc.org/documents/scientific/Terminology_and_Information_on_Drugs-E_3rd_edition.pdf

Global estimates of individual drug prevalence are reported by the UN Office on Drugs and Crime (UNODC) (2019). In adults aged 15–64 years, the highest rates were seen for marijuana 188 million past year users (PYU), followed by opioids 53 million PYU, amphetamines 29 million PYU, ecstasy 21 million PYU and cocaine 18 million PYU. Polysubstance use is however common with many users reported to take more than one substance (Forray et al. 2015).

A greater number of men than women were reported to be using drugs, but women are more likely to use prescription drugs (Center for Substance Abuse Treatment 2015). In the United Kingdom and United States, the number of women misusing substances, including cocaine, marijuana and opioids, has dramatically increased over the past 30 years, with many being in their childbearing years (Center for Substance Abuse Treatment 2015; NICE 2020b). It is reported that of the 600,000 pregnancies recorded in the UK each year, 30,000 involve substance abuse

(NICE 2020b). In the United States, between 2004 and 2014, there was a reported fivefold increase of babies born with neonatal abstinence syndrome (NAS) (National Institute on Drug Abuse (NIH) 2020). Many were seen in the 15–25 age group and this higher prevalence is consistent across most countries highlighting the importance of targeting young people (Peacock et al. 2018).

Prevalence of drug use may reflect multifactorial and complex socioeconomic circumstances which rarely exist in isolation. Poverty, poor housing, mental health conditions and domestic violence lead to vulnerability and the need to consider issues of equity and reproductive justice (United Nations Office on Drugs and Crime 2019).

8.4.3   Effect of Psychoactive Drug Dependency on Reproductive Health

Most illicit and new psychoactive drugs can induce dependency syndrome whereby a strong desire to take the drug together with tolerance results in increasing use and higher doses despite harmful consequences. Globally, cannabis and opioid dependence are the most common types of illicit drug dependence with amphetamine and cocaine dependence being less prevalent (Peacock et al. 2018).

Gender differences are evident in drug dependence. Men have higher rates overall, but women appear to be more sensitive than men to even small amounts of illicit drugs. This is possibly due to their hormonal profile, and this can lead to dependency, even if substances are taken for a short period of time (Cotto et al. 2010). Women frequently describe their initiation of drug use as self-medication to cope with pain, mental health problems and tiredness, and there is risk of inadvertent substance dependency (National Institute on Drug Abuse (NIH) 2020). The current rise in opioid use amongst women of childbearing age is of concern with an increased risk of adverse pregnancy outcomes and neonates born with NAS (Centers for Disease Control and Prevention 2020).

In men, illicit drug use has been shown to affect hormone profiles, sperm health and fertility in human and animal studies. Impairment in the structure, number and quality of sperm has been found and with opioids a decrease in testosterone concentration, potentially reducing fertility (Sansone et al. 2018).

Table 8.3 presents common drugs and their effect on fertility, pregnancy and the fetus/neonate. In addition to the direct detrimental effect on reproductive health, drug users are more likely to have medical comorbidities such as mental health conditions, sexually transmitted infections, blood-borne viruses (Floyd et al. 2008), poor nutrition, anaemia and low body mass index (Sebastiani et al. 2018). Socioeconomic disadvantage associated with drug use infers higher risk for domestic abuse, relationship difficulties and unintentional pregnancies (Lundsberg et al. 2018).

Environmental factors, including maternal and paternal use of drugs in the periconception period, have been identified to affect the long-term health of offspring and that of future generations through epigenetic effects (Fleming et al. 2018). Management of psychoactive illicit drugs before pregnancy is therefore vital not only to prevent poor pregnancy outcomes, neonatal abstinence syndrome (NAS) and socioeconomic breakdown but to promote the health of future generations.

8.4.4   Assessment and Screening

Assessment and identification of risk is integral to reducing the detrimental effects of illicit drug use on reproductive health and pregnancy. There is a lack of awareness by women (Stephenson et al. 2014) and men (Bodin et al. 2017; Shawe et al. 2019) of the importance of PCC as they often do not see themselves at risk or consider 'planning' pregnancy (Ricks et al. 2017). Healthcare providers also have been found to lack knowledge and time for PCC (Stephenson et al. 2014).

Table 8.3 Common psychoactive drugs and effect on reproductive health

Drug name (FRANK 2020)	Action (National Institute on Drug Abuse (NIH) 2020)	Effect on fertility	Effect on pregnancy	Effect on fetus/ neonate
Cannabis, marijuana, hashish, weed, grass, dope, skunk, resin, sinsemilla, sensi, puff, pot, herb, hash, ganja, draw, bud, bhang, pollen	Hallucinogenic and sedative euphoria, relaxation, heightened senses, increased hunger Dependence common Indicator of poly substance use	Suppression of ovulation (Center for Substance Abuse Treatment 2015) Reduced sperm count (Sansone et al. 2018)	Miscarriage (Center for Substance Abuse Treatment 2015) Mood and mental health disorders (Center for Substance Abuse Treatment 2015) Sleep disorder (Center for Substance Abuse Treatment 2015)	2–3 × risk of stillbirth (NIH Sex and Gender Differences in Substance Use 2020) Hyperactivity disorder (Behnke and Smith 2013) Low birth weight (NIH Sex and Gender Differences in Substance Use 2020) SIDS (NIH Sex and Gender Differences in Substance Use 2020) Impaired neurological development in young children (Behnke and Smith 2013)

Table 8.3 (continued)

Drug name (FRANK 2020)	Action (National Institute on Drug Abuse (NIH) 2020)	Effect on fertility	Effect on pregnancy	Effect on fetus/neonate
Cocaine derived from coca plant (*Erythroxylum coca*) Crack, coke, blow, Charlie, white, wash, toot, flake, stones, sniff, snow, rocks, Percy, pebbles, freebase, Ching, Chang	CNS stimulant Dependence common	Reduced male fertility (Sansone et al. 2018) Suppression of ovulation (Center for Substance Abuse Treatment 2015)	Raised blood pressure (Center for Substance Abuse Treatment 2015) Decreased uterine blood flow (Wilson and Thorp Jr 2008) Miscarriage (Wilson and Thorp Jr 2008) Placental abruption (Wilson and Thorp Jr 2008)	Poor oxygenation, increased BP and heart rate (Gouin et al. 2010) Structural and other abnormalities (Behnke and Smith 2013) Low birth weight (Gouin et al. 2010) Poor fetal growth (Behnke and Smith 2013) Premature labour (Gouin et al. 2010)
Amphetamine, speed, whizz, sulph, paste, Billy, base, amphetamine sulphate Methamphetamine, yaba, Tina and Christine, meth, crystal meth, ice, glass, crank	CNS stimulant Stimulant mental health risk Dependence common	Male erectile dysfunction (McKay 2005)	Preeclampsia (Center for Substance Abuse Treatment 2015)	Low birth weight (Wright et al. 2015) Premature birth (Wright et al. 2015)
Prescription opioids Morphine Codeine Fentanyl Derivatives from the opium poppy (*Papaver somniferum*)	Relieve pain, produce euphoria, may cause respiratory depression Dependence common	Reduced male fertility (Sansone et al. 2018)	Miscarriage (FRANK 2020) Still birth (Centers for Disease Control and Prevention 2020) Constipation (FRANK 2020)	NAS (Behnke and Smith 2013) Neurological behaviour changes (Behnke and Smith 2013)

(continued)

Table 8.3 (continued)

Drug name (FRANK 2020)	Action (National Institute on Drug Abuse (NIH) 2020)	Effect on fertility	Effect on pregnancy	Effect on fetus/neonate
Heroin, diamorphine, smack, skag, H, gear, brown derivatives from the opium poppy	Sedative Dependence common	Amenorrhoea and menstrual irregularities (Center for Substance Abuse Treatment 2015) Danger of overdose (FRANK 2020)	Maternal mortality (Centers for Disease Control and Prevention 2020)	Congenital abnormalities (Centers for Disease Control and Prevention 2020), Low birth weight, small for gestational age SGA (Centers for Disease Control and Prevention 2020), NAS (Centers for Disease Control and Prevention 2020) Neonatal mortality (Centers for Disease Control and Prevention 2020)
Methadone, mixture, linctus, physeptone **Buprenorphine**	Synthetic opioids alternative to heroin. Sedative effect, anti—anxiety	Amenorrhoea (Center for Substance Abuse Treatment 2015)	Miscarriage (FRANK 2020)	NAS (Centers for Disease Control and Prevention 2020) Stillbirth (Centers for Disease Control and Prevention 2020)
Ecstasy (pill), **MDMA** (powder), Mandy, Molly, dizzle, XTC, superman, crystal, brownies, beans, MD, E, dolphins **LSD** trips acid micro dot	Hallucinogens—Mental health effects	Reduced male fertility (Sansone et al. 2018)	Motor problems (Singer et al. 2012)	Learning and motor problems (Center for Substance Abuse Treatment 2015)
New psychoactive substances, PlantFood, Nps, Mdat, Eric3, Dimethocaine, Bath salts	Formally known as legal highs. A variety of chemical substances that produce similar effects to drugs such as cocaine, cannabis and ecstasy	No research found	No research found	No research found

Current policy mainly focuses on universal or risk-based screening for women who are pregnant (Ricks et al. 2017). In order to promote preconception health and identify risk *before* conception in both women and men, different approaches are needed which consider the wider determinants of health that reflect real life. The complex and chaotic nature of the lives of some drug users may mean that they do not routinely attend health services and are unlikely to plan pregnancy (NIH Sex and Gender Differences in Substance Use 2020). Men in general may need specifically targeting as they are less likely to access healthcare (Shawe et al. 2019). Community services and those for sexual health, drugs and alcohol may provide opportunities for screening for infection and blood-borne viruses as sexually transmitted infections (STIs) are higher in women and men who have a history of substance use (Substance Abuse and Mental Health Services Administration (SAMHSA) 2018).

Any contact with healthcare professionals is an opportunity for assessment and health professionals can start a conversation by asking one key question: 'are you planning to have a baby in the next year?' (Bellanca and Stranger 2013) which can identify need for either contraception or preconception care. History taking and using a non-judgemental and open-questioning approach has been found to identify perinatal substance use in women (Hinderliter and Zelenak 1993). Risk can be identified by taking a complete history to include medical, psychiatric, obstetric and social factors and prescribed medication and illicit drug use (Wong et al. 2011). Questions that may be sensitive can be normalised; 'we ask all people about substance use' and if concerns are highlighted referral can be made for further assessment.

There are few validated instruments available to screen childbearing age women specifically for illicit drug use (Floyd et al. 2008) as most screening tools have focused on the perceived more commonly used alcohol and tobacco. However, the use of generic instruments for any substance use such as the NIDA Quick Screen (National Institute on Drug Abuse (NIH) (2020) or the 4Ps test (Chasnoff et al. 2007) may help in screening. NIDA Quick Screen is based on three open-ended questions about tobacco smoking, use of alcohol or drugs. It includes the question 'How many times in the past year have you used an illegal drug or used a prescription medication for nonmedical reasons?' which, in primary care, has been found to be 100% sensitive and 73.5% specific for the detection of a substance use disorder (Smith et al. 2010). The 4Ps asks about any substance use in the Past, the Present, by Parents or by Partner, and a positive result can lead to referral for appropriate intervention. With increasing rates of illicit and prescription drug misuse healthcare providers need to be alert for any potential opportunity to identify risk and to refer for support and treatment.

Toxicologic drug testing by urine or blood sample used in pregnancy by some clinicians for substance use disorder is not routinely recommended in the preconception period or in primary care settings (Floyd et al. 2008). This is due to complex issues relating to the reliability of testing, and ethical concerns found to lead to lack of engagement with services by women and partners at a time when a trusting relationship with health professionals is vital (Wong et al. 2011; Wright 2017).

8.4.5   Interventions

The preconception period is an ideal time for interventions to promote healthy life behaviours as women and partners are often highly motivated to make changes (Solomon and Quinn 2004). Women and men should be informed of the effects that drug use can have on pregnancy and counselled about their own risk prior to conception, and the support and treatment available to reduce adverse outcomes. Interventions need to be tailored to address the appropriate level of risk and may need to differ according to gender and cultural circumstances (Ricks et al. 2017). Wright et al. (2016) developed a pyramid model to stratify risk for drug use into 'zones' of low, medium and high risk in pregnant women, and this model could potentially be used prior to pregnancy. It provides recommendation for interventions at each level of risk. Counselling and advice for low risk; brief interventions for medium risk; referral to specialist addiction services for those deemed high risk.

The Screening, Brief Intervention, Referral to Treatment (SBIRT) approach (Wright et al. 2016) has been found to be effective in primary care and can be delivered by a range of health professionals for any substance use. Screening includes assessment of risk as discussed above with information and advice for those of low risk. Brief intervention such as motivational interviewing teaches behaviour change skills, focusing on goal setting and a step approach to reach the goals to reduce harm. Referral to treatment for those identified as requiring specialist care allows appropriate interventions to be provided, including behavioural, pharmacological, self-help and community support.

Intervention studies for alcohol and drug use have demonstrated that contraceptive consultation and services in conjunction with brief interventions reduced consumption and increased contraceptive use (Floyd et al. 2008). Contraception counselling and services are important in providing reliable contraceptive methods to prevent high risk unintended pregnancies and in offering choice to develop a reproductive life plan which may involve delaying pregnancy until free from drug use. Practitioners should be well informed to enable counselling about available methods including long-acting reversible contraception such as intrauterine devices, sub-dermal implants and injectables that may be especially suitable for people with chaotic lifestyles associated with substance use.

8.4.6   Recommendations for Clinical Practice

- Non-judgemental counselling regarding risk of substance use along with support for behavioural change can modify health behaviours and optimise preconception wellbeing.
- Ensure access to effective contraceptive counselling, choice and provision.
- Asking one key question 'are you planning a baby in the next year' can highlight pregnancy intention or the need for contraception.

- In women and men planning pregnancy who are known drug users offer information about the potential effects of substance misuse on unborn children and referral to integrated care services with substance misuse programmes.

8.4.7 Conclusion

Misuse of illicit substances and prescription medication by women and men of childbearing age is rising and reflects multifactorial and complex socioeconomic circumstances rarely existing in isolation. Misuse poses significant risk to health and poor health outcomes such as mental health conditions, addiction and overdose. In addition, there is an associated rise in social issues such as intimate partner violence, unintended pregnancy and child safeguarding issues. Access to non-judgemental services for counselling, support and treatment programmes is essential to promote preconception health and to prevent adverse events for future children across the life course.

References

Amaro H, Larson MJ, Gampel J, Richardson E, Savage A, Wagler D. Racial/Ethnic differences in social vulnerability among women with co-occurring mental health and substance abuse disorders: implications for treatment services. J Community Psychol. 2005;33(4):495–511.

American Society for Reproductive Medicine. Smoking and infertility: a committee opinion. Fertil Steril. 2018;110(4):611–8. https://www.fertstert.org/article/S0015-0282(18)30492-8/pdf. Accessed 1 Feb 2020.

Australian guidelines to reduce health risks from drinking alcohol. NHMRC. 2009. https://www.nhmrc.gov.au/about-us/publications/australian-guidelines-reduce-health-risks-drinking-alcohol. Accessed 1 Feb 2020.

Bakhireva LN, Wilsnack SC, Kristjanson A, Yevtushok L, Onishenko S, Wertelecki W, et al. Paternal drinking, intimate relationship quality, and alcohol consumption in pregnant Ukrainian women. J Stud Alcohol Drugs. 2011;72(4):536–44. https://doi.org/10.15288/jsad.2011.72.536.

Balachova T, Bonner B, Chaffin M, Bard D, Isurina G, Tsvetkova L, et al. Women's alcohol consumption and risk for alcohol-exposed pregnancies in Russia. Addiction. 2012;107(1):109–17. https://doi.org/10.1111/j.1360-0443.2011.03569.x.

Behnke M, Smith VC. Prenatal substance abuse: short- and long-term effects on the exposed fetus. Pediatrics. 2013;131(3):e1009–24.

Bellanca HK, Stranger HM. One key question: preventive reproductive health is part of high quality primary care. Contraception 2013; 88(1): 3-6. doi https://doi.org/10.1016/j.contraception.2013.05.003. Accessed 1 Feb 2020.

Bodin M, Käll L, Tydén T, Stern J, Drevin J, Larsson M. Exploring men's pregnancy-planning behaviour and fertility knowledge: a survey among fathers in Sweden. Ups J Med Sci. 2017;122(2):127–35. https://doi.org/10.1080/03009734.2017.1316531.

Bush K, Kivlahan DR, McDonell MB, Fihn SD, Bradley KA. The AUDIT alcohol consumption questions (AUDIT-C): an effective brief screening test for problem drinking. Ambulatory care quality improvement project (ACQUIP). Alcohol use disorders identification test. Arch Intern Med. 1998;158:1789–95.

Cao S, Gan Y, Dong X, Liu J, Lu Z. Association of quantity and duration of smoking with erectile dysfunction: a dose-response meta-analysis. J Sex Med. 2014;11:2376–84.

Carson G, Cox LV, Crane J, Croteau P, Graves L, Kluka S, et al. Alcohol use and pregnancy consensus clinical guidelines.; Society of Obstetricians and Gynaecologists of Canada. J Obstet Gynaecol Can. 2010;32(8 Suppl 3):S1–31.

Cecil CA, Walton E, Smith RG, Viding E, McCrory EJ, Relton CL, et al. DNA methylation and substance-use risk: a prospective, genome-wide study spanning gestation to adolescence. Transl Psychiatry. 2016;6(12):e976. https://doi.org/10.1038/tp.2016.247.

Center for Substance Abuse Treatment. Substance abuse treatment: addressing the specific needs of women. Treatment improvement Protocol (TIP) Series, No. 51. HHS Publication No. (SMA) 15-4426. Rockville, MD: Substance Abuse and Mental Health Services Administration; 2015.

Centers for Disease Control and Prevention. Opioid use during pregnancy. 2020. https://www.cdc.gov/pregnancy/opioids/basics.html. Accessed 1 Feb 2020.

Chasnoff IJ, Wells AM, McGourty RF, Bailey LK. Validation of the 4P's plus screen for substance use in pregnancy. J Perinatol. 2007;27:744–8.

Chastain LG, Sarkar DK. Alcohol effects on the epigenome in the germline: role in the inheritance of alcohol-related pathology. Alcohol. 2017;60:53–66. https://doi.org/10.1016/j.alcohol.2016.12.007.

Chiodo LM, da Costa DE, Hannigan JH, Covington CY, Sokol RJ, Janisse J, et al. The impact of maternal age on the effects of prenatal alcohol exposure on attention. Alcohol Clin Exp Res. 2010;34(10):1813–21. https://doi.org/10.1111/j.1530-0277.2010.01269.x.

Chuang CH, Hillemeier MM, Dyer AM, Weisman CS. The relationship between pregnancy intention and preconception health behaviors. Prev Med. 2011;53(1–2):85–8. https://doi.org/10.1016/j.ypmed.2011.04.009.

Cotto JH, Davis E, Dowling GJ, Elcano JC, Staton AB, Weiss SR. Gender effects on drug use, abuse, and dependence: a special analysis of results from the National Survey on Drug Use and Health. SR Gend Med. 2010;7(5):402–13. NIH PubMed

Danish Health and Medicines Authority. 2007. http://www.sst.dk/publ/Publ2007/CFF/Alkohol_graviditet/Alk_grav.pdf. Accessed 1 Feb 2020.

Degenhardt L, Hall W. Extent of illicit drug use and dependence, and their contribution to the global burden of disease. Lancet. 2012;379:55–70.

Denny CH, Floyd RL, Green PP, Hayes DK. Racial and ethnic disparities in preconception risk factors and preconception care. J Women's Health (Larchmt). 2012;21(7):720–9. https://doi.org/10.1089/jwh.2011.3259.

DOH. 2016 UK Chief Medical Officers' Low Risk Drinking Guidelines. 2016. https://assets.publishing.service.gov.uk/government/uploads/system/uploads/attachment_data/file/545937/UK_CMOs__report.pdf. Accessed 1 Feb 2020.

Ekpu VU, Brown AK. The economic impact of smoking and of reducing smoking prevalence: review of evidence. Tob Use Insights. 2015;8:1–35. https://doi.org/10.4137/TUI.S15628.

Elsinga J, de Jong-Potjer LC, van der Pal-de Bruin KM, le Cessie S, Assendelft WJ, Buitendijk SE. The effect of preconception counselling on lifestyle and other behaviour before and during pregnancy. Womens Health Issues. 2008;18(6 Suppl):S117–25. https://doi.org/10.1016/j.whi.2008.09.003.

European Drug Report. 2019. http://www.emcdda.europa.eu/edr2019. Accessed 1 Feb 2020.

Fan D, Liu L, Xia Q, Wang W, Wu S, Tian G, et al. Female alcohol consumption and fecundability: a systematic review and dose-response meta-analysis. Sci Rep. 2017;7(1):13815. https://doi.org/10.1038/s41598-017-14261-8.

Farrell-Carnahan L, Hettema J, Jackson J, Kamalanathan S, Ritterband LM, Ingersoll KS. Feasibility and promise of a remote-delivered preconception motivational interviewing intervention to reduce risk for alcohol-exposed pregnancy. Telemed J E Health. 2013;19(8):597–604. https://doi.org/10.1089/tmj.2012.0247.

Fleming TP, Watkins AJ, Velazquez MA, Mathers JC, Prentice AM, Stephenson J, et al. Origins of lifetime health around the time of conception: causes and consequences. Lancet. 2018;391(10132):1842–52. https://doi.org/10.1016/S0140-6736(18)30312-X.

Floyd RL, Sobell M, Velasquez MM, et al. Preventing alcohol-exposed pregnancies: a randomized controlled trial. Am J Prev Med. 2007;32:1–10.

Floyd RL, Jack BW, Cefalo R, Atrash H, Mahoney J, Herron A, et al. The clinical content of pre-conception care: alcohol, tobacco, and illicit drug exposures. Am J Obstet Gynecol. 2008;199(6 Suppl 2):S333–9. https://doi.org/10.1016/j.ajog.2008.09.018.

Fonseca-Moutinho JA. Smoking and cervical cancer. ISRN Obstet Gynecol. 2011;2011:847684. https://doi.org/10.5402/2011/847684.

Forray A, Merry B, Lin H, Ruger JP, Yonkers KA. Perinatal substance use: a prospective evaluation of abstinence and relapse. Drug Alcohol Depend. 2015;150:147–55. https://doi.org/10.1016/j.drugalcdep.2015.02.027.

FRANK. 2020. https://www.talktofrank.com/drugs-a-z. Accessed 1 Feb 2020.

Fullston T, McPherson NO, Zander-Fox D, Lane M. The most common vices of men can damage fertility and the health of the next generation. J Endocrinol. 2017;234(2):F1–6. https://doi.org/10.1530/JOE-16-0382.

Furtwängler N, de Visser R. Lack of international consensus in low risk drinking guidelines. Drug Alcohol Rev. 2012;32(1):11–8. ISSN: 0959-5236

Goodchild M, Nargis N, d'Espaignet ET. Global economic cost of smoking-attributable diseases. Tob Control. 2018;27:58–64. https://doi.org/10.1136/tobaccocontrol-2016-053305.

Goossens J, Beeckman D, Van Hecke A, Delbaere I, Verhaeghe S. Preconception lifestyle changes in women with planned pregnancies. Midwifery. 2018;56:112–20. https://doi.org/10.1016/j.midw.2017.10.004.

Gouin K, Murphy K, Shah PS. Effects of cocaine use during pregnancy on low birthweight and preterm birth: systematic review and metaanalyses. Am J Obstet Gynecol. 2010;204(4):340. e1-12. https://doi.org/10.1016/j.ajog.2010.11.013.

Grewal J, Carmichael SL, Ma C, Lammer EJ, Shaw GM. Maternal periconceptional smoking and alcohol consumption and risk for select congenital anomalies. Birth Defects Res A Clin Mol Teratol. 2008;82(7):519–26. https://doi.org/10.1002/bdra.20461.

Hajek P, Phillips-Waller A, Przulj D, Pesola F, Myers Smith K, Bisal N, et al. A randomized trial of e-cigarettes versus nicotine-replacement therapy. N Engl J Med. 2019;380(7):629–37. https://doi.org/10.1056/NEJMoa1808779.

Hammiche F, Laven JS, van Mil N, de Cock M, de Vries JH, Lindemans J, et al. Tailored precon-ceptional dietary and lifestyle counselling in a tertiary outpatient clinic in The Netherlands. Hum Reprod. 2011;26(9):2432–41. https://doi.org/10.1093/humrep/der225.

Hartmann-Boyce J, Chepkin SC, Ye W, Bullen C, Lancaster T. Nicotine replacement therapy ver-sus control for smoking cessation. Cochrane Database Syst Rev. 2018;5:CD000146. https://doi.org/10.1002/14651858.CD000146.pub5.

Henriksen TB, Hjollund NH, Jensen TK, Bonde JP, Andersson AM, Kolstad H, et al. Alcohol consumption at the time of conception and spontaneous abortion. Am J Epidemiol. 2004;160(7):661–7.

Heyes T, Long S, Mathers N. Preconception care: practice and beliefs of primary care workers. Fam Pract. 2004;21(1):22–7.

Hinderliter SA, Zelenak JP. A simple method to identify alcohol and other drug use in pregnant adults in a prenatal care setting. J Perinatol. 1993;13(2):93–102.

Huang L, Wang Y, Zhang L, Zhu T, Qu Y, Mu D. Maternal smoking and attention-deficit/hyper-activity disorder in offspring: a meta-analysis. Pediatrics. 2018;141(1):2017–465. https://doi.org/10.1542/peds.2017-2465.

Ingersoll KS, Ceperich SD, Hettema JE, Farrell-Carnahan L, Penberthy JK. Preconceptional moti-vational interviewing interventions to reduce alcohol-exposed pregnancy risk. Subst Abuse Treat. 2013;44(4):407–16. https://doi.org/10.1016/j.jsat.2012.10.001.

Iversen ML, Sørensen NO, Broberg L, Damm P, Hedegaard M, Tabor A, et al. Alcohol con-sumption and binge drinking in early pregnancy. A cross-sectional study with data from the Copenhagen Pregnancy Cohort. BMC Pregnancy Childbirth. 2015;15:327. https://doi.org/10.1186/s12884-015-0757-z.

Jayes L, Haslam PL, Gratziou CG, Powell P, Britton J, Vardavas C, et al. SmokeHaz: system-atic reviews and meta-analyses of the effects of smoking on respiratory health. Chest. 2016;150(1):164–79. https://doi.org/10.1016/j.chest.2016.03.060.

Jenkins TG, James ER, Alonso DF, Hoidal JR, Murphy PJ, Hotaling JM, et al. Cigarette smoking significantly alters sperm DNA methylation patterns. Andrology. 2017;5(6):1089–99. https://doi.org/10.1111/andr.12416.

Joelsson LS, Berglund A, Wånggren K, Lood M, Rosenblad A, Tydén T. Do subfertile women adjust their habits when trying to conceive? Ups J Med Sci. 2016;121(3):184–91. https://doi.org/10.1080/03009734.2016.1176094.

Kovac JR, Labbate C, Ramasamy R, Tang D, Lipshultz LI. Effects of cigarette smoking on erectile dysfunction. Andrologia. 2015;47(10):1087–92. https://doi.org/10.1111/and.12393.

Krulewitch CJ. Alcohol consumption during pregnancy. Annu Rev Nurs Res. 2005;23:101–34.

La Vignera S, Condorelli RA, Balercia G, Vicari E, Calogero AE. Does alcohol have any effect on male reproductive function? A review of literature. Asian J Androl. 2013;15(2):221–5. https://doi.org/10.1038/aja.2012.118.

Landgraf MN, Albers L, Rahmsdorf B, Vill K, Gerstl L, Lippert M, et al. Fetal alcohol spectrum disorders (FASD)—what we know and what we should know—the knowledge of German health professionals and parents. Eur J Paediatr Neurol. 2018;22(3):507–15. https://doi.org/10.1016/j.ejpn.2018.02.010.

Lange S, Probst C, Gmel G, Rehm J, Burd L, Popova S. Global prevalence of Fetal alcohol Spectrum disorder among children and youth: a systematic review and meta-analysis. JAMA Pediatr. 2017;171(10):948–56. https://doi.org/10.1001/jamapediatrics.2017.1919.

Lange S, Probst C, Rehm J, Popova S. National, regional, and global prevalence of smoking during pregnancy in the general population: a systematic review and meta-analysis. Lancet Glob Health. 2018;6(7):E769–76.

Lee LJ, Lupo PJ. Maternal smoking during pregnancy and the risk of congenital heart defects in offspring: a systematic review and metaanalysis. Pediatr Cardiol. 2013;34(2):398–407. https://doi.org/10.1007/s00246-012-0470-x.

Levin ED, Conners CK, Sparrow E, Hinton SC, Erhardt D, Meck J, et al. Nicotine effects on adults with attention- deficit/hyperactivity disorder. Psychopharmacology. 1996;123:55.

Lum KJ, Sundaram R, Buck Louis GM. Women's lifestyle behaviors while trying to become pregnant: evidence supporting preconception guidance. Am J Obstet Gynecol. 2011;205(3):203. e1-7. https://doi.org/10.1016/j.ajog.2011.04.030.

Lundsberg LS, Peglow S, Qasba N, Yonkers KA, Gariepy AM. Is preconception substance use associated with unplanned or poorly timed pregnancy? J Addict Med. 2018;12(4):321–8. https://doi.org/10.1097/ADM.0000000000000409.

Luton D, Forestier A, Courau S, Ceccaldi PF. Preconception care in France. Int J Gynaecol Obstet. 2014;125(2):144–5. https://doi.org/10.1016/j.ijgo.2013.10.019.

Mahnke AH, Miranda RC, Homanics GE. Epigenetic mediators and consequences of excessive alcohol consumption. Alcohol. 2017;60:1–6. https://doi.org/10.1016/j.alcohol.2017.02.357.11.

Mallard SR, Connor JL, Houghton LA. Maternal factors associated with heavy periconceptional alcohol intake and drinking following pregnancy recognition: a post-partum survey of New Zealand women. Drug Alcohol Rev. 2013;32(4):389–97. https://doi.org/10.1111/dar.12024.

Mazurek JM, England LJ. Cigarette smoking among working women of reproductive age—United States, 2009–2013. Nicotine Tob Res. 2016;18(5):894–9.

McBride N, Johnson S. Fathers' role in alcohol-exposed pregnancies: systematic review of human studies. Am J Prev Med. 2016;51(2):240–8. https://doi.org/10.1016/j.amepre.2016.02.009.

McBride N, Carruthers S, Hutchinson D. Reducing alcohol use during pregnancy: listening to women who drink as an intervention starting point. Glob Health Promot. 2012;19(2):6–18. https://doi.org/10.1177/1757975912441225.

McCormack C, Hutchinson D, Burns L, Wilson J, Elliott E, Allsop S, et al. Prenatal alcohol consumption between conception and recognition of pregnancy. Alcohol Clin Exp Res. 2017;41(2):369–78. https://doi.org/10.1111/acer.13305.

McDonnell BP, Regan C. Smoking in pregnancy: pathophysiology of harm and current evidence for monitoring and cessation. Obstet Gynaecol. 2019;21:169–75. https://doi.org/10.1111/tog.12585. Accessed 1 Feb 2020.

McKay A. Sexuality and substance use: the impact of tobacco, alcohol, and selected recreational drugs on sexual function. Can J Hum Sex. 2005;14(1-2):47–56.

Meneses-Gaya C, Zuardi AW, Loureiro SR, Hallak JE, Trzesniak C, de Azevedo Marques JM, et al. Is the full version of the AUDIT really necessary? Study of the validity and internal construct of its abbreviated versions. Alcohol Clin Exp Res. 2010;34(8):1417–24. https://doi. org/10.1111/j.1530-0277.2010.01225.x.

Morley R, Halliday JL, Donath SM. A review of policies on alcohol use during pregnancy in Australia and other English-speaking countries. Med J Aust. 2007;187(5):315.

Mullally A, Cleary BJ, Barry J, Fahey TP, Murphy DJ. Prevalence, predictors and perinatal outcomes of peri-conceptional alcohol exposure—retrospective cohort study in an urban obstetric population in Ireland. BMC Pregnancy Childbirth. 2011;11:27. https://doi. org/10.1186/1471-2393-11-27.

Mund M, Louwen F, Klingelhoefer D, Gerber A. Smoking and pregnancy—a review on the first major environmental risk factor of the unborn. Int J Environ Res Public Health. 2013;10:6485–99.

Naimi TS, Lipscomb LE, Brewer RD, Gilbert BC. Binge drinking in the preconception period and the risk of unintended pregnancy: implications for women and their children. Pediatrics. 2003;111(5 Pt 2):1136–41.

National Institute on Drug Abuse (NIH). 2020. https://www.drugabuse.gov/national-survey-drug-use-health. Accessed 1 Feb 2020.

Naughton F, Cooper S, Foster K, Emery J, Leonardi-Bee J, Sutton S, et al. Large multi-centre pilot randomized controlled trial testing a low-cost, tailored, self-help smoking cessation text message intervention for pregnant smokers (MiQuit). Addiction. 2017;112(7):1238–49. https://doi. org/10.1111/add.13802.

NICE. Stop-Smoking Interventions. 2018. https://www.nice.org.uk/guidance/ng92/resources/ stop-smoking-interventions-and-services-pdf-1837751801029. Accessed 1 Feb 2020.

NICE. British National Formulary. 2020a. https://bnf.nice.org.uk/. Accessed 1 Feb 2020.

NICE. Pregnancy and complex social factors: a model for service provision for pregnant women with complex social factors Clinical guideline [CG110]. 2020b. https://www.nice.org.uk/guid-ance/cg110. Accessed 1 Feb 2020.

NIH. National Institute on Alcohol Abuse and Alcoholism. 2020. https://pubs.niaaa.nih.gov/publi-cations/arh28-2/78-79.htm. Accessed 1 Feb 2020.

NIH Sex and Gender Differences in Substance Use. 2020. https://www.drugabuse.gov/publica-tions/drugfacts/substance-use-in-women. Accessed 1 Feb 2020.

Nykjaer C, Alwan NA, Greenwood DC, Simpson NA, Hay AW, White KL, et al. Maternal alcohol intake prior to and during pregnancy and risk of adverse birth outcomes: evidence from a British cohort. J Epidemiol Community Health. 2014;68(6):542–9. https://doi.org/10.1136/ jech-2013-202934.

Opuwari CS, Henkel RR. An update on oxidative damage to spermatozoa and oocytes. Biomed Res Int. 2016;2016:9540142. https://doi.org/10.1155/2016/9540142.

Ouko LA, Shantikumar K, Knezovich J, Haycock P, Schnugh DJ, Ramsay M. Effect of alcohol consumption on CpG methylation in the differentially methylated regions of H19 and IG-DMR in male gametes: implications for fetal alcohol spectrum disorders. Alcohol Clin Exp Res. 2009;33(9):1615–27. https://doi.org/10.1111/j.1530-0277.2009.00993.x.

Passey ME, Sanson-Fisher RW, D'Este CA, Stirling JM. Tobacco, alcohol and cannabis use during pregnancy: clustering of risks. Sci Direct. 2014;134:44–50.

Peacock A, Leung J, Larney S, Colledge S, Hickman M, Rehm J, et al. Global statistics on alcohol, tobacco and illicit drug use: 2017 status report. Addiction. 2018;113:1905–26. https://doi. org/10.1111/add.14234.

Pineles BL, Park E, Samet JM. Systematic review and meta-analysis of miscarriage and maternal exposure to tobacco smoke during pregnancy. Am J Epidemiol. 2014;179(7):807–23. https:// doi.org/10.1093/aje/kwt334.

Poels M, van Stel HF, Franx A, Koster MPH. Actively preparing for pregnancy is associated with healthier lifestyle of women during the preconception period. Midwifery. 2017;50:228–34. https://doi.org/10.1016/j.midw.2017.04.015.

Poole N, Schmidt RA, Green C, Hemsing N. Prevention of fetal alcohol spectrum disorder: current Canadian efforts and analysis of gaps. Subst Abus. 2016;10:1–11. https://doi.org/10.4137/SART.S34545.

Porto PN, Borges SAC, de Souza Araújo AJ, de Oliveira JF, Almeida MS, Pereira MN. Factors associated with the use of alcohol and drugs by pregnant women. Rev Red Enfermag Nordest. 2018; https://doi.org/10.15253/2175-6783.2018193116.

Pourmand G, Alidaee MR, Rasuli S, Maleki A, Mehrsai A. Do cigarette smokers with erectile dysfunction benefit from stopping? A prospective study. BJU Int. 2004;94(9):1310–3. https://doi.org/10.1111/j.1464-410X.2004.05162.x.

Raisanen S, Sankilampi U, Gissler M, Ktamer MR, Hakulinen-Viitanen T, Saari J, et al. Smoking cessation in the first trimester reduces most obstetric risks, but not the risks of major anomalies and admission to antenatal care: a population-based cohort study of 1164953 singleton pregnancies in Finland. J Epidemiol Community Health. 2014;68(2):159–64. https://doi.org/10.1136/jech-2013-202991.

Ricks N, Comer L, Liu F, DeGrande H, Adeniran O. Substance use and preconception care: a review of the literature. Int J Women's Health Reproduct Sci. 2017;5(1):3–10.

Rogers JM. Smoking and pregnancy: epigenetics and developmental origins of the metabolic syndrome. Birth Defects Res. 2019;111(17):1259–69. https://doi.org/10.1002/bdr2.1550.

Sansone A, Di Dato C, de Angelis C, Menafra D, Pozza C, Pivonello R, et al. Smoke, alcohol and drug addiction and male fertility. Reprod Biol Endocrinol. 2018;16(1):3. https://doi.org/10.1186/s12958-018-0320-7.

Sarokhani M, Veisani Y, Mohamadi A, Delpisheh A, Sayehmiri K, Direkvand-Moghadam A, et al. Association between cigarette smoking behavior and infertility in women: a case-control study. Biomed Res Therap. 2017;4(10):1705–15. https://doi.org/10.15419/bmrat.v4i10.376.

Saunders JB, Aasland OG, Babor T, de la Fuente JR, Grant M. Development of the alcohol use disorders identification test (AUDIT): WHO collaborative project on early detection of persons with harmful alcohol consumption–II. Addiction. 1993;88:791–804.

Schoenaker DA, Jackson CA, Rowlands JV, Mishra GD. Socioeconomic position, lifestyle factors and age at natural menopause: a systematic review and meta-analyses of studies across six continents. Int J Epidemiol. 2014;43(5):1542–62. https://doi.org/10.1093/ije/dyu094.

Schoenborn CA, Gindi RM. Electronic cigarette use among adults: United States. 2014. https://www.cdc.gov/nchs/data/databriefs/db217.pdf. Accessed 1 Feb 2020.

Sebastiani G, Borrás-Novell C, Casanova MA, Pascual Tutusaus M, Ferrero Martínez S, Gómez Roig M, et al. The effects of alcohol and drugs of abuse on maternal nutritional profile during pregnancy. Nutrients. 2018;10(8):1008. https://doi.org/10.3390/nu10081008.

Shannon GD, Alberg C, Nacul L, Pashayan N. Preconception health care and congenital disorders: mathematical modelling of the impact of a preconception care programme on congenital disorders. BJOG. 2013;120(5):555–66. https://doi.org/10.1111/1471-0528.12116.

Shawe J, Patel D, Joy M, Howden B, Barrett G, Stephenson J. Preparation for fatherhood: a survey of men's preconception health knowledge and behaviour in England. PLoS One. 2019;14(3):e0213897. https://doi.org/10.1371/journal.pone.0213897.

Singer LT, Moore DG, Min MO, Goodwin J, Turner JJ, Fulton S, et al. One-year outcomes of prenatal exposure to MDMA and other recreational drugs. Pediatrics. 2012;130(3):407–13. https://doi.org/10.1542/peds.2012-0666.

Siu AL, for the U.S. Preventive Services Task Force. Behavioral and Pharmacotherapy Interventions for Tobacco Smoking Cessation in Adults, Including Pregnant Women: U.S. Preventive Services Task Force Recommendation Statement. Ann Intern Med. 2015;163:622–34. https://doi.org/10.7326/M15-2023.

Skagerström J, Häggström-Nordin E, Alehagen S. The voice of non-pregnant women on alcohol consumption during pregnancy: a focus group study among women in Sweden. BMC Public Health. 2015;15:1193. https://doi.org/10.1186/s12889-015-2519-2.

Smith PC, Schmidt SM, Allensworth-Davies D, Saitz R. A single-question screening test for drug use in primary care. Arch Intern Med. 2010;170(13):1155–60. https://doi.org/10.1001/archinternmed.2010.140.

Smith L, Savory J, Couves J, Burns E. Alcohol consumption during pregnancy: cross-sectional survey. Midwifery. 2014;30(12):1173–8. https://doi.org/10.1016/j.midw.2014.04.002.

Smoking Cessation. A Report of the Surgeon General. 2020. https://www.hhs.gov/sites/default/files/2020-cessation-sgr-full-report.pdf. Accessed 1 Feb 2020.

Soares SR, Simon C, Remohi J, Pellicer A. Cigarette smoking affects uterine receptiveness. Hum Reprod. 2007;22(2):543–7. https://doi.org/10.1093/humrep/del394.

Sokol RJ, Martier SS, Ager JW. The T-ACE questions: practical prenatal detection of risk-drinking. Am J Obstet Gynecol. 1989;160(4):863–8; discussion 868-70

Solomon LJ, Quinn VP. Spontaneous quitting: self-initiated smoking cessation in early pregnancy. Nicotine Tob Res. 2004;6(Suppl_2):S203–16. https://doi.org/10.108 0/14622200410001669132.

Stade BC, Bailey C, Dzendoletas D, Sgro M, Dowswell T, Bennett D. Psychological and/or educational interventions for reducing alcohol consumption in pregnant women and women planning pregnancy. Cochrane Database Syst Rev. 2009;2:CD004228. https://doi.org/10.1002/14651858. CD004228.pub2.

Stark KD, Beblo S, Murthy M, Whitty JE, Buda-Abela M, Janisse J, et al. Alcohol consumption in pregnant, black women is associated with decreased plasma and erythrocyte docosahexaenoic acid. Jr Alcohol Clin Exp Res. 2005;29(1):130–40.

Statistics on Drug Misuse England. 2019. https://digital.nhs.uk/data-and-information/publications/statistical/statistics-on-drug-misuse/2019/part-3-drug-use-among-adults. Accessed 1 Feb 2020.

Steegers-Theunissen RP, Twigt J, Pestinger V, Sinclair KD. The periconceptional period, reproduction and long-term health of offspring: the importance of one-carbon metabolism. Hum Reprod Update. 2013;19(6):640–55. https://doi.org/10.1093/humupd/dmt041.

Stephenson J, Patel D, Barrett G, Howden B, Copas A, Ojukwu O, et al. How do women prepare for pregnancy? Preconception experiences of women attending antenatal services and views of health professionals. PLoS One. 2014;9(7):e103085. https://doi.org/10.1371/journal.pone.0103085.

Stephenson J, Heslehurst N, Hall J, et al. Before the beginning: nutrition and lifestyle in the preconception period and its importance for future health. Lancet. 2018;391:1830–41. https://doi.org/10.1016/S0140-6736(18)30311-8.

Substance Abuse and Mental health Services Administration (SAMHSA). National Survey on Drug Use and Health. 2018. http://www.samhsa.gov/data/data-we-collect/nsduh-national-survey-drug-use-and-health. Accessed 1 Feb 2020.

Symon A, Rankin J, Sinclair H, Butcher G, Smith L, Gordon R, et al. Peri-conceptual and mid-pregnancy alcohol consumption: a comparison between areas of high and low deprivation in Scotland. Birth. 2016;43(4):320–7. https://doi.org/10.1111/birt.12252.

Tobacco Advisory Group of the Royal College of Physicians. Harm reduction in nicotine addiction: helping people who can't quit. Royal College of Physicians of London. 2007.

Toivonen KI, Oinonen KA, Duchene KM. Preconception health behaviours: a scoping review. Prev Med. 2017;96:1–15. https://doi.org/10.1016/j.ypmed.2016.11.022.

Tolstrup JS, Kjaer SK, Munk C, Madsen LB, Ottesen B, Bergholt T, et al. Does caffeine and alcohol intake before pregnancy predict the occurrence of spontaneous abortion? Hum Reprod. 2003;18(12):2704–10.

Tough S, Tofflemire K, Clarke M, Newburn-Cook C. Do women change their drinking behaviors while trying to conceive? An opportunity for preconception counseling. Clin Med Res. 2006;4(2):97–105.

Traversy G, Chaput JP. Alcohol consumption and obesity: an update. Curr Obes Rep. 2015;4(1):122–30. https://doi.org/10.1007/s13679-014-0129-4.

United Nations Office on Drugs and Crime. World Drug Report. 2019. https://wdr.unodc.org/wdr2019/. Accessed 1 Feb 2020.

United Nations Terminology and Information on Drugs. 2016. https://www.unodc.org/documents/scientific/Terminology_and_Information_on_Drugs-E_3rd_edition.pdf. Accessed 1 Feb 2020.

US. Food & Drug Administration (FDA). Tobacco Products. 2019. https://www.fda.gov/tobacco-products. Accessed 1 Feb 2020.

van Dijk MR, Oostingh EC, Koster MPH, Willemsen SP, Laven JSE, Steegers-Theunissen RPM. The use of the mHealth program smarter pregnancy in preconception care: rationale, study design and data collection of a randomized controlled trial. BMC Pregnancy Childbirth. 2017;17:46. https://doi.org/10.1186/s12884-017-1228-5

VandeVoort CA, Grimsrud KN, Midic U, Mtango N, Latham KE. Transgenerational effects of binge drinking in a primate model: implications for human health. Fertil Steril. 2015;103(2):560–9. https://doi.org/10.1016/j.fertnstert.2014.10.051.

Velasquez MM, von Sternberg KL, Floyd RL, Parrish D, Kowalchuk A, Stephens NS, et al. Preventing alcohol and tobacco exposed pregnancies: CHOICES plus in primary care. Am J Prev Med. 2017;53(1):85–95. https://doi.org/10.1016/j.amepre.2017.02.012.

Wang M, Wang ZP, Zhang M, Zhao ZT. Maternal passive smoking during pregnancy and neural tube defects in offspring: a meta-analysis. Arch Gynecol Obstet. 2014;289:513. https://doi.org/10.1007/s00404-013-2997-3.

WHO. Report on the Global Tobacco Epidemic. 2019. https://www.who.int/tobacco/global_report/en/. Accessed 1 Feb 2020.

Wiklund P, Karhunen V, Richmond RC, Parmar P, Rodriguez A, De Silva M, et al. DNA methylation links prenatal smoking exposure to later life health outcomes in offspring. Clin Epigenetics. 2019;11:97. https://doi.org/10.1186/s13148-019-0683-4.

Wilson J, Thorp J Jr. Substance abuse in pregnancy. Glob Libr Women's Med. 2008; https://doi.org/10.3843/GLOWM.10115. (ISSN: 1756-2228)

Witt WP, Mandell KC, Wisk LE, Cheng ER, Chatterjee D, Wakeel F, et al. Predictors of alcohol and tobacco use prior to and during pregnancy in the US: the role of maternal stressors. Arch Womens Ment Health. 2015;18(3):523–37. https://doi.org/10.1007/s00737-014-0477-9.

Wong S, Ordean A, Kahan M, Gagnon R, Hudon L, Basso M, et al. Substance use in pregnancy. J Obstet Gynaecol Can. 2011;33(4):367–84. https://doi.org/10.1016/S1701-2163(16)34855-1.

World Health Organisation. Global report on trends in prevalence of tobacco smoking 2000–2025, second edition. Geneva: World Health Organization; 2018a. https://www.who.int/tobacco/publications/surveillance/trends-tobacco-smoking-second-edition/en/. Accessed 1 Feb 2020.

World Health Organisation. Global status report on Alcohol and Health. 2018b. https://apps.who.int/iris/bitstream/handle/10665/274603/9789241565639-eng.pdf?ua=1. Accessed 1 Feb 2020.

World Health Organisation. Tobacco key facts. 2019. https://www.who.int/news-room/fact-sheets/detail/tobacco. Accessed 1 Feb 2020.

World Health Organization. Recommendations for the prevention and management of tobacco use and second-hand smoke exposure in pregnancy. 2013. https://www.who.int/tobacco/publications/pregnancy/guidelinestobaccosmokeexposure/en/. Accessed 9 Jan 2020.

Wright TE. Screening, brief intervention, and referral to treatment for opioid and other substance use during infertility treatment. Fertil Steril. 2017;108:2.

Wright TE, Schuetter R, Tellei J, Sauvage L. Methamphetamines and pregnancy outcomes. J Addict Med. 2015;9(2):111–7. https://doi.org/10.1097/ADM.0000000000000101.

Wright TE, Terplan M, Ondersma SJ, Boyce C, Yonkers K, Chang G, et al. The role of screening, brief intervention, and referral to treatment in the perinatal period. Am J Obstet Gynecol. 2016;215:539–47. https://doi.org/10.1016/j.ajog.2016.06.038.

Zuccolo L, DeRoo LA, Wills AK, Davey Smith G, Suren P, Roth C, et al. Pre-conception and prenatal alcohol exposure from mothers and fathers drinking and head circumference: results from the Norwegian mother-child study (MoBa). Sci Rep. 2016;7:39535. https://doi.org/10.1038/srep39535.

Mental Health Conditions

9

Abigail Easter, Heather Hopper, Louise M. Howard,
and Maddalena Miele

9.1   Introduction

Mental health conditions, which include depression, anxiety, schizophrenia and bipolar disorder, are common among women and men prior to or during pregnancy, as well as in the postnatal period. It's estimated that approximately 18% of parents will have a preconception common mental disorder (e.g. depression and anxiety) in adolescence and young adulthood (Spry et al. 2020). Furthermore, the prevalence of psychotic disorders and bipolar disorder is estimated to be around 0.4% and 2.8%, respectively, among women in the year prior to pregnancy (Jones et al. 2014; Vesga-Lopez et al. 2008). Women may be especially vulnerable in terms of their reproductive health and often experience stigma from healthcare professionals towards their desire for motherhood (Dolman et al. 2013; 2016). They are more likely have additional needs, such as pre-existing health risks, including increased rates of smoking and obesity, and social care vulnerabilities including domestic abuse, homelessness

A. Easter (✉)
Section of Women's Mental Health, Department of Health Service and Population Research, Institute of Psychiatry, Psychology & Neuroscience King's College, London, UK

David Goldberg Centre, Denmark Hill, London, UK
e-mail: abigail.easter@kcl.ac.uk

H. Hopper
Faculty of Health, University of Plymouth, Plymouth, Devon, UK

L. M. Howard
King's College London, Institute of Psychiatry, Psychology and Neuroscience, Section of Women's Mental Health, London, UK

M. Miele
Perinatal Psychiatry and Perinatal Mental Health Clinical Lead, CNWL Perinatal Mental Health Services, The Paterson Cabin—St Mary's Hospital, Imperial College Healthcare NHS Trust, London, UK
e-mail: maddalena.miele@nhs.net

© Springer Nature Switzerland AG 2020   159
J. Shawe et al. (eds.), *Preconception Health and Care: A Life Course Approach*,
https://doi.org/10.1007/978-3-030-31753-9_9

and child removal (Frieder 2010; McCracken et al. 2017). In the short term, these can adversely impact on fertility and pregnancy and have long-term implications for maternal and child health and wellbeing (Stein et al. 2014). Ensuring access to ethical preconception care, which incorporates and promotes positive mental health, is therefore particularly important to helping women achieve their desired fertility.

Prescribing psychotropic medication to women of childbearing age also presents unique challenges related to concerns for teratogenic harm if a pregnancy occurs and infant exposure through breastmilk (McAllister-Williams et al. 2017). Many women stop taking medication for a mental illness when they discover they are pregnant, often without advice from a practitioner (Margulis et al. 2014; Taylor et al. 2016), which can have major adverse consequences, including relapse.

The consensus is that the use of medication in the periconception period and during pregnancy is indicated when risk from exposure to is outweighed by the risks of untreated illness in the mother (McAllister-Williams et al. 2017; Howard et al. 2014a). Yet, current evidence on the risks and benefits is inconclusive, and healthcare decisions are inherently individual, as such profound uncertainty about medication use during pregnancy and for women planning a pregnancy remains.

The remits of preconception care extend beyond the dilemma of prescribing and should incorporate psychological health and wellbeing, as well as a sensitive exploration of the potential impact of mental health on pregnancy, childbirth and parenting. Given the increased rate of unplanned pregnancies among women with mental health conditions, a life course approach to preconception care and family planning is vital to discuss contraception and medication use and address preconception interrelated issues such smoking and obesity at an early stage (Catalao et al. 2020). Providing preconception advice should therefore be an integral component in the universal care of all individuals of childbearing age with mental health conditions, irrespective of pregnancy planning.

This chapter provides a brief overview of the epidemiology of mental health conditions and the effect on fertility, family planning and pregnancy. It provides a discussion of the specific needs and concerns related to mental health, including decisions around use of psychotropic medication, and considers the clinical implications for providing preconception care. The evidence base to guide recommendations for the preconception care of women with mental health conditions is limited and evolving. This chapter will therefore refer to relevant guidelines on prescribing psychotropic medication to women of childbearing age but will not detail the evidence on the association between the exposure of specific class of psychotropics and adverse outcomes. It will focus on general principles of care and the need for individualised discussions on the risks and benefits of different options to support decision-making, but should be considered within the context of current research evidence and clinical guidance.

9.2   Definitions and Epidemiology

Mental health conditions, also referred to as mental or psychiatric disorders, include a wide range of diagnoses characterised by clinically significant disturbance in cognition, emotional regulation or behaviour, usually associated with substantial distress or disability (Association AP 2013). The severity of symptoms associated with these conditions can range from mild-moderate to severe and often vary over time.

Nonpsychotic or common mental health conditions include depressive disorders, anxiety disorders, eating disorders and personality disorders (Howard et al. 2014b). Schizophrenia, affective psychosis and psychotic and nonpsychotic forms of bipolar disorder are often referred to as severe mental illness, due to their enduring nature and level of functional impairment (Jones et al. 2014).

Increasing evidence suggests that perinatal mental health problems often begin before pregnancy; however robust statistics on the epidemiology of preconception mental illness are lacking. Population statistics from the UK suggest that mental health conditions, such as depression and anxiety, are very common during adolescent and young adulthood. Between the ages of 16 and 24 years, 9% of males and 26% of females reported symptoms suggestive of a common mental health disorder. Among 25–34-year-olds, 15% of males and 19% of females had a likely common mental health disorder (McManus et al. 2016). In one of the few studies to investigate, rates on common mental disorders among individuals who went on to become parents reported that 18% of parents had preconception common mental disorders in adolescence and young adulthood (Spry et al. 2020). A US population-based study found the prevalence of any anxiety disorder (including panic disorder, social anxiety disorder, specific phobia and generalized anxiety disorder) in the previous year to be 13% in women who were currently pregnant or post-partum (Vesga-Lopez et al. 2008). Depression and anxiety disorders continue to be common during pregnancy, affecting approximately 11% and 17% during early pregnancy, respectively (Howard et al. 2014b, 2018; Nath et al. 2018). The rate of severe mental disorders has been less well studied; however recent US epidemiological studies have estimated the prevalence of psychotic disorder and bipolar disorder to be 0.4% and 2.8% among women in the year prior to pregnancy, similar to rates of these disorders in non-pregnant women (Jones et al. 2014; Vesga-Lopez et al. 2008).

Mental health conditions during pregnancy have been associated with several adverse pregnancy and birth outcomes, including gestational diabetes, low birth weight and prematurity (Stein et al. 2014). In part these outcomes arise from preventable factors, including poor nutrition, tobacco, drug and alcohol use as well as a lack of prenatal care, which should be addressed as part of preconception care for this group of women. However, there is increasing evidence to suggest a direct impact via increased stress and activation of the hypothermic-pituitary-adrenal (HPA) axis (Glover et al. 2010), emphasising the importance of integrating good mental healthcare and increasing access to psychological therapies for women during the preconception period.

Nevertheless, it is important to recognise that women with different mental health conditions will have distinct preconception needs related to their severity of symptoms, social situations and lifestyle factors. An individualised woman-centred approach to preconception assessments and care is therefore paramount.

9.3   Fertility and Family Planning

Infertility and difficulties conceiving have been associated with a range of mental health conditions, including anxiety, depression and eating disorders in a number of studies (Anderson et al. 2003; Klemetti et al. 2010; Easter et al. 2011). The underlying physiology of mental health conditions such as depression may directly affect a woman's fertility via mechanisms which include elevated prolactin levels, disruptions to the hypothalamic-pituitary-adrenal axis and thyroid regulation (Schweiger et al. 2018). Furthermore, depression and anxiety in males has been linked to decreased semen volume and sperm density, associated with lower secretion of sex hormone-binding globulin (SHBG) and dehydroepiandrosterone sulphate (DHEA-S), as well as higher secretion of cortisol and prolactin (Wdowiak et al. 2017). Other associated factors such as decreased libido, obesity, smoking and alcohol use may also contribute indirectly to the reduced fertility observed in this group. As such, the causal role of mental health in the development of infertility remains unclear as many studies have been unable to adequately control for the range of contributing factors.

Some psychotropic medications may also lead to reduced fertility in both women and men. Most notably, use of all first-generation or typical antipsychotics and some second-generation or atypical antipsychotics (such as risperidone and amisulpride) can cause impaired fertility resulting from hyperprolactinaemia (McAllister-Williams et al. 2017; Haddad and Wieck 2004). Although there is no current evidence to suggest that antidepressant medications or lithium impacts on a woman's chances of conceiving, use of selective serotonin reuptake inhibitors (SSRIs) or lithium may adversely affect semen parameters, including as reduced sperm count and morphology (McAllister-Williams et al. 2017; Nørr et al. 2016; Akasheh et al. 2014). However, confounding by indication, attributable to associations with the underlying depression, cannot be ruled out.

The chance of unplanned and unwanted pregnancies is also increased among this group of women, which may be attributed to inconsistent contraceptive use and increased numbers of sexual partners (Hall et al. 2015; Kaltenthaler et al. 2014; Miller 1997). A growing evidence base has highlighted reduced contraceptive use, misuse and discontinuation among women with schizophrenia, depression and anxiety disorders (Frieder 2010; Hall et al. 2015). The differences in contraceptive behaviour in this group are unclear but may arise from differences in knowledge and beliefs about contraceptive methods and their side effects. Additional barriers, including more risky sexual behaviours, unplanned sexual encounters and lack of access to contraception, may also contribute and need to be considered as part of any preconception counselling.

In light of this evidence, healthcare professionals should not assume impaired fertility, and it is recommended that discussions about contraception methods should be integrated into routine appointments with all women of childbearing age with mental health conditions (McAllister-Williams et al. 2017). This should include a non-judgemental empathetic approach discussion about sexual activity and pregnancy plans. Routine monitoring of use and adherence to contraception is also recommended to reduce occurrence of unintended and unplanned pregnancies.

9.4 Decisions About Motherhood

Qualitative studies have emphasised the importance of motherhood to women with bipolar disorder and the negative impact of feelings of failure and loss when they are unable to fulfil this role (Dolman et al. 2013). Women have a basic human right to make decisions around the number and spacing of children and a right to adequate information about planning a pregnancy (Freedman and Isaacs 1993). However, stigma surrounding reproductive issues is a common experience for this group of women particularly towards their capacity to be a 'good mother' (Dolman et al. 2013; Krumm et al. 2014). Supporting reproductive decisions for women with severe mental illness can create complex ethical dilemmas for healthcare professionals, who need to simultaneously consider the needs and autonomy of the woman planning a pregnancy alongside the needs of the developing foetus and unborn child (Miller 2009). Findings from a survey of women with bipolar disorder attending a preconception clinic found that almost half had been advised to actively avoid pregnancy by a friend or healthcare professional (Nguyen et al. 2015). In order to support women's reproductive choices, preconception care for women needs to encourage ethical reflection of these complex issues.

For women with mental health problems, particularly those with severe and enduring symptoms, decisions about motherhood can be especially challenging and extend beyond considerations of medication use (Dolman et al. 2016; Frieder 2010). Women commonly express concerns which include their child's genetic susceptibility, the risk of perinatal relapse and fears of loss of child custody, which should be assessed and discussed as part of preconception care and future planning.

Pregnancy is not protective against poor mental health, and fear of relapse when women are considering starting or extending their family is a common concern. A study of women with a history of depression found 43% experienced a relapse during pregnancy, although this was more common among women who had discontinued their antidepressant medication (26% vs. 68%) (Cohen et al. 2006). The risk of relapse for women with non-affective psychoses during pregnancy has been reported to be 24% and 12% in women with affective psychotic or bipolar disorders (Taylor et al. 2018). Women on no regular medication throughout the first trimester were also at greater risk of relapse in pregnancy. Concerns about the risk of intergenerational transmission of mental health conditions may also be particularly pervasive for women considering a pregnancy (Stevenson et al. 2016). There is evidence that some mental health conditions have a strong genetic loading, with the genetic risk being higher for more severe mental illnesses. For example, bipolar disorder has been found to be a highly heritable disorder, with heritability estimates from twin studies of 89–93% (Craddock and Sklar 2013). Good preconception care should therefore include consideration of genetic counselling prior to conception (Frieder 2010).

9.5 Use of Psychotropic Medication

Decisions concerning psychotropic medication use in women of childbearing age are complex, and much of the preconception literature has focused on how to manage medication plans for women planning a pregnancy. Psychotropic medication use (including antidepressants, anxiolytic/sedative-hypnotics, antiepileptics, antipsychotics, lithium, stimulants) is not uncommon in women of childbearing age, and there is evidence that the mean number of medications taken during or in the months prior to pregnancy has substantially increased (Jimenez-Solem et al. 2013; Leong et al. 2017). Findings from a Canadian cohort study of approximately 225,000 pregnancies found the use of psychotropics in the 3–12 months prior to pregnancy had increased 1.6-fold (from 6.4 to 10.5%) between 2001 and 2013, highlighting increasing importance of considering the safety of prescribing to women of childbearing age (Leong et al. 2017).

Clinicians and women often face challenging decisions about the use of psychotropic medication in pregnancy, resulting from inconsistencies in the evidence base about the safety and effectiveness of medications during pregnancy and for breastfeeding mothers (McAllister-Williams et al. 2017; Khalifeh et al. 2019). Given these uncertainties, women with pre-existing mental health conditions often discontinue medication once they decide to start or extend their family or discover they are pregnant, increasing the risk of relapse (McAllister-Williams et al. 2017).

Women describe the complexity of decisions about medication use preconceptionally and perinatally and the lack of definitive evidence leaving them to feel they are taking a gamble with their health and that of their unborn child (Stevenson et al. 2016). The evidence suggests that untreated (or suboptimally treated) maternal mental health conditions are associated with an increased risk of adverse obstetric outcomes, childhood emotional and behavioural problems (Stein et al. 2014; Howard et al. 2014b; Jablensky et al. 2005), although it is unclear if this is secondary to health behaviours or social circumstances or is a direct effect of maternal mental health. In rare circumstances sudden changes or discontinuation in medication may contribute to an increased risk of maternal suicide (Knight et al. 2018).

Clinical guidelines regarding the use of psychotropic medication during preconception, pregnancy and postpartum exist, such as the National Institute for Health and Care Excellence (NICE) and the British Association for Psychopharmacology Consensus Guideline, which should be consulted along with current research evidence and recommendation of UK Teratology Information Service (McAllister-Williams et al. 2017; National Institute for Health and Care Excellence 2014). Guidance for clinical practice is generally in agreement that the use of medication during for women who have recently conceived or are planning a pregnancy is indicated when risk to the foetus from in utero exposure is outweighed by the risks of untreated maternal psychiatric illness. However, health professionals can be apprehensive about prescribing to women planning a pregnancy, possibly on account of the paucity of high-quality research evidence and lack of training in this area (Stevenson et al. 2016; Watanabe 2014).

Discussions about medication options should start early in the preconception period for women who are planning a pregnancy and be integrated into routine healthcare appointments for all women of childbearing age who are prescribed psychotropic medication (Catalao et al. 2020). This is particularly important when women are being prescribed medications with known adverse effects on foetal development, such as valproate or carbamazepine (McAllister-Williams et al. 2017). Prescribing patterns of valproate and carbamazepine have decreased considerably since 1994 (Man et al. 2012). Interestingly, this study showed that pregnant women with epilepsy were three times as likely to stop receiving antiepileptic drugs compared to women with bipolar disorder, suggesting a potential disparity in the perception of risk of relapse for these conditions among prescribing clinicians (Man et al. 2012).

There is very limited data to guide clinicians in dosing strategies women who are planning a pregnancy, as pregnant women are often excluded from pharmaceutical trials. Clinicians must therefore rely on what is known about pharmacokinetic in pregnancy and the critical stages of foetal development. Consideration should be given to continuation of current medication plans, switching to a medication that has less known adverse maternal or foetal effects or discontinuing medication (Miele et al. 2019). Basic principles of prescribing to women who are planning a pregnancy include using the lowest beneficial dose, considering a slow discontinuation of medication, closely and responsively monitoring of mental state and avoidance of polypharmacy (Miele et al. 2019). Mental health conditions and the associated risks should not be downplayed, but a transparent risk-benefit analysis balanced by the inclusion of protective factors as well as information on accessing specialist professional help is likely to empower women and couples to make the best choice. An unbiased shared decision-making approach, which weighs up the potential risks of psychotropic medication use among women of childbearing potential, with the effects of untreated mental health conditions, alongside women's concerns and needs can be beneficial (Khalifeh et al. 2019).

9.6 Social Support Needs

Mental health conditions are associated with increased social vulnerability, including unemployment, unstable relationships, housing and poverty (Murali and Oyebode 2004), and likely to reflect a bidirectional relationship between mental health and social circumstances. Social support and secure partner relationships are therefore an important aspect of perception care. Women may have more limited social support or unstable partner relationships, and preconception consultations can provide an opportunity to enhance and mobilise these where possible.

Severe or enduring mental illness can also result in poor socioeconomic circumstances particularly when individuals have had long periods of unemployment due to poor health resulting in a lack of financial resources, housing and poverty (Murali and Oyebode 2004). It is therefore recommended that preconception care should include a comprehensive assessment of a woman's housing and financial situation, environmental safety and access to care and healthy nutrition (Frieder 2010). Preconception care provides an opportunity for open discussions about a woman and her families' socioeconomic situation and to work with women to overcome barriers to accessing additional support and financial resources prior to conception where possible.

Domestic violence is a pervasive public health problem and an important determinant of women and children's health. Research suggests a bidirectional and causal relationship between domestic violence and abuse and mental health, in that poor mental health has been associated with subsequent episodes of violence and abuse and interpersonal violence and abuse can have an adverse effect on mental health (Devries et al. 2013). Furthermore, studies have indicated that over 10% of postnatal depression may be attributed to domestic abuse or violence (Howard et al. 2013a). Healthcare professionals have a responsibility to facilitate identification and prevention and sensitively respond to domestic abuse and sexual violence (Oram et al. 2017). This is particularly important as rates of domestic violence are known to escalate during pregnancy and can negatively affect obstetric and neonatal outcomes. Women, particularly those with severe mental illness, may have lost previous children to foster care or have intermittent contact (McCracken et al. 2017). Preconception care provides an address a woman's fears about the involvement of children's services, by providing information tailored to their needs. Where there are safeguarding concerns for a woman planning a pregnancy or her unborn child, it is important that this is discussed sensitively and supportively at the earliest opportunity and need for involvement of social care services explored.

9.7   Integrating Physical Health

Women with mental health conditions, particularly severe mental illnesses such as schizophrenia, have higher morbidity and mortality related to physical illness than the general population (Firth et al. 2019). The chance of having a healthy pregnancy and birth may be impacted upon by several factors such as weight, diet, smoking, substance abuse, misuse environmental pollutants, infections, medical conditions, medications and family medical history. Higher rates of smoking and alcohol and drug use than the general population have been reported and are more likely to continue throughout pregnancy (Richardson et al. 2019; Howard et al. 2013b). An Australian study of women with severe mental illness referred to preconception counselling found all women were taking psychotropic medication, 40% were over 35 years, 36% smoked daily and 52% were overweight/obese at the time of referral (Nguyen et al. 2015). Smoking is a leading cause of foetal and neonatal morbidity, and therefore access to smoking cessation programmes is an important part of preconception care.

Identification of people contemplating pregnancy provides a window of opportunity to improve physical and mental health before conception, whilst population-level initiatives to reduce the determinants of preconception risks irrespective of pregnancy planning are essential to improve outcomes (Stevenson et al. 2016). As such, preconception care provides women and couples the opportunity to discuss physical health, including vitamins, macronutrient supplementation (e.g. folic acid) and nutrition prior to pregnancy, and to review smoking status, alcohol consumption and weight (Stevenson et al. 2016). Furthermore, physical adaptation in pregnancy can lead to changes in drugs pharmacokinetics, i.e. absorption, distribution, metabolism and elimination, with implications for prescribing. Therefore, the approach to preconception advice cannot preclude from the integration of reproductive health and physical health.

The evidence suggests that untreated (or suboptimally treated) mental health conditions are associated with an increased risk of adverse obstetric outcomes (Stein et al. 2014), although it is unclear if this is secondary to health behaviour or is a direct effect of maternal mental health. The susceptibility to factors affecting foetal development varies throughout the different stages of pregnancy. Teratogens are especially damaging in the first 12 weeks of gestation because it is a critical period in perinatal development. Therefore, timely assessment and support to access effective interventions can be crucial to addressing modifiable risk factors such as weight and smoking at an early stage is crucial.

9.8 Considerations for the Postnatal Period

9.8.1 Infant Feeding

The subject of infant feeding can be highly emotive; whilst most people are aware of the benefits of breastfeeding, many families have not breastfed or have tried and not succeeded, which can be traumatic and upsetting (Unicef 2016a). Considering options before conception may therefore be helpful, especially since there is evidence of reduced initiation and decreased breastfeeding duration in women with depression (Dennis and McQueen 2009).

Preconception discussions about infant feeding should include the evidence-based information that breastfeeding can be beneficial for both mothers and babies (Victora et al. 2016). This includes evidence from a large cohort study in the UK that breastfed babies had improved emotional development and there was a significant association between breastfeeding and good maternal mental health (Del Bono and Rabe 2012). Other studies have shown that breastfeeding can help women feel empowered and confident (Brown and Lee 2011), help reduce the impact of stress and sleep deprivation and help reduce the risk of depression (Cong et al. 2011).

For some women, however, breastfeeding can be challenging to establish, and women with difficulties need a positive experience of support to reduce the risk of postpartum depression (de Lauzon-Guillain et al. 2012; Chaput et al. 2016). Identifying sources of support, such as a local peer support group, is therefore recommended so parents know where to go for help when they need it.

Medication is not always a contraindication for breastfeeding, although current evidence is limited as pregnant and breastfeeding women are often excluded from clinical trials. Evidence shows that the health benefits of continued breastfeeding significantly outweigh the perceived risks to the baby from taking antidepressants, and some medications are only found in low levels in breast milk; sertraline, for example, is the antidepressant of choice when breastfeeding (Oystein Berle and Spigset 2011). Whilst there is limited information on the effects of exposure to anti-psychotic medication during breastfeeding, decisions should be made on an individual basis, in conjunction with guidance relating to specific drugs; polypharmacy should be avoided and infants should be monitored for sedation, poor feeding and behavioural effects. Access to specialist expert advice from mental health teams about the risks and benefits of breastfeeding is recommended for women who are prescribed psychotropic medications (National Institute for Health and Care Excellence 2014).

For women who choose to bottle-feed, it is important to note that the mechanism for findings linking breastfeeding with an improvement in child emotional development and good maternal mental health is still unclear (Del Bono and Rabe 2012). Responsive bottle-feeding should be recommended, since this includes skin-to-skin contact with the infant and responsive feeding patterns that support the development of close and loving relationships (Unicef UK 2016b). An awareness of this before conception will be reassuring for women who know they will not breastfeed.

9.8.2 Parenting

Perinatal mental health disorders are associated with an increased risk of a range of psychological and developmental disturbances in children (Stein et al. 2014). Whilst this is likely to be concerning in the preconception period however, these outcomes are not inevitable, and the effect sizes are mostly moderate or small. Stein et al. explore factors that can ameliorate the risk of psychological and developmental disturbances in children, highlighting that both mothers' and fathers' mental health can contribute to their child's development (Stein et al. 2014). Exploring parenting concerns in the preconception period is therefore important so that actions can be identified to ameliorate the risk, reduce any potential negative impact on future children and empower women and couples for parenthood.

Mechanisms contributing to psychological and developmental disturbances in children include genetics (an inherited genotype from either or both parents) and epigenetics (modification of gene expression), although there is restricted knowledge about both of these (Stein et al. 2014). There is ample evidence, however, that effective early sensitive parenting can promote the development of secure attachment, resilience and emotional wellbeing in children (Stein et al. 2014; Slade 2005). Exploring aspects of effective early parenting in the preconception period can therefore be helpful and empowering, since interventions to enhance sensitivity have also been shown to have a positive impact on the child (Bakermans-Kranenburg and Van Ijzendoorn 2014).

Emotional and social support during pregnancy and the postnatal period should also be discussed before conception, since this is another moderating factor (Frieder 2010; Stein et al. 2014; McManus and Poehlmann 2012) that can be explored, and plans put in place for when additional support is most likely to be needed. Socioeconomic factors have been repeatedly shown to moderate the effects of depression and other mental health problems (Frieder 2010; Stein et al. 2008; 2014). Having a plan in place is, in itself, a protective factor that may help reduce parental anxiety.

9.9   Principles of Providing Preconception Care

Evidence on the effectiveness of preconception care and targeted interventions for women and couples with mental health difficulties is lacking, and there no single guideline about what preconception advice should be offered. Nevertheless, there is a strong need and clear potential for benefit of providing preconception care tailored for this group of women.

Where possible, pregnancy should be planned to coincide with time of emotional wellbeing and stability (Frieder 2010). It has been recommended that a woman with severe mental illnesses should be in remission for at least one year prior to planning a pregnancy (Romans and Seeman 2006), although this will be very personalised to a women and her family circumstances. For example, access to psychological interventions and enhanced support systems can help women manage symptoms and prepare for pregnancy. Healthcare professionals play a key role in identifying and providing adequate diagnosis, treatment and support prior to conception, by incorporating preconception care into all healthcare encounters with women of reproductive age (Catalao et al. 2020). Preconception care should encourage reflection on the frequency and severity of episodes of mental illness, experiences of current and previous treatments, the impact of the mental health on daily functioning and relationships and social circumstances and support (Green et al. 2013).

9.9.1   Setting the Tone

Many women and couples affected by a mental health conditions often face the prospect of a pregnancy with profound apprehension. They are concerned about the intrauterine exposure to psychotropic medication, the risk of a relapse precipitated by the physical adaptation to pregnancy and parenthood and the impact of psychiatric symptoms on their ability to care for their baby. Women may harbour fears and beliefs that they will never be able to have children, fear removal of a child from their care. A thoughtful and well-informed preconception consultation can empower women and their partners to make informed choices and plan for a pregnancy knowing that their mental health will receive equal consideration to their physical health.

Healthcare professionals need to be mindful of the language used to explore sensitive areas during consultations and formulate the relevant recommendations. Women may feel overwhelmed discussions of medication use, risk of relapse and adverse outcomes. Consultations should take a strengths-based approach and seek to empower women and couples to feel confident that they will be supported in their decisions, whatever these may be (Miele et al. 2019). Judgements should about parenting potential based on a particular diagnosis or symptoms should not be made (Green et al. 2013). Clinicians should avoid placing blame and the potential unintended consequences of messages about the impact of mental health on fertility and pregnancy outcomes, which may further exacerbate feelings of depression or anxiety.

9.9.2 Whole Systems Approach

Preconception care for individuals with mental health conditions requires a collaborative whole systems approach, with involvement across professional disciplines and across settings (Catalao et al. 2020). This is particularly important for this population, who can face substantial barriers accessing healthcare. A Collaborative model of care, using a strengths-based formulation which incorporates integrated assessments and discussions about physical and mental health, social circumstances is crucial to addressing the issues outlined above. Discussions should actively incorporate protective factors as well as triggers and maintaining factors in order to help women to make positive changes and improve their reproductive choices and the chances of having a healthy pregnancy outcome (Miele et al. 2019).

Individuals may not be in contact with specialist mental health services. Routine appointments with general practitioners provide opportunity to raise awareness of preconception health and wellbeing and depending on need signpost to specific preconception services and integrate discussions about family planning, use of contraception, vitamin intake and health promotion for those with low awareness or not actively considering pregnancy (Public Health England 2018). Healthcare services should be aware of the specific needs and risks associated with perinatal mental health conditions and facilitate referrals to mental health teams where appropriate.

For those under the care of mental health services, routine appointments, such as care planning meetings and medication reviews, can be a chance to discuss plans for pregnancy, decisions about medication use and symptom management. For individuals who are actively planning a pregnancy more in-depth, preconception counselling is required to provide a holistic discussions and treatment plans. It is important that they are offered preconception counselling by a psychiatrist, ideally a perinatal psychiatrist, particularly if they have severe mental illness or currently being prescribed psychotropic medication (Miele et al. 2019). Preconception care should involve an exploration of all treatment options and consideration of how to improve a woman's mental health and social situation prior to conception. Women and couples may benefit from psychological therapies or support from community-based voluntary organisations.

Barriers to accessing care exist, and this has been particularly highlighted for women during pregnancy (Bye et al. 2018). Women are often fearful of accessing statutory services, due to fear of stigma and concerns about child removal. A sensitive approach to engaging with women and families with mental health conditions and complex social needs is therefore paramount to helping women seek and engage in treatment. Where possible, preconception care for this group should aim to involve partners and significant others whilst being mindful of the increased social vulnerability women may face. A strengths-based approach, tailored to the individual mental health needs and social circumstances, is likely to be crucial to empowering individuals to make informed reproductive health decisions and improving more long-term maternal and child health outcomes. However, further research is vitally needed to inform and evaluate models of preconception care that incorporate mental health and are tailored to the specific needs of individuals experiencing mental health conditions.

References

Akasheh G, Sirati L, Kamran ARN, Sepehrmanesh Z. Comparison of the effect of sertraline with behavioral therapy on semen parameters in men with primary premature ejaculation. Urology. 2014;83(4):800–4.

Anderson K, Sharpe M, Rattray A, Irvine D. Distress and concerns in couples referred to a specialist infertility clinic. J Psychosom Res. 2003;54(4):353–5.

Association AP. Diagnostic and statistical manual of mental disorders (DSM-5®): American Psychiatric Pub; 2013.

Bakermans-Kranenburg MJ, Van Ijzendoorn MH. A sociability gene? Meta-analysis of oxytocin receptor genotype effects in humans. Psychiatr Genet. 2014;24(2):45–51.

Brown A, Lee M. An exploration of the attitudes and experiences of mothers in the United Kingdom who chose to breastfeed exclusively for 6 months postpartum. Breastfeed Med. 2011;6(4):197–204.

Bye A, Shawe J, Bick D, Easter A, Kash-Macdonald M, Micali N. Barriers to identifying eating disorders in pregnancy and in the postnatal period: a qualitative approach. BMC Pregnancy Childbirth. 2018;18(1):114.

Catalao R, Howard LM, Mann S, Wilson C. Preconception care in mental health services: planning for a better future. Br J Psychiatry. 2020;216(4):180–1.

Chaput KH, Nettel-Aguirre A, Musto R, Adair CE, Tough SC. Breastfeeding difficulties and supports and risk of postpartum depression in a cohort of women who have given birth in Calgary: a prospective cohort study. CMAJ Open. 2016;4(1):E103.

Cohen LS, Altshuler LL, Harlow BL, Nonacs R, Newport DJ, Viguera AC, et al. Relapse of major depression during pregnancy in women who maintain or discontinue antidepressant treatment. JAMA. 2006;295(5):499–507.

Cong Z, Hale T, Kendall-Tackett K. The effect of feeding method on sleep duration, maternal well. Being, and Pospartum depression. Clin Lactat. 2011;2(2):22–6.

Craddock N, Sklar P. Genetics of bipolar disorder. Lancet. 2013;381(9878):1654–62.

Del Bono E, Rabe B. Breastfeeding and child cognitive outcomes: evidence from a hospital-based breastfeeding support policy. ISER Working Paper Series; 2012.

Dennis C-L, McQueen K. The relationship between infant-feeding outcomes and postpartum depression: a qualitative systematic review. Pediatrics. 2009;123(4):e736–e51.

Devries KM, Mak JY, Bacchus LJ, Child JC, Falder G, Petzold M, et al. Intimate partner violence and incident depressive symptoms and suicide attempts: a systematic review of longitudinal studies. PLoS Med. 2013;10(5):e1001439.

Dolman C, Jones I, Howard LM. Pre-conception to parenting: a systematic review and meta-synthesis of the qualitative literature on motherhood for women with severe mental illness. Arch Womens Ment Health. 2013;16(3):173–96.

Dolman C, Jones IR, Howard LM. Women with bipolar disorder and pregnancy: factors influencing their decision-making. BJPsych Open. 2016;2(5):294–300.

Easter A, Treasure J, Micali N. Fertility and prenatal attitudes towards pregnancy in women with eating disorders: results from the Avon Longitudinal Study of Parents and Children. BJOG Int J Obstet Gynaecol. 2011;118(12):1491–8.

Firth J, Siddiqi N, Koyanagi A, Siskind D, Rosenbaum S, Galletly C, et al. The lancet psychiatry commission: a blueprint for protecting physical health in people with mental illness. Lancet Psychiatry. 2019;6(8):675–712.

Freedman LP, Isaacs SL. Human rights and reproductive choice. Stud Fam Plan. 1993;24:18–30.

Frieder A. Preconception counseling for women with schizophrenia. Curr Women's Health Rev. 2010;6(1):12–6.

Glover V, O'Connor T, O'Donnell K. Prenatal stress and the programming of the HPA axis. Neurosci Biobehav Rev. 2010;35(1):17–22.

Green L, Vais A, Harding K. Preconception care for women with mental health conditions. Br J Hosp Med. 2013;74(6):319–21.

Haddad PM, Wieck A. Antipsychotic-induced hyperprolactinaemia. Drugs. 2004;64(20):2291–314.

Hall KS, Steinberg JR, Cwiak CA, Allen RH, Marcus SM. Contraception and mental health: a commentary on the evidence and principles for practice. Am J Obstet Gynecol. 2015;212(6):740–6.

Howard LM, Oram S, Galley H, Trevillion K, Feder G. Domestic violence and perinatal mental disorders: a systematic review and meta-analysis. PLoS Med. 2013a;10(5):e1001452.

Howard L, Bekele D, Rowe M, Demilew J, Bewley S, Marteau T. Smoking cessation in pregnant women with mental disorders: a cohort and nested qualitative study. BJOG Int J Obstet Gynaecol. 2013b;120(3):362–70.

Howard LM, Megnin-Viggars O, Symington I, Group GD. Antenatal and postnatal mental health: summary of updated NICE guidance. BMJ. 2014a;349:g7394.

Howard LM, Molyneaux E, Dennis C-L, Rochat T, Stein A, Milgrom J. Non-psychotic mental disorders in the perinatal period. Lancet. 2014b;384(9956):1775–88.

Howard LM, Ryan EG, Trevillion K, Anderson F, Bick D, Bye A, et al. Accuracy of the Whooley questions and the Edinburgh Postnatal Depression Scale in identifying depression and other mental disorders in early pregnancy. Br J Psychiatry. 2018;212(1):50–6.

Jablensky AV, Morgan V, Zubrick SR, Bower C, Yellachich L-A. Pregnancy, delivery, and neonatal complications in a population cohort of women with schizophrenia and major affective disorders. Am J Psychiatr. 2005;162(1):79–91.

Jimenez-Solem E, Andersen JT, Petersen M, Broedbaek K, Andersen NL, Torp-Pedersen C, et al. Prevalence of antidepressant use during pregnancy in Denmark, a nation-wide cohort study. PLoS One. 2013;8(4):e63034.

Jones I, Chandra PS, Dazzan P, Howard LM. Bipolar disorder, affective psychosis, and schizophrenia in pregnancy and the post-partum period. Lancet. 2014;384(9956):1789–99.

Kaltenthaler E, Pandor A, Wong R. The effectiveness of sexual health interventions for people with severe mental illness: a systematic review. Health Technol Assess. 2014;18(1):1–74.

Khalifeh H, Molyneaux E, Brauer R, Vigod S, Howard LM. Patient decision aids for antidepressant use in pregnancy: a pilot randomised controlled trial in the UK. BJGP Open. 2019.

Klemetti R, Raitanen J, Sihvo S, Saarni S, Koponen P. Infertility, mental disorders and well-being—a nationwide survey. Acta Obstet Gynecol Scand. 2010;89(5):677–82.

Knight M, Bunch K, Tuffnell D, Jayakody H, Shakespeare J, Kotnis R, et al. Saving lives, improving mothers' care—lessons learned to inform maternity are from the UK and Ireland confidential enquiries into maternal deaths and morbidity 2014–16, vol. 2018. University of Oxford; 2018.

Krumm S, Checchia C, Badura-Lotter G, Kilian R, Becker T. The attitudes of mental health professionals towards patients' desire for children. BMC Med Ethics. 2014;15(1):18.

de Lauzon-Guillain B, Wijndaele K, Clark M, Acerini CL, Hughes IA, Dunger DB, et al. Breastfeeding and infant temperament at age three months. PLoS One. 2012;7(1):e29326.

Leong C, Raymond C, Château D, Dahl M, Alessi-Severini S, Falk J, et al. Psychotropic drug use before, during, and after pregnancy: a population-based study in a Canadian cohort (2001–2013). Can J Psychiatry. 2017;62(8):543–50.

Man S-L, Petersen I, Thompson M, Nazareth I. Antiepileptic drugs during pregnancy in primary care: a UK population based study. PLoS One. 2012;7(12):e52339.

Margulis AV, Kang EM, Hammad TA. Patterns of prescription of antidepressants and antipsychotics across and within pregnancies in a population-based UK cohort. Matern Child Health J. 2014;18(7):1742–52.

McAllister-Williams RH, Baldwin DS, Cantwell R, Easter A, Gilvarry E, Glover V, et al. British Association for Psychopharmacology consensus guidance on the use of psychotropic medication preconception, in pregnancy and postpartum 2017. J Psychopharmacol. 2017;31(5):519–52.

McCracken K, Priest S, FitzSimons A, Bracewell K, Torchia K, Parry W, et al. Evaluation of pause: research report. Children's Social Care Innovation Programme evaluation report; 2017. p. 49.

McManus BM, Poehlmann J. Parent–child interaction, maternal depressive symptoms and preterm infant cognitive function. Infant Behav Dev. 2012;35(3):489–98.

McManus S, Bebbington P, Jenkins R, Brugha T. Mental health and wellbeing in England: Adult Psychiatric Morbidity Survey 2014. A survey carried out for NHS Digital by NatCen Social Research and the Department of Health Sciences, University of Leicester. 2016.

Miele M, Jayarajah C, Kabacs N, Arulkumaran S. Pre-conception advice: best practice toolkit for perinatal mental health services. 2019.

Miller LJ. Sexuality, reproduction, and family planning in women with schizophrenia. Schizophr Bull. 1997;23(4):623–35.

Miller LJ. Ethical issues in perinatal mental health. Psychiatr Clin. 2009;32(2):259–70.

Murali V, Oyebode F. Poverty, social inequality and mental health. Adv Psychiatr Treat. 2004;10(3):216–24.

Nath S, Ryan EG, Trevillion K, Bick D, Demilew J, Milgrom J, et al. Prevalence and identification of anxiety disorders in pregnancy: the diagnostic accuracy of the two-item Generalised Anxiety Disorder scale (GAD-2). BMJ Open. 2018;8(9):e023766.

National Institute for Health and Care Excellence. Clinical guideline: CG192. Antenatal and postnatal mental health: clinical management and service guidance. 2014.

Nguyen T, Brooks J, Frayne J, Watt F, Fisher J. The preconception needs of women with severe mental illness: a consecutive clinical case series. J Psychosom Obstet Gynecol. 2015;36(3):87–93.

Nørr L, Bennedsen B, Fedder J, Larsen ER. Use of selective serotonin reuptake inhibitors reduces fertility in men. Andrology. 2016;4(3):389–94.

Oram S, Khalifeh H, Howard LM. Violence against women and mental health. Lancet Psychiatry. 2017;4(2):159–70.

Oystein Berle J, Spigset O. Antidepressant use during breastfeeding. Curr Women's Health Rev. 2011;7(1):28–34.

Public Health England. Making the case for preconception care: planning and preparation for pregnancy to improve maternal and child health outcomes. London, UK; 2018.

Richardson S, McNeill A, Brose LS. Smoking and quitting behaviours by mental health conditions in Great Britain (1993–2014). Addict Behav. 2019;90:14–9.

Romans SE, Seeman MV. Women's mental health: a life-cycle approach. Philadelphia: Lippincott Williams & Wilkins; 2006.

Schweiger U, Schweiger JU, Schweiger JI. Mental disorders and female infertility. Arch Psychol. 2018;2(6):1–14

Slade A. Parental reflective functioning: an introduction. Attach Hum Dev. 2005;7(3):269–81.

Spry E, Olsson CA, Hearps SJ, Aarsman S, Carlin JB, Howard LM, et al. The Victorian Intergenerational Health Cohort Study (VIHCS): study design of a preconception cohort from parent adolescence to offspring childhood. Paediatr Perinat Epidemiol. 2020;34(1):86–98.

Stein A, Malmberg LE, Sylva K, Barnes J, Leach P. The influence of maternal depression, caregiving, and socioeconomic status in the post-natal year on children's language development. Child Care Health Dev. 2008;34(5):603–12.

Stein A, Pearson RM, Goodman SH, Rapa E, Rahman A, McCallum M, et al. Effects of perinatal mental disorders on the fetus and child. Lancet. 2014;384(9956):1800–19.

Stevenson F, Hamilton S, Pinfold V, Walker C, Dare CR, Kaur H, et al. Decisions about the use of psychotropic medication during pregnancy: a qualitative study. BMJ Open. 2016;6(1):e010130.

Taylor CL, Van Ravesteyn LM, van denBerg MP L, Stewart RJ, Howard LM. The prevalence and correlates of self-harm in pregnant women with psychotic disorder and bipolar disorder. Arch Womens Ment Health. 2016;19(5):909–15.

Taylor CL, Broadbent M, Khondoker M, Stewart RJ, Howard LM. Predictors of severe relapse in pregnant women with psychotic or bipolar disorders. J Psychiatr Res. 2018;104:100–7.

UNICEF. Protecting health and saving lives: a call to action. London: UNICEF; 2016a.

UNICEF. Responsive feeding: supporting close and loving relationships. Unicef UK Baby Friendly Initiative infosheet. 2016b. www.unicef.org.uk

Vesga-Lopez O, Blanco C, Keyes K, Olfson M, Grant BF, Hasin DS. Psychiatric disorders in pregnant and postpartum women in the United States. Arch Gen Psychiatry. 2008;65(7):805–15.

Victora CG, Bahl R, Barros AJ, França GV, Horton S, Krasevec J, et al. Breastfeeding in the 21st century: epidemiology, mechanisms, and lifelong effect. Lancet. 2016;387(10017):475–90.

Watanabe O. Current evaluation of teratogenic and fetotoxic effects of psychotropic drugs. Psychiatr Neurol Jpn. 2014;116(12):996–1004.

Wdowiak A, Bien A, Iwanowicz-Palus G, Makara-Studzińska M, Bojar I. Impact of emotional disorders on semen quality in men treated for infertility. Neuroendocrinol Lett. 2017;38(1):50–8.

Chronic Medical Conditions

10

Karl Neff, Kate Hunt, and Jill Shawe

10.1 Introduction

Chronic medical conditions are increasingly common in women of reproductive age. There are a number of disease-specific factors that can explain this phenomenon. The increasing incidence and prevalence of diabetes, for example, is associated with an increase in rates of obesity worldwide, which on a population level increases the risk of developing diabetes (Wild et al. 2004). In rheumatological conditions such as lupus, the increased incidence and prevalence is likely to be due to greater access to screening and improving medical assessment, resulting in more accurate diagnoses (Uramoto et al. 1999). In cystic fibrosis, the increased prevalence is largely due to greater survival into adulthood as a result of improved multidisciplinary care (Edenborough et al. 2008).

While chronic medical conditions are more common than ever, and while many are associated with poor maternal and fetal outcomes in pregnancy, it is the case that in most conditions appropriate disease-specific individualised preconception care plans can optimise outcomes. Good preconception care often results in normalisation of risk, so that any increased risk of complications in pregnancy associated with the chronic medical condition is reduced back to that of the reference population.

It should be noted that in tandem with an increased prevalence and incidence of chronic medical conditions in reproductively active women, some developed countries, and in particular the United States, have seen an increase in the incidence of

K. Neff (✉)
King's College Hospital NHS Foundation Trust, London, UK
e-mail: karl.neff@nhs.net

K. Hunt
Diabetes Consultant at King's College Hospital, London, UK

J. Shawe
Faculty of Health, School of Nursing and Midwifery, University of Plymouth, Plymouth, UK

© Springer Nature Switzerland AG 2020
J. Shawe et al. (eds.), *Preconception Health and Care: A Life Course Approach*,
https://doi.org/10.1007/978-3-030-31753-9_10

175

pregnancy-related deaths (Creanga et al. 2015, 2017; Berg et al. 2010). Cardiovascular conditions account for at least 25% of these deaths, and this number is increasing over time (Creanga et al. 2015, 2017; Berg et al. 2010). An increasing number are attributed to non-cardiovascular chronic medical conditions (Creanga et al. 2015, 2017; Berg et al. 2010).

It seems possible that the increased complexity of pre-pregnancy and antenatal care in women with chronic medical conditions is contributing to an increase in maternal mortality. However, we cannot be definitive about this based on the current evidence base. The two phenomena may not be causally linked. It should also be noted that while in many chronic medical conditions, there is evidence that appropriate preconception and antenatal care reduce maternal mortality, it is not known if this is the case in cardiovascular disease.

In the absence of definitive evidence, it is prudent to optimise chronic medical conditions prior to pregnancy and to actively manage them during pregnancy. Therefore, everybody with chronic medical conditions should receive the information and support they need to plan for pregnancy, if that is something they wish to achieve. It is important to identify and address any risks associated with chronic medical conditions early in preconception care. Once the condition and risks have been identified, it is essential to develop an individualised care plan that will reduce risk and optimise outcomes. All people with chronic disease should receive quality care and have the resources they need to live a healthy life, which includes assistance in achieving their best health prior to conception to minimize the risk of pregnancy on their long-term wellbeing.

This chapter outlines some of the chronic diseases that clinicians regularly encounter in preconception care. Given their prevalence, diabetes and thyroid disease receive particular attention. Each section includes a summary of the major points that need to be considered in preconception assessment and how any associated risks can be remediated. Women of reproductive age with chronic conditions are often not asked about their pregnancy intentions, or if asked, with the assumption that they should not become pregnant. Providers must consider their own bias, ask their patients about their desire to have a family, and be prepared to offer patient-centred strategies and referrals for those who choose to become pregnant.

10.2 Contraception for Women with Chronic Medical Conditions

Women with chronic medical conditions are at a higher risk of complications in pregnancy. However, many of these risks can be remediated with good preconception care. To optimise pregnancy outcomes, women with chronic medical conditions should avoid pregnancy until preconception care is in place, and they are meeting their disease-specific individualised treatment targets.

It is sometimes assumed that chronic medical conditions reduce fertility. In general this is not the case. Aside from specific conditions such as cystic fibrosis, reproductive capacity is not directly affected by chronic medical conditions, and so it must be assumed that there is no limitation in reproductive capacity. A comprehensive contraception plan is therefore essential in the preconception care of any woman with a chronic medical condition.

This is to allow time for women planning pregnancy to achieve their treatment targets with respect to their chronic medical condition. The choice of contraceptive will depend on the woman and her medical history with guidance available through published Medical Eligibility Criteria for Contraceptive Use (WHO 2015; FSRH 2016; CDC 2016). Generally, many options are available to women with chronic medical conditions (WHO 2015), but estrogen-containing oral contraceptives should be used with caution in women with a medical or family history that suggests an increased risk of thromboembolic disease (Curtis et al. 2016; WHO 2015). When counselling women with a history of cardiovascular disease, cardiovascular risk factors, or rheumatological diseases that are associated with thrombosis (such as lupus), an individualised assessment must be made to determine the risk-benefit ratio of an estrogen-containing regimen.

Women with chronic medical conditions may be on chronic medical therapy, sometimes incorporating multiple agents. Some medications will reduce the efficacy of hormonal contraception by altering the metabolism of the contraceptive. This can occur in any woman using any chronic medical therapy, but women on anticonvulsant or antiseizure therapy for epilepsy or seizure disorders are especially likely to be on an agent that might interfere with their contraceptive plan (Voinescu and Pennell 2017). Therefore, care should be taken when selecting a contraceptive plan to ensure that the woman's ongoing medical therapy will not interfere with the contraception itself. When in doubt about the potential for medication and contraceptive interactions, a pharmacist should be consulted.

10.3   Preconception Diabetes Care

Diabetes mellitus, commonly termed diabetes, is a group of conditions characterised by high blood glucose and defects in insulin production or action. Insulin is the major hormone responsible for maintaining blood glucose concentrations within normal limits. In normal physiology, as blood glucose concentrations rise, following a meal, for example, insulin is secreted. Insulin then acts to allow the circulating glucose to be metabolised throughout the body, moving the glucose from the bloodstream into the cells, thereby reducing blood glucose concentrations. In diabetes, due to either a lack of insulin or an inability of circulating insulin to act as normal, blood glucose concentrations rise.

Pre-gestational diabetes (diabetes diagnosed prior to pregnancy) is common and is associated with an increased risk of adverse pregnancy outcomes for both the mother and baby as well as health problems for the women regardless of pregnancy (NICE 2015a). The risk of adverse outcomes can be reduced with good care (NICE 2015a). Therefore, the importance of preconception care, and avoiding unplanned pregnancy, should be an integral part of standard clinical care for reproductively capable women with diabetes.

There are two main types of pre-gestational diabetes: type 1 diabetes and type 2 diabetes. Type 1 diabetes (T1D) is due to autoimmune destruction of the insulin-producing beta cells in the pancreas, so that the pancreas produces little or no insulin. Therefore T1D is a state of absolute insulin deficiency and can only be treated with insulin replacement (IDF 2017). T1D can develop at any age, but peak onset is in childhood and adolescence. People with T1D always need insulin treatment, even when fasting or unwell, and so insulin therapy should never be discontinued for any reason in people with T1D.

Type 2 diabetes (T2D) is due to a combination of insulin resistance and inadequate production of insulin by the pancreas. In T2D, the body is resistant to the action of insulin, and so more insulin is needed to maintain blood glucose concentrations within normal limits (IDF 2017). However, even though the pancreas can produce more insulin (at least in the early stages of T2D), it is unable to overcome the intrinsic resistance to insulin and so hyperglycaemia (high blood glucose) develops.

T2D is the most common type of diabetes, accounting for around 90% of all cases (IDF 2017). T2D is more common in older adults but is increasingly seen in children, adolescents, and younger adults. The causes of T2D are not completely understood, but there is a strong association between T2D and obesity, increasing age, ethnicity, and a family history of T2D. Maternal diabetes status may also be important. Babies exposed to maternal hyperglycaemia during pregnancy are at increased risk of developing T2D as they grow up (Damm et al. 2016).

Other types of diabetes are less common and include monogenic diabetes and diabetes secondary to other medical problems (such as pancreatitis or endocrine conditions) or medications (such as corticosteroids) (IDF 2017). Gestational diabetes (GDM) is raised blood glucose detected during pregnancy (IDF 2017). In GDM, the raised blood glucose usually normalises on delivery. However, about half of women with GDM will develop diabetes (usually, but not always, T2D) within 5–10 years after delivery (Damm et al. 2016). Therefore, a history of GDM should prompt diabetes screening in preconception care and periodically during well woman preventive visits over the lifecourse.

People with T1D will always need insulin treatment to treat their diabetes. People with T2D usually, but not always, need to take medication to help control glucose levels. Many people with T2D will also need to use insulin. It should be noted that this does not mean that their diabetes is now T1D (a popular misconception is some regions). The use of insulin does not define the type of diabetes. People with T2D using insulin still have T2D and should be treated as such.

Lifestyle modification, including maintaining a healthy diet, is central to the management of diabetes but is of particular importance in T2D as it can have a major impact on how well or not the individual's diabetes is controlled. However, pharmacotherapy will usually be needed at some point. In T2D there are many pharmacotherapeutic options, with a total of eight classes of medication now available to achieve glycaemic control: biguanides (metformin), sulphonylureas, acarbose, thiazolidinediones, DPP-4 (dipeptidyl peptidase 4) inhibitors, SGLT2 (sodium-glucose cotransporter-2) inhibitors, GLP-1 (glucagon-like peptide-1) receptor agonists, and insulins (Davies et al. 2018a, b). Metabolic (bariatric) surgery is also used to treat T2D, particularly in those with obesity who are not meeting treatment targets with medical therapy alone (Davies et al. 2018a, b).

As well as needing to control glucose concentrations, people with diabetes are more likely to have associated medical problems such as hypertension, dyslipidaemia, and obesity (IDF 2017). These conditions will need additional medical therapy. Therefore, people with diabetes are often treated for multiple medical conditions. Given the likelihood of concurrent medical conditions, preconception care of women with diabetes can be complex, and women with diabetes and their healthcare professionals should plan carefully for pregnancy (Forde 2019; Yamamoto et al. 2018).

In diabetes, the risk of adverse pregnancy outcomes can be reduced with effective preconception care focused on achieving excellent blood glucose control prior to conception, folic acid supplementation, adjusting medication appropriately, and optimising the preconception management of associated conditions (NICE 2015a). With respect to glycaemic control, the aim in preconception care is to maintain blood glucose concentrations as close to normal as possible. Therefore, premeal and fasting capillary blood glucose targets in the preconception care setting are generally 5–7 mmol/L (90–126 mg/dL), with a HbA1c target of 6.5% (48 mmol/mol) or less (American Diabetes Association 2019; Blumer et al. 2013). This is not standard diabetes care, as this level of glycaemic control is expected to significantly increase the risk of hypoglycaemia. However, given the risk associated with any hyperglycaemia in pregnancy, the risk of hypoglycaemia is justified in the specific setting of preconception and antenatal diabetes care.

As diabetes care in the preconception setting is complex, women with diabetes who are planning a pregnancy should ideally be seen in a specialist clinical setting where diabetes can be optimised prior to conception (Yamamoto et al. 2018). In cases of unplanned pregnancy, women should inform their diabetes team as soon as possible after confirmation of pregnancy so that early intensive intervention can be put in place to optimise pregnancy outcomes.

10.3.1 Prevalence

Diabetes is common and increasing in prevalence. Worldwide there are 425 million adults with diabetes (1 in 11 adults), and this number is predicted to increase to 629 million by 2045 (IDF 2017). Up to 6% of pregnancies are now complicated by pregestational diabetes, although the prevalence may be higher in low- and middle-income countries given the tendency to limited access to diagnosis in these countries (Deputy et al. 2018; Goldenberg et al. 2016).

However, even in developed economies with free healthcare, as few as 1 in 12 women with pre-gestational diabetes are well prepared for pregnancy (defined as a first trimester HbA1c of less than 48 mmol/mol (6.5%), taking folic acid 5 mg and stopping adverse medication) (NHS_Digital 2017). Therefore it seems that there is still much work to be done in raising awareness about the important of preconception care in women with diabetes.

10.3.2 Associated Morbidity and Mortality

Diabetes is a complex condition that can affect all aspects of women's health. Vascular complications, such as diabetic retinopathy, chronic kidney disease, and neuropathy, can develop over time; however reducing hyperglycaemia can significantly reduce the risk of these complications (Diabetes Control and Complications Trial Research Group 1993; UK Prospective Diabetes Study (UKPDS) Group 1998). Cardiovascular disease is also associated with diabetes. In women with type 1 diabetes, excellent glycaemic control may reduce the risk of cardiovascular disease (Nathan et al. 2005). In women with type 2 diabetes, a multimodal approach is needed to reduce cardiovascular risk, so that associated risk factors such as blood pressure are managed, as well as hyperglycaemia (Gaede et al. 2003).

Aside from physical health complications, diabetes can also impact mental health, social health, and economic health. Women with diabetes are more likely to suffer from mental health issues, including depression and eating disorders (Jones et al. 2000; Kan et al. 2013; Mannucci et al. 2005). Social and economic health can be negatively affected by diabetes, with higher rates of unemployment and limitation of socio-economic opportunity in some cohorts (Tunceli et al. 2005).

These comorbidities need to be considered in all women, irrespective of reproductive status or plans. However, in preconception care, the focus is on hyperglycaemia, as this is the risk factor that has been most associated with complications in pregnancy. Pre-gestational diabetes is associated with an increased risk of adverse pregnancy outcomes that include an increased risk of congenital malformations, miscarriage, pre-eclampsia, preterm delivery, large for gestational age, birth injury (to the mother and baby), induction of labour, caesarean section, neonatal morbidity (including hypoglycaemia, hyperbilirubinaemia, and respiratory distress), and neonatal death (NICE 2015a). In the United Kingdom, the current National Pregnancy in Diabetes Audit reports rates of congenital anomaly 47.6/1000 (T1D) and 44.8/1000 (T2D); preterm delivery 43% (T1D) and 21% (T2D); and large for gestational age (≥90th centile) 48% (T1D) and 23% (T2D) (NHS_Digital 2017). Stillbirth rates were 10.4 per 1000, more than twice that seen in the general population, and neonatal death rates were 6.6 per 1000 (T1D) and 13.8 per 1000 (T2D), almost four times that seen in the general population (NHS_Digital 2017).

Women's health may also be affected by progression of diabetic complications during pregnancy. Pregnancy may precipitate a deterioration in maternal retinopathy and diabetic kidney disease (NICE 2015a). In women with T1D, pregnancy increases the risk of maternal hypoglycaemia, particularly in the first trimester, and increases the risk of diabetic ketoacidosis (NHS_Digital 2017). As many as 1 in 10 pregnant women with T1D have at least 1 hospital admission for severe hypoglycaemia, and diabetic ketoacidosis occurs in at least 1 in 40 pregnancies (NHS_Digital 2017).

The future health of offspring of mothers with pre-gestational diabetes can be affected by maternal hyperglycaemia in pregnancy. Children born to women with either pre-gestational diabetes or GDM have an increased risk of obesity and T2D

(NICE 2015a; Damm et al. 2016). The magnitude of this effect and how much of the effect is due to other environmental, genetic, and epigenetic factors (rather than maternal hyperglycaemia alone) remains a matter of debate (Donovan and Cundy 2015).

10.3.3 Blood Glucose Control

Establishing good blood glucose control (glycaemic control) before conception and maintaining this throughout pregnancy reduces the risk of adverse pregnancy outcomes in women with pre-gestational diabetes, and so is a principle focus of diabetes care (NICE 2015a). Glycated haemoglobin (HbA1c) is currently the best-validated risk marker with respect to glycaemic control. HbA1c is a measure of the proportion of haemoglobin that is glycated and indicates blood glucose concentrations over the 12 weeks preceding the blood sample (assuming normal haemoglobin structure and metabolism).

Higher first trimester HbA1c concentrations are associated with higher rates of congenital abnormality and, in women with T1D, higher rates of stillbirth and neonatal death (NHS_Digital 2017). HbA1c should be measured at least once every 3 months in women with pre-gestational diabetes who are planning pregnancy, with an aim of maintaining HbA1c below 48 mmol/mol (6.5%) while avoiding problematic hypoglycaemia (NICE 2015a; American Diabetes Association 2019; Blumer et al. 2013).

It should be noted that any reduction in HbA1c reduces the risk of congenital malformations, and so if women are unable to meet the HbA1c treatment target of 48 mmol/mol (6.5%), but have reduced HbA1c concentrations from baseline, then they can be reassured that the risk of adverse outcomes has been reduced (NICE 2015a). Women with HbA1c concentrations over 86 mmol/mol (10%) should be advised to avoid pregnancy until glycaemic control has been improved, given the high risk of poor outcomes at this range of hyperglycaemia (NICE 2015a).

As HbA1c is a haemoglobin-based measurement, it can only be used in women that have normal red cell turnover. This means in women with any kind of anaemia, thalassaemia, or any condition requiring regular blood transfusions, HbA1c cannot be used as a marker of glycaemic control. Likewise, in women who regularly donate blood, or who require regular venesection for any reason, HbA1c is not a reliable marker of glycaemic control. In these women, care providers should use either capillary blood glucose measurements or other blood markers such as glycated albumin or fructosamine to evaluate glycaemic control.

If capillary blood glucose measurements are being used as markers of glycaemic control, then the targets for women with pre-gestational diabetes planning pregnancy are (NICE 2015a):

- Fasting (on waking) 5–7 mmol/L.
- Before meals at other times of the day 4–7 mmol/L.
- Two hours after meals 5–9 mmol/L.

As soon as pregnancy is confirmed, these targets change to (NICE 2015a):

- Premeals 4.0–5.3 mmol/L.
- After meals.
  - 1 h after meals 4.0–7.8 mmol/L
  - 2 h after meals 4. 0–6.4 mmol/L.

Women treated with insulin should test capillary blood glucose on waking in the morning, before meals, 2 h after meals, and before bed. For women with diabetes that does not require insulin therapy, frequency of testing depends on whether treatment intensification is required or not. Therefore, in women not using insulin, monitoring schedules can be individualised in collaboration between the woman and her diabetes care team.

Real-time continuous glucose monitoring (RT-CGM) is a technology that measures glucose in the interstitial fluid just below the skin. This allows the RT-CGM device to relay continuous information about glucose concentrations (albeit with a time lag of at least 15 min) and trends in glucose concentrations (i.e. tendency for glucose concentrations to move above or below treatment targets at different times of day) to women and their diabetes care team. This technology can improve glucose control and neonatal outcomes in selected populations (Feig et al. 2017). However, the evidence of the use of this technology in preconception care is not of sufficient strength to recommend its routine use. For now, RT-CGM is only expected to have benefit in women with T1D not meeting treatment targets in preconception care. However, RT-CGM will not be useful in all of these women, so the use of this technology should only be considered following an individualised assessment with a specialised diabetes care team.

10.3.4 Folic Acid

Offspring of women with pre-gestational diabetes are at higher risk of neural tube defects than offspring of women without diabetes (Becerra et al. 1990). Therefore, the general recommendation for women with pre-gestational diabetes who are planning pregnancy is to take folic acid at a dose of at least 4 mg daily until 12 weeks' gestation to reduce the risk of neural tube defects (NICE 2015a; Moussa et al. 2016). It is recognised that there is a dearth of good randomised controlled data to inform us on the optimal dose of folic acid needed to reduce the risk of neural tube defects in women with diabetes. In the absence of such data, given the risk-benefit ratio associated with folic acid supplementation, it is reasonable to continue to recommend higher doses of folic acid (i.e. 4–5 mg daily) in women with diabetes in preconception care (Moussa et al. 2016). Given high rates of unplanned pregnancy, all women of reproductive age should be counselled to take a daily multivitamin with folic acid.

10.3.5 Medication Review

Diabetes pharmacotherapy can be complex. All women with T1D will need insulin therapy, and this can be delivered in a number of ways. Women with T2D may not need medication. If they do, then it may be non-insulin pharmacotherapy, insulin therapy only, or any number of combinations of insulin and non-insulin pharmacotherapy. As well as glycaemic therapy, many women with diabetes will also require antihypertensive therapy, statin therapy, and other medical therapies for diabetic complications.

For women with T1D, or any women using insulin to treat their diabetes, insulin doses will likely need to be adjusted to meet preconception treatment targets while avoiding significant hypoglycaemia. Insulin therapy is usually delivered as multiple daily injections (MDI) or continuous subcutaneous insulin infusion (CSII: also called insulin pump therapy). MDI in women with T1D usually involves injection of long-acting insulin once or twice per day and injection of rapid-acting insulin before meals containing carbohydrate. In some women with T1D, mixed insulin (injections of insulin that contain both rapid- and long- or intermediate-acting insulin) may be used instead of classic MDI regimens. Mixed insulins are given up to three times a day, usually with the largest meals of the day. Given the relative inflexibility of mixed insulin regimens, which is expected to limit the ability to achieve preconception treatment targets, women using these insulins should be converted to a standard MDI regimen or CSII if planning pregnancy.

CSII uses a battery operated, portable, programmable pump that delivers a continuous infusion of rapid-acting insulin via an infusion set that is inserted subcutaneously (ABCD-DTN-UK 2018). The continuous infusion of rapid-acting insulin acts as the basal insulin requirement (i.e. the insulin needed to maintain normal blood glucose concentrations when not eating). Women using CSII can adjust the amount of basal insulin on an hour-by-hour basis to accommodate changes in metabolic requirements that occur throughout the day, during exercise, for example. This is done by adjusting the infusion rate (termed the 'basal rate') on the CSII pump device.

When eating, women give boluses of rapid-acting insulin via their CSII. This can be done by simply inputting a number of units of insulin into the pump device that will then inject an extra bolus of insulin (in addition to the ongoing 'basal rate' infusion of insulin) to accommodate the ingestion of carbohydrates. As well as simply manually inputting insulin units, women can programme the pump to give a bolus of rapid-acting insulin before meals containing carbohydrate depending on the carbohydrate content (ABCD-DTN-UK 2018; NICE 2008). They will do this by using a ratio of carbohydrate (measured in grams or 'exchanges') to insulin. This ratio can be preprogrammed into the CSII device, and so women will input the carbohydrate content into the device, which will then calculate the appropriate amount of insulin to give for that particular meal. Women will often refer to this as their 'ratio' and will quote numbers like 1:10. In this example, the ratio 1:10 means that the woman would take one unit of insulin for every 10 g of carbohydrate ingested. If women use carbohydrate ratios, then how they are using their ratios will need to be clarified in preconception care to allow titration of insulin doses. Carbohydrate ratios (as part of carbohydrate counting) can be used by both CSII users and women on MDI regimen.

Insulin has a narrow therapeutic range, meaning that there is a small difference between too small a dose, resulting in glucose levels above the target range, and too large a dose, resulting in glucose levels below the target range or hypoglycaemia (Lamont et al. 2010). Furthermore, many factors influence insulin requirements including carbohydrate content of meals, exercise, stress, illness, and the menstrual cycle. Therefore, most women using insulin will self-adjust their insulin doses based on meal content, activity, etc. Structured education programmes inform women on how to adjust insulin doses to match requirements, and the use of these types or programmes can optimise glycaemic control and general diabetes care (Hopkins et al. 2012). Women with T1D planning pregnancy should be encouraged to attend structured T1D education if available (NICE 2015a). It should be noted that in many regions, access to structured education can be severely limited or non-existent.

Given the individualised nature of diabetes care, there is no standard insulin dose change recommended in preconception care. Instead, preconception care providers should work with the women to optimise basal insulin control, before then optimising prandial insulin therapy. This is an individualised process and needs to be done in collaboration with the woman herself and her primary diabetes care team.

Women with T2D may be on a range of glucose-lowering treatments. Metformin can be used in women planning pregnancy and during pregnancy (NICE 2015a). All other oral glucose-lowering treatments and GLP-1 receptor agonists (which are given by injection) should be discontinued in women planning pregnancy. Given that other agents are discontinued prior to conception, insulin is often required in women with T2D planning pregnancy in order to achieve their glycaemic treatment targets. If this is the case, then a MDI regimen should be used and adjusted as needed to achieve the blood glucose targets mentioned above.

In women with T2D that require insulin, a full MDI regimen similar to that used in T1D may already be in use prior to pregnancy, but many women will be using a combination of non-insulin pharmacotherapy with basal insulin alone or non-insulin pharmacotherapy with a mixed insulin regimen. These women should be converted to MDI prior to pregnancy. CSII use is uncommon in women with T2D, but if in place, then it can continue throughout pregnancy.

Women with diabetes may also be on medications for associated conditions, such as hypertension and dyslipidaemia, or on medical therapy for diabetic complications. Antihypertensive medications and lipid therapy should be reviewed in women planning pregnancy as discussed later. The blood pressure treatment target in people with diabetes is 140/80 mmHg if there are no associated complications such as retinopathy, kidney disease, or coronary artery disease and 130/80 mmHg if there are such complications (NICE 2015b).

10.3.6 Review of Diabetes Complications

Microvascular (small vessel) diabetes complications include retinopathy, nephropathy (diabetic kidney disease), and neuropathy. Pregnancy may precipitate a deterioration in the mother's diabetes complications, so women with diabetes planning pregnancy should be assessed for diabetes complications during preconception care.

People with diabetes should be screened, at least annually, for retinopathy. Ideally, this would be completed using digital retinal imaging as part of a systematic screening programme. However, in many regions, this may not be available. Women planning pregnancy should be offered retinal assessment during preconception care unless they have had an assessment in the last 6 months (NICE 2015a). If no retinopathy is found, they should continue to have annual screening while in preconception care.

Women with significant retinopathy should be referred to an ophthalmologist for assessment and treatment as necessary and should be advised to defer pregnancy until treatment has been completed. This is important as rapid optimisation of blood glucose may result in a deterioration in retinopathy and result in permanent loss of vision (NICE 2015a).

Neuropathy is detected by specialist examination and should be included in the first diabetes evaluation in preconception care (NICE 2015a). As with retinopathy, rapid improvement in glycaemic control can precipitate a deterioration in neuropathy. Therefore, women with advanced neuropathy should avoid rapid improvements in glycaemic control and will need a more gradual reduction in blood glucose concentrations during preconception care.

People with diabetes should have an annual renal assessment including measurement of serum creatinine and measurement of urinary albumin-creatinine ratio. In women with diabetes in preconception care, this renal assessment should be completed at first visit. If significant renal disease is identified, then pregnancy should be deferred, and the woman should be referred to a nephrologist for assessment. Significant renal disease includes a serum creatinine of 120 micromol/L or greater and/or an estimated glomerular filtration rate (eGFR) of 45 mL/min/1.73 m^2 or less (NICE 2015a).

Macrovascular (large vessel) diabetes complications include cardiovascular disease. The management of these conditions in preconception care is discussed later.

10.3.7 Hypoglycaemia

Hypoglycaemia means low blood glucose. In day-to-day management of diabetes, a capillary blood glucose of less than 3.5 mmol/L (63 mg/dL) is considered to be hypoglycaemia, although some apply a higher threshold of 4.0 mmol/L (72 mg/dL). Hypoglycaemia does not occur because of diabetes itself. Hypoglycaemia occurs as a result of the treatment of diabetes, usually in the context of insulin or sulphonylurea use.

Hypoglycaemia is important because the brain is dependent on blood glucose (or ketones) to provide energy. Profound, untreated hypoglycaemia can result in seizures, coma, brain damage, or death. Hypoglycaemia is classified as mild, when the person is able to treat the hypoglycaemia themselves, or severe, when the person is unable to treat themselves because of cognitive incapacity as a result of the hypoglycaemia (Choudhary et al. 2015).

Hypoglycaemia warning symptoms and signs may be 'autonomic' (such as tremor, sweating, palpitations), 'neuroglycopenic' (such as poor concentration, confusion, behaviour change), and non-specific (such as hunger or headache). People with diabetes who develop such symptoms should test their capillary blood glucose immediately, and, if hypoglycaemia is confirmed, they should treat the hypoglycaemia immediately with oral fast-acting carbohydrate.

Some people with diabetes have impaired awareness of hypoglycaemia and are at increased risk of severe hypoglycaemia (Gold et al. 1994). The risk of impaired awareness of hypoglycaemia increases with longer durations of diabetes and with repeated exposure to hypoglycaemia (Pedersen-Bjergaard et al. 2004). Problematic hypoglycaemia is more likely in people with T1D than those with T2D. This is because most people with T2D retain some endogenous insulin and glucagon secretion and function, so as glucose falls, insulin secretion falls, and glucagon secretion increases, protecting against hypoglycaemia. People with T1D have an absolute insulin deficiency and an impaired glucagon response, so they are more exposed to the onset of hypoglycaemia than people with T2D.

It is important that optimisation of blood glucose control in women with T1D planning pregnancy is achieved through careful matching of insulin doses to requirements, supported by structured education and frequent glucose testing to minimise the risk of hypoglycaemia (NICE 2015a). Women should be reminded to treat hypoglycaemia promptly and effectively, and they should be having no more than two episodes of mild hypoglycaemia per week in order to minimise exposure to hypoglycaemia and the risk of developing reduced awareness.

Hypoglycaemia awareness should be assessed in women with diabetes in preconception care. This is essential to determine the risk of severe hypoglycaemia during the period of glycaemic optimisation in preconception care. Hypoglycaemia awareness should be evaluated using a validated tool such as the Gold score. The Gold score asks, 'Do you know when hypoglycaemia is happening?' The response is on a scale of 1 (always aware) to 7 (never aware) (Gold et al. 1994). The higher the score, the more likely the person is to have impaired hypoglycaemic awareness. In people with impaired hypoglycaemic awareness, the risk of severe hypoglycaemia is elevated.

People with impaired awareness of hypoglycaemia or with a history of severe hypoglycaemia should be strongly advised to attend structured education if they have not already done so, as this reduces rates of severe hypoglycaemia and improves hypoglycaemia awareness (Hopkins et al. 2012; Choudhary et al. 2015). Diabetes technology such as RT-CGM or CSII should also be considered, as these interventions can also reduce hypoglycaemia frequency and improve awareness of hypoglycaemia (ABCD-DTN-UK 2018; NICE 2008; Choudhary et al. 2015).

Women with T1D, or any diabetes with impaired awareness of hypoglycaemia, should be prescribed glucagon and taught, with a partner, how to administer it in the event of severe hypoglycaemia. For those who drive, the legal requirements for driving for people with diabetes treated with insulin should be discussed with reference to local guidelines and law.

10.4 Thyroid and Endocrine Care

Thyrotoxicosis (also known as hyperthyroidism or overactive thyroid disease) will affect approximately 1% of the population at some stage in their lives (Aoki et al. 2007). Thyrotoxicosis is defined by an elevation in free thyroxine concentrations to above normal levels and suppression (reduction) in thyroid-stimulating hormone (TSH) concentrations to below normal, usually undetectable, levels.

Primary hypothyroidism is defined as low free thyroxine concentrations and elevated TSH concentrations. In this disease state, the thyroid gland fails to produce sufficient quantities of hormone to maintain health, and therefore thyroid hormone replacement is needed. This condition affects approximately 1% of the population (Aoki et al. 2007; Vanderpump et al. 1995).

Subclinical hypothyroidism is defined as elevated TSH concentrations with normal free thyroxine concentrations. In this condition, the thyroid gland is functioning, and producing normal quantities of hormone, but requires additional stimulation to maintain normal output. Subclinical hypothyroidism affects up to 4% of the total population (and 3% of women of reproductive age) (Aoki et al. 2007; Vanderpump et al. 1995). This condition does not always require treatment, but in preconception care hormonal supplementation is recommended, as there may be a benefit in terms of a reduction in miscarriage risk.

Thyroid status is only proven to require monitoring and treatment in preconception care in women. In general, treatment of thyroid disorders in men is not proven to enhance preconception health or fertility outcomes. However, for their own health and wellbeing, appropriate treatment of thyroid disease in men is recommended.

10.4.1 Prevalence of Adrenal Insufficiency, Polycystic Ovarian Syndrome, and Hyperprolactinaemia in Reproductively Active Women

For normal adrenal function, functioning adrenal glands and a functioning pituitary gland are needed. In normal physiology, adrenocorticotrophic hormone (ACTH) is secreted from the pituitary and acts on the adrenal glands to stimulate cortisol secretion. Adrenal insufficiency can be due to either primary adrenal failure (usually as a result of Addison's disease) where the pituitary is normal, but the adrenal glands are unable to respond to ACTH stimulation, or ACTH deficiency, in which the pituitary is no longer able to secrete sufficient ACTH to generate cortisol production from the adrenal glands. ACTH deficiency is most often a result of previous pituitary surgery, radiotherapy, or long-term steroid use. Adrenal insufficiency is very uncommon in women of reproductive age (Yuen et al. 2013).

Polycystic ovarian syndrome (PCOS) is a relatively common condition that affects at least 5% of women (Bozdag et al. 2016). The prevalence varies significantly between regions and populations, potentially as a result of variation in access to screening and diagnosis (Bozdag et al. 2016). PCOS can be defined in a number of ways but usually includes oligomenorrhoea. Hyperandrogenism causing excessive hair growth, hair loss, or acne is part of PCOS, but not all affected women will have clinically obvious hyperandrogenism. As part of PCOS, there are usually multiple cysts obvious on transvaginal ultrasound examination, but to fit the criteria for diagnosis, a specific number of cysts at a specified volume are required (Bozdag et al. 2016).

Hyperprolactinaemia affects up to 1% of the population at any one time, and prevalence has been increasing over time (Soto-Pedre et al. 2017). Prolactin is a hormone primarily involved in lactation in pregnant and breastfeeding women, but in some women excessive quantities of prolactin will be secreted as a result of medication use, pituitary dysfunction, or a pituitary tumour. Hyperprolactinaemia is associated with pituitary tumours in approximately 25% of cases. These tumours are almost always benign adenomata (Soto-Pedre et al. 2017).

10.4.2 Associated Morbidity and Mortality

Thyroid disease, both thyrotoxicosis (hyperthyroidism) and hypothyroidism, has a severe effect on health and wellbeing. Thyrotoxicosis results in a hypermetabolic state. This usually produces weight loss, tachycardia, and tremor. However, the presentation can vary, and so not all symptoms may be present. Untreated thyrotoxicosis is associated with atrial fibrillation and stroke and mental health disorders such as anxiety (De Leo et al. 2016). Hypothyroidism is associated with a wider range of symptoms that can affect almost any organ in the body, as well as mental health effects such as depression (Chaker et al. 2017). Untreated thyroid disease is expected to result in a progressive loss of health and wellbeing, and so treatment is essential.

This is important in all women, but extra attention is needed in pregnancy and in preconception care. Untreated thyrotoxicosis is associated with an increased risk of serious antenatal complications, including miscarriage, preterm labour, and fetal growth restriction (Luewan et al. 2011). Women can develop heart failure and stroke if thyrotoxicosis is left untreated. However, the treatment of thyrotoxicosis itself can also increase the risk of maternal and fetal complications. Therefore, preconception optimisation of thyroid disease and antithyroid therapy is essential in women planning pregnancy. There is no convincing evidence that adjusting thyrotoxicosis therapy is needed in men with respect to preconception health.

For women with either primary or subclinical hypothyroidism, optimising TSH concentrations prior to pregnancy is recommended in order to minimise the risk of antenatal complications (Alexander et al. 2017; De Groot et al. 2012). While there have been concerns around a number of antenatal maternal and fetal complications, the most consistently observed complication of untreated hypothyroidism is first trimester miscarriage (Alexander et al. 2017; Taylor et al. 2014). There is also an increased risk of miscarriage in women with normal thyroid function but detectable TPO antibodies (Thangaratinam et al. 2011; Chen and Hu 2011). Best practice on how to manage this risk is not yet defined.

While untreated adrenal insufficiency will result in high maternal mortality, appropriately treated disease is not associated with significant morbidity or mortality (Yuen et al. 2013; Lindsay and Nieman 2005). Given the physiological stress of labour, women will need additional steroid replacement while giving birth (Lindsay and Nieman 2005). If additional steroid is not given, then an adrenal crisis may ensue during labour, resulting in maternal shock and fetal compromise.

PCOS can result in menstrual disturbance and hyperandrogenism (including excessive facial or body hair, loss of hair, and acne). The associated oligomenorrhoea can complicate attempts to conceive, with attendant negative effects on mental health and wellbeing (Greenwood et al. 2018). PCOS is also associated with an increased risk of pre-gestational and gestational diabetes (Ehrmann et al. 1999; Qin et al. 2013). In pregnancy, a diagnosis of PCOS is associated with an increased risk of complications including miscarriage and preterm birth, although how much of this risk is as a result of PCOS itself and how much is related to associated obesity and metabolic disease is not entirely clear (Qin et al. 2013).

Hyperprolactinaemia is associated with oligomenorrhoea, and therefore treatment is often needed in preconception care to regularise menses and increase the likelihood of conception (Soto-Pedre et al. 2017). While the condition itself is not associated with any significant complications in pregnancy, hyperprolactinaemia can be associated with a pituitary tumour. The pituitary tumour may increase in size during pregnancy, resulting in visual disturbance and other neurological compromise (Soto-Pedre et al. 2017). The risk of this is dependent on the nature of the pituitary lesion, if present, and so an individualised risk assessment should be made during preconception care by the woman's primary endocrinologist.

10.4.3 Treatment Targets for Thyroid and Endocrine Disease

Untreated or incompletely treated thyrotoxicosis is associated with an increased risk of fetal and maternal complications in pregnancy. Similarly, the treatment of thyrotoxicosis is associated with fetal complications including malformation and fetal hypothyroidism. Therefore, it is recommended that women fully complete their treatment for thyrotoxicosis prior to conception.

Women who receive radioactive iodine therapy as treatment for their thyrotoxicosis are advised to avoid conception for at least the first 6 months following treatment (De Groot et al. 2012). If women conceive in the first year after receiving radioiodine therapy for thyrotoxicosis, then they should be advised of the risk of fetal hypothyroidism.

In women who conceive while thyrotoxic or while on treatment for thyrotoxicosis, antithyroid therapy should be adjusted so that the minimum dose of antithyroid treatment is used to maintain free thyroxine concentrations at the upper end or just above the upper end of the normal range on the local assay (De Groot et al. 2012). The aim is to avoid free T4 concentrations that are excessively elevated (the exact concentration depends on the assay used) while minimising fetal exposure to anti-thyroid therapy. Exact free T4 targets (with reference to the local assay) can be set with the woman's primary endocrinologist.

In women with pre-existing hypothyroidism, thyroid hormone replacement (usually given as Levothyroxine) should be adjusted as needed to maintain TSH concentrations of between 2.5 mIU/L and the lower limit of normal on the local assay (De Groot et al. 2012). TSH suppression (i.e. TSH concentrations lower than 0.1 mIU/L) should be avoided. There is no good evidence to guide the use of lio-thyronine (T3) or dessicated thyroid extract, in treating hypothyroidism in pregnancy, but if these agents are used, then it is reasonable to apply the same TSH targets.

Routine administration of levothyroxine in women with positive TPO antibodies but normal thyroid function is not strongly supported by the current evidence base. However, it may be reasonable to consider levothyroxine supplementation in women with additional risk factors for miscarriage or a history of miscarriage. The use of levothyroxine therapy in women with normal thyroid function to reduce miscarriage risk has been suggested based on data from randomised trials (Negro et al. 2005, 2006). However, more recent larger randomised controlled trials in this population of women have not detected any reduction in miscarriage risk in as a result of levo-thyroxine use (Dhillon-Smith et al. 2019; Wang et al. 2017). If given to women with normal thyroid function, a levothyroxine dose of 50mcg daily is sufficient in almost all women, but this should be adjusted as needed to maintain TSH concentrations within treatment targets.

In adrenal insufficiency, there are no specific biochemical targets. Preconception care in women with adrenal insufficiency is aimed at ensuring that adequate steroid replacement is ongoing, and that there is a perinatal care plan in place, as women will need additional steroid replacement during labour. Both women and men should be on sufficient steroid replacement and should be compliant with therapy. Annual review with an endocrinologist should be up to date in order to screen for comorbid conditions such as thyroid disease that could complicate pregnancy.

All people with adrenal insufficiency need additional steroid supplementation in times of increased physiological stress. Women will need to at least double the dose of steroids while in labour (Lindsay and Nieman 2005). Individualised care plans should be prepared in advance of labour with the woman's primary endocrinologist.

In PCOS, specialist endocrine advice may be needed prior to conception in women with severe oligomenorrhoea, or amenorrhoea, as they may require medical therapy to regularise menses. Assisted fertility may also be needed. There are no specific biochemical treatment targets. The treatment targets are to ensure that menses are sufficiently regular to enhance the likelihood of conception and that general metabolic health is safe for pregnancy. Given the association between some PCOS phenotypes and diabetes, preconception screening for diabetes should be considered (Ehrmann et al. 1999).

In hyperprolactinaemia, the treatment target is to facilitate regular menses using dopamine agonist therapy. The treatment dose should be kept as low as possible while maintaining regular menses and controlling tumour growth (if the hyperprolactinaemia is associated with a pituitary tumour). If menses are regular, then biochemical surveillance is not necessary.

On initiation of preconception care, the cause of the hyperprolactinaemia should be clear, as pituitary tumours may grow during pregnancy causing neurological compromise including visual impairment. The need for pituitary imaging prior to conception should be discussed with the woman's primary endocrinologist.

10.4.4 Medication Review: Altering Medications Appropriately in the Preconception Phase

The ambition in the preconception care of thyrotoxicosis should be to complete treatment prior to conception. However, if a woman is on long-term therapy, or plans to conceive while on treatment for thyrotoxicosis, then the aim is to minimise exposure to antithyroid treatment while maintaining free thyroxine concentrations at the upper end of normal, or just over the upper end of normal, on the local assay (De Groot et al. 2012). Given a slightly increased (but still very low) risk of maternal liver failure associated with antithyroid medical therapy, the use of propylthiouracil is recommended in preconception care and through the first trimester (De Groot et al. 2012). If women are on other agents, then they should convert to propylthiouracil in preconception care unless contraindicated. In the second trimester, and for the remainder of pregnancy, propylthiouracil should be discontinued, and carbimazole or methimazole should be used.

In hypothyroidism, thyroid supplementation may need to be increased in order to optimise TSH concentrations prior to pregnancy (as outlined above) to minimise the risk of complications (Alexander et al. 2017; De Groot et al. 2012). Levothyroxine is the only thyroid replacement that is proven to be safe in pregnancy. Other forms of thyroid replacement such as liothyronine and desiccated thyroid extract are yet to be established as safe in pregnancy.

In adrenal insufficiency, steroid replacement does do not need to be adjusted prior to conception or at conception.

In PCOS, specific treatment adjustments will likely be needed as many women will use hormonal contraceptives to regularise menses. When contraception is discontinued, oligomenorrhoea or amenorrhoea may resume. Therefore, additional medical therapy may be needed to regularise menses or assist with conception. Sometimes this can be achieved with metformin. In women who are on metformin as part of the treatment of PCOS, it can be continued in preconception care without dose adjustment and then discontinued on diagnosis of pregnancy, unless another indication for metformin exists, such as diabetes.

Hyperprolactinaemia is associated with oligomenorrhoea, and therefore treatment with dopamine agonist therapy such as cabergoline or bromocriptine is often needed in preconception care to regularise menses (Soto-Pedre et al. 2017). In hyperprolactinaemia, adjustment of dopamine agonist therapy to minimise dosage while maintaining regular menses should be considered prior to conception.

Dopamine agonists are not proven to be safe in pregnancy, and so ideally would be discontinued in pregnancy if possible. However, they may need to be continued if the hyperprolactinaemia is associated with a large pituitary tumour, as without treatment the tumour could grow and cause visual loss, seizures, or other neurological compromise. The decision on the need to continue treatment in pregnancy should be made with the woman's primary endocrinologist.

10.4.5 Monitoring Disease in the Preconception Phase

Thyroid function tests should be checked at least every 3 months while attempting to conceive and treatment adjusted as needed to achieve treatment targets.

Ongoing review with the treating endocrinologist should be in place prior to conception to monitor adrenal insufficiency. Specific biochemical monitoring above and beyond standard care is not necessarily required, but in women with Addison's disease, it would be reasonable to measure serum electrolytes, thyroid function tests, and vitamin B12 concentrations every 6 months while in preconception care.

Ongoing review with the woman's treating endocrinologist should be in place prior to conception for hyperprolactinaemia. The primary aim is to ensure regular menses. If menses are regular, then no particular disease monitoring is needed in preconception care. In women who do not have regular menses, then measurement of serum prolactin is needed to adjust dopamine agonist therapy. In this case, serum prolactin should be measured every 6 weeks, while therapy is adjusted to ensure normalisation of prolactin concentrations. Once prolactin concentrations have normalised, then further biochemical monitoring is only needed if clinically indicated by oligomenorrhoea or galactorrhoea.

In some women with hyperprolactinaemia due to a macroprolactinoma, additional MRI surveillance or visual field assessment may need to be arranged prior to conception. The need for these assessments will depend on the nature of the pituitary tumour and the disease history. Therefore, the decision to proceed with these assessments will need to be made with the treating endocrinologist.

In women with PCOS, the main focus of preconception care is ensuring menses are as regular as possible. If menses are insufficiently regular to facilitate conception, then endocrine or fertility specialist review is needed. Given the association with metabolic disease, it would be prudent to screen for diabetes and hypertension prior to conception (Ehrmann et al. 1999).

10.5 Cardiovascular Risk and Disease: Modifying Therapy in Preparation for Pregnancy

Heart disease in general, and cardiovascular disease in particular, is very uncommon in women of reproductive age. However, heart disease remains a major cause of death in reproductively capable women in developed economies (Weindling 2003). The major physiological changes associated with pregnancy can precipitate deterioration in pre-existing heart disease. Therefore it is important to consider the possibility of heart disease in women attending for preconception care.

If heart disease is detected, then specialist advice should be sought. This will be targeted advice in the context of potential pregnancy. However, it is also important to give advice on good cardiac care that can be applied over the woman's lifetime (Weindling 2003).

There is very little good data on cardiovascular morbidity and mortality in the preconception care population. Fewer than 1% of women of reproductive age have a history of myocardial infarction (Kannel and Abbott 1984; Wilson et al. 2004). Therefore, the risk of clinically significant cardiovascular disease itself in women of reproductive age remains very low. However, if present, then an individualised care plan should be put in place in collaboration with a specialised cardiac care team.

While cardiovascular disease itself remains very uncommon in women of reproductive age, risk factors for cardiovascular disease, in particular hypertension and dyslipidaemia, are increasingly common (Wilson et al. 2004; Bramham et al. 2014; Laz et al. 2013; Mendelson et al. 2016; Hayes et al. 2011). Depending on the population, up to 10% of pregnancies are complicated by chronic hypertension (i.e. hypertension that predates pregnancy or is diagnosed before 20 weeks' gestation) (Bramham et al. 2014; Hayes et al. 2011). Dyslipidaemia can affect over 10% of the pregnant population, although this is not always treated (Hayes et al. 2011). This increase in the prevalence of metabolic diseases such as dyslipidaemia and hypertension in pregnancy may be related to increasing maternal age and the concurrent increase in the prevalence of obesity (Bramham et al. 2014; Yoder et al. 2009; Callaway et al. 2009).

Cardiovascular risk factors are associated with adverse outcomes in pregnancy.

Hypertension is associated with pre-eclampsia, preterm birth, and an increased risk of perinatal death (Bramham et al. 2014). There is also an increased risk of low birth weight and caesarean delivery (Bramham et al. 2014). The treatment of hypertension is also associated with an increased risk of complications in pregnancy. All antihypertensive medications cross the placenta, and some agents are associated with an increased risk of congenital malformations (Fitton et al. 2017).

Dyslipidaemia is associated with other metabolic diseases such as gestational diabetes and pre-eclampsia (Baumfeld et al. 2015). Statin therapy is the first-line treatment for hypercholesterolaemia, the most common dyslipidaemia, but statin therapy is currently contraindicated in pregnancy due to concerns with regard to a risk of congenital malformation. The magnitude of this risk is not clear. While some studies have reported an increased risk of fetal malformation, others have not identified any increased risk (Karalis et al. 2016).

10.5.1 Treatment Targets for Cardiovascular Risk Factors

Antihypertensive therapy will need to be reviewed prior to conception. The aim is to maintain adequate control of hypertension while minimising exposure to pharmacotherapy. Treatment targets need to be individualised. In women with hypertension alone, a blood pressure of less than 150/90 mmHg is reasonable (ACOG Practice Bulletin No. 203 2019; NICE 2011). In women with coexisting cardiovascular or renal disease, a blood pressure target of 140/90 mmHg is acceptable (Sibai 2002). However, individual treatment targets should be set with the woman's treating physicians.

In general, dyslipidaemia does not need to be monitored prior to conception. The exception would be women with severe hypertriglyceridaemia (>10 mmol/L or >886 mg/dL) as they may be at risk of pancreatitis. In these women, individualised treatment targets should be set in collaboration with their treating physician.

10.5.2 Medication Review: Altering Medications Appropriately in the Preconception Phase

All antihypertensive therapy will need to be reviewed. Many commonly used antihypertensive agents will need to be discontinued prior to conception. In particular, ACE inhibitors, angiotensin receptor antagonists, and potassium-sparing diuretics (such as spironolactone) are contraindicated in pregnancy.

The favoured approach is to convert preconception antihypertensive therapy to preferred agents such as beta-blockers and methyldopa (Yakoob et al. 2013; Magee et al. 2016). Calcium channel antagonists can also be used, although there is potential for increased fetal complications based on results from some small studies (Fitton et al. 2017). Nifedipine is the calcium channel antagonist of choice as it appears to be as efficacious and safe as labetalol in pregnancy (Firoz et al. 2014; Shekhar et al. 2016).

Statins are contraindicated in pregnancy and should be discontinued for 3 months prior to conception (Thorogood et al. 2009). Similarly, fibrates and other lipid therapies should not be used in pregnancy. In the rare circumstances where women have severe dyslipidaemia, individual preconception care plans should be developed with their treating physician.

While coronary artery disease requiring percutaneous intervention (such as coronary artery stents) is very uncommon in women of reproductive age, if a woman has recently had coronary artery stenting, then medical therapy including statin therapy, anti-platelet agents such as aspirin or clopidogrel, and ACE inhibitors will likely be prescribed. Many of these agents will need to be stopped prior to conception, but given the potential for recurrent cardiovascular disease in pregnancy, an individualised care plan needs to be made with the woman's treating cardiologist.

10.5.3 Monitoring Disease in the Preconception Phase

Everyone with hypertension should attend for regular blood pressure checks to ensure that they are at their treatment targets and are therefore protecting themselves from the associated risks of hypertension such as heart disease and stroke. In women with hypertension in preconception care, blood pressure should be monitored regularly prior to conception. The optimal monitoring schedule is not defined with reference to an evidence base, but measurements every 3 months prior to conception seem reasonable. More frequent testing will be needed in women who are not meeting their treatment targets.

Women with a history of high cholesterol should have a single measurement of their cholesterol after discontinuing their lipid therapy in preconception care. Ongoing monitoring during preconception care is not required. In women with severe hypertriglyceridaemia (>10 mmol/L or >886 mg/dL), triglycerides should be monitored as there may be an increased risk of pancreatitis if concentrations rise significantly. In these women, individualised monitoring schedules should be set in collaboration with their treating physician.

10.6 Epilepsy and Seizure Disorders: Key Points in Preconception Care

Epilepsy and seizure disorders are routinely encountered in preconception care. Point prevalence for epilepsy is currently estimated at 6 per 1000 women, and up to 1% of pregnancies are complicated by a diagnosis of epilepsy (Fiest et al. 2017; Edey et al. 2014). While the numbers of women affected by epilepsy and seizure disorders are low, neurological diseases such as epilepsy produce significant morbidity and mortality in pregnancy and are a common cause of maternal death in high-income countries (Kelso AaWA 2014).

While the vast majority of women with seizure disorders have uncomplicated pregnancies, the diagnosis and treatment of epilepsy is associated with a significant risk of maternal and fetal complications, including miscarriage and fetal malformation (Viale et al. 2015). Women may encounter greater rates of seizure in pregnancy, due to changes to medications, potential lapses in compliance with therapy due to fears about congenital malformations, and changes associated with pregnancy, such as sleep disturbance (Harden et al. 2009a).

The medical treatment of seizure disorders is associated with fetal malformation. In women with epilepsy, congenital malformation occurs at a rate of up to 3% (Artama et al. 2005). Some medications can increase this risk, while some appear to be safe in pregnancy (Tomson et al. 2011). Fetal malformations associated with the medical treatment of epilepsy include neural tube defects and congenital cardiac malformations (Tomson et al. 2011; Meador et al. 2008).

Given the risk of serious complications, preconception care is essential in all reproductively capable women with epilepsy or seizure disorder. These women are advised to plan for pregnancy in association with a dedicated preconception care team including a neurologist. There is no clear association between paternal diagnosis and treatment of epilepsy or seizure disorder and risks of complications in pregnancy.

10.6.1 Treatment Targets

The treatment target in preconception care is to avoid maternal seizures by using an appropriate pharmacotherapeutic regimen that will enable control of the underlying seizure disorder while minimising the risk of fetal malformation. The optimal pharmacotherapeutic regimen will need to be individualised in collaboration between the woman, her neurologist, and her preconception care team.

All reproductively capable women with epilepsy or seizure disorder should take folic acid supplementation. There is no evidence from randomised controlled trials to inform the optimal dose of folic acid supplementation in women with epilepsy or seizure disorder, but the dose should be at least 400 mcg daily (Harden et al. 2009b). Some authorities recommend giving doses of up to 5 mg of folic acid daily.

Pregnancy should be delayed until medical therapy has been optimised. It should be noted that many antiseizure drugs will affect the metabolism of hormonal contraception and therefore result in unplanned pregnancies. Commonly used agents such as carbamazepine and phenytoin induce hepatic enzymes resulting in rapid metabolism of hormonal contraceptives (Voinescu and Pennell 2017). When deciding on a contraceptive strategy, liaison with the woman's pharmacist and neurologist is recommended to optimise the care plan and minimise drug interactions.

10.6.2 Medication Review: Altering Medications Appropriately in the Preconception Phase

While care needs to be individualised, there are some basic principles that apply in the preconception care of women with epilepsy or seizure disorder. The first is to avoid the use of sodium valproate if at all possible. While there is an increased risk of fetal malformation with many antiseizure drugs, valproate has been consistently identified as the agent with the highest associated risk (Meador et al. 2008). Valproate is also associated with neurocognitive developmental delay in the offspring (Bromley et al. 2014). Therefore, if clinically feasible with respect to the woman's seizure disorder, valproate should be withdrawn prior to conception.

Another general principle is to minimise exposure to medication as much as possible. This means rationalising antiseizure therapy to a single agent if possible and minimising the dose of the agent used. Single-agent pharmacotherapy of epilepsy is associated with a lower risk of fetal malformation than regimens that include multiple agents (Tomson et al. 2011; Mawhinney et al. 2013). Similarly, lower doses of some antiseizure drugs are associated with lower rates of fetal malformation (Tomson et al. 2011).

If rationalising therapy, the antiseizure medications associated with the lowest risk of fetal malformation include lamotrigine, levetiracetam, and carbamazepine (Tomson et al. 2011; Mawhinney et al. 2013). The evidence base is incomplete at this point, and the ultimate decision on medication changes needs to be made in collaboration with the woman and her neurologist.

10.7 Disease-Modifying Therapy and Anti-inflammatory Therapy in Rheumatological and Gastrointestinal Disease: Important Points

Rheumatological disease and gastrointestinal disease are found with increasing frequency in women of reproductive age. Inflammatory bowel disease affects up to 1% of reproductively aged women and men, with an emerging trend for increasing prevalence (Kappelman et al. 2007; Ng et al. 2018). In the case of rheumatoid arthritis, up to 1% of women of reproductive age are affected (Dugowson et al. 1991). Vasculitides are less prevalent, but conditions such as lupus are becoming more common and primarily affect women of reproductive age (Danchenko et al. 2006).

This increase in prevalence of rheumatological and gastrointestinal disease is likely due to a combination of factors, including improved detection and diagnosis (Uramoto et al. 1999). Other factors such as dietary changes and environmental factors have been suggested as causal or contributory. However, while there is a clear trend towards increased incidence and prevalence, there is no clear indicator as to why these conditions are becoming more common (Molodecky et al. 2012).

The morbidity and mortality associated with disease-modifying therapy and anti-inflammatory therapy in rheumatological and gastrointestinal disease vary significantly between treatments. Some therapies are relatively low risk or are not known to impair fertility or increase the risk of antenatal complications. In some cases, risks are dose dependent. In all cases, a primary aim is to ensure that maternal disease remains controlled. Therefore, individualised preconception care is the only appropriate approach in people using disease modifying therapy or anti-inflammatory therapy.

Inflammatory bowel disease is the most common class of gastrointestinal disease requiring disease-modifying therapy. In inflammatory bowel disease, both the disease itself and the treatment can complicate preconception care. Fertility can be impaired in both men and women by both disease activity and previous surgical interventions such as proctocolectomy (Mahadevan et al. 2019; Van Assche et al. 2010; Waljee et al. 2006; Narendranathan et al. 1989), Active inflammatory bowel disease at the time of conception or during pregnancy is associated with an increased risk of complications during pregnancy (Norgard et al. 2007).

The term 'rheumatological disease' encompasses a wide range of conditions that include rheumatoid arthritis, lupus, and other vasculitic disorders. In some of these conditions, fertility can be impaired, and pregnancy complications can be more common due to an increased risk of thrombosis (Ostensen et al. 2015). Therefore, the specific preconception care plan for a woman with rheumatological disease will depend entirely on the type of disease she has and the type of disease-modifying therapy used.

10.7.1 Treatment Targets

Preconception care in the context of rheumatological and gastrointestinal disease is complicated, and treatment targets need to be individualised. In general, the treatment target is to minimise the risk of disease flare in the women and men who are planning pregnancy while minimising risk of impaired fertility and complications in pregnancy by adjusting medical therapy. This should be done following an individualised assessment in collaboration with the woman, her preconception care team, and her primary rheumatology or gastroenterology teams.

All women on disease-modifying agents should be on folic acid supplementation. In the case of rheumatological disease, the woman's rheumatology team should be involved in preconception care. In general, sulphasalazine and hydroxychloroquine are not associated with a significant risk of complications in pregnancy and can be continued. Steroids, non-steroidal anti-inflammatory analgesia, and tumour necrosis factor inhibitors are not associated with a significantly elevated risk of complications in pregnancy, but doses should be reduced as much as possible by the woman's primary rheumatology team to minimise drug exposure during pregnancy (Flint et al. 2016a, b).

Some agents are strongly associated with severe adverse events in pregnancy and should be discontinued prior to conception by the woman's primary rheumatology team. Methotrexate, leflunomide, and mycophenolate mofetil are all associated with a very high risk of complications including miscarriage and fetal anomalies (Flint et al. 2016a, b; Gotestam Skorpen et al. 2016; Buckley et al. 1997; Ostensen et al. 2006). The evidence base of mycophenolate mofetil-associated complications is underdeveloped, but the current advice is to discontinue mycophenolate mofetil completely prior to pregnancy (Ostensen et al. 2006). Methotrexate should be discontinued for at least 3 months prior to conception in both men and women given its longer half-life (Flint et al. 2016a, b; Gotestam Skorpen et al. 2016).

In inflammatory bowel disease, men should discontinue sulphasalazine if planning pregnancy, as this agent impairs sperm function and is associated with oligospermia (Wu et al. 1989). As with the use of disease-modifying therapy in rheumatological conditions, steroids, thiopurines, and tumour necrosis factor inhibitors should be dose reduced as much as possible but can be continued in pregnancy as clinically indicated (Nguyen et al. 2016). Methotrexate should be discontinued prior to conception for at least 3 months in both men and women (Flint et al. 2016b; Gotestam Skorpen et al. 2016).

10.8 Cystic Fibrosis and Respiratory Disease

Cystic fibrosis (CF) is a condition that affects at least 1 in 3200 people with white European ancestry (Hamosh et al. 1998). It is less common in other ethnic groups. Historically, CF resulted in death in childhood or early adulthood. However, with improved multidisciplinary care focused on optimising nutrition and respiratory function, most people with CF now live into adulthood, and rates of pregnancy, though low, have increased over time (Edenborough et al. 2008; Heltshe et al. 2017).

Men and women with CF have impaired fertility due to inhibition of sperm transport, menstrual disturbance, and changes in cervical secretions (Sueblinvong and Whittaker 2007). Most men and some women with CF will need assisted conception in order to become pregnant. However, with good preconception care, many people with CF can conceive, and the majority of pregnancies have a good outcome, with live birth rates comparable to the non-CF population (Heltshe et al. 2017; Boyd et al. 2004; Frangolias et al. 1997; Gilljam et al. 2000).

In women with CF, pregnancy produces a physiological deterioration in respiratory function, with a small but significant increased risk of respiratory failure and death (Boyd et al. 2004; Frangolias et al. 1997; Gilljam et al. 2000; Patel et al. 2015). In most women, the respiratory deterioration associated with pregnancy is transitory, and there is no persistent change in lung function postpartum as a result of pregnancy (Edenborough et al. 2008). However, given the reduction in lung capacity during pregnancy, woman should be counselled as to the risk of respiratory decline in pregnancy prior to conception. This is especially important in women with worse than average lung function parameters at baseline, as they are at a greater risk of critical decline during pregnancy (Boyd et al. 2004; Frangolias et al. 1997; Gilljam et al. 2000; Lau et al. 2011).

The risk of miscarriage, preterm labour, and other complications in pregnancy is generally more common in women with CF (Heltshe et al. 2017; Gilljam et al. 2000; Edenborough et al. 1995; Thorpe-Beeston et al. 2013). However, the degree of risk associated with pregnancy does appear to vary depending on genotype and preconception lung function (Edenborough et al. 2008; Heltshe et al. 2017). Therefore, preconception counselling does need to be individualised based on the woman's genotype and clinical phenotype.

Operative delivery and induction of labour can be more common, but in some series women with CF have caesarean rates comparable to the non-CF population (Girault et al. 2016). Therefore, it is entirely possible, with good preconception and antenatal care, for women to have a healthy pregnancy and a vaginal delivery.

Cystic fibrosis is associated with a specific form of diabetes termed cystic fibrosis-related diabetes, which is characterised by coexistent defects in insulin secretion with fluctuating insulin resistance. Cystic fibrosis-related diabetes affects up to 50% of women with CF (Moran et al. 2009). Interestingly, the diagnosis of diabetes does not appear to increase the risk of complications in pregnancy, although the evidence base at present is underdeveloped (Reynaud et al. 2017). However, as with any woman with diabetes, glycaemic control should be optimised, and retinal screening should be up to date, prior to conception.

10.8.1 Treatment Targets: Nutrition and Medical Therapy

In preparation for pregnancy, women with CF should have their nutritional status assessed and optimised by a specialist dietician within their primary CF team. Preconception malnutrition is associated with poor maternal and fetal outcomes, but optimising a woman's nutritional status prior to conception can improve these outcomes (Cheng et al. 2006). A focus on macronutrients is important, as higher maternal weight prior to pregnancy is associated with better antenatal and postnatal outcomes (Lau et al. 2011; Edenborough et al. 1995). However, micronutrient assessment and folic acid supplementation should also be part of the nutritional assessment (Edenborough et al. 2008).

Enhanced medical therapy and physiotherapy are recommended prior to conception to optimise respiratory capacity as much as possible. As outlined above, reduced respiratory capacity prior to pregnancy is associated with worse antenatal outcomes (Boyd et al. 2004; Frangolias et al. 1997; Gilljam et al. 2000; Lau et al. 2011). Therefore, maximising respiratory function prior to pregnancy may improve pregnancy outcomes and mitigate against clinically important respiratory decline during pregnancy.

Genetic counselling should be offered to people with CF planning pregnancy (Edenborough et al. 1995). This will involve testing of partners. As genetic counselling will determine the risk to the fetus of having CF, the offer of counselling should be made sensitively. Due consideration should be given to cultural and social sensitivities that may apply.

10.8.2 Medication Review: Altering Medications Appropriately in the Preconception Phase

In general, the medical therapy used in CF is safe in pregnancy and so adjustments do not need to be made prior to conception (Edenborough et al. 2008). However, people with CF do develop regular respiratory infections, and certain antibiotic therapy may need to be avoided during pregnancy. Pharmacy review of the individual's medical therapy is recommended as part of preconception care, and plans made for respiratory infection management in pregnancy, so that antimicrobial treatment is effective and safe.

10.9 Conclusion

Managing chronic medical conditions in pregnancy is becoming increasingly common. While chronic medical conditions are often associated with poor maternal and fetal outcomes in pregnancy, with good preconception care, the risk of poor outcomes can be reduced and even normalised in some cases.

Unfortunately, despite the risks associated with chronic medical conditions, it remains the case that most women with these conditions do not plan their pregnancy and are not well prepared for pregnancy. Therefore, there is a clear need to increase awareness among women and healthcare providers about the importance of preconception care and pregnancy planning when there is a coexistent chronic medical condition. Providers should routinely ask their patients about their desire to become pregnant in the future, be prepared to provide supportive care to women who wish to conceive, and encourage open conversations about this important topic.

Management of chronic medical conditions is individualised, and so while we can apply some broad principles to the approach taken in preconception care (as in Table 10.1), we must always remember to individualise our care plans. Some of the broad recommendations made are suitable for many or most women, but will be entirely unsuitable, or even detrimental, to some women. Therefore, it is vital to keep the woman at the centre of the care plan, by setting targets and adjusting therapy in collaboration with the woman and her primary specialist team. Additionally, the woman's environmental, economic, and social context should be taken into

Table 10.1 Reference guide for the preconception management of chronic medical conditions

Condition	Treatment targets	Medication adjustment

Pre-gestational diabetes	• Glycaemic control
	  – HbA1c 48 mmolmol (6.5%) or less.
	  – Capillary blood glucose concentrations
	  Fasting (on waking) 5–7 mmol/L
	  Before meals 4–7 mmol/L
	  Two hours after meals 5–9 mmol/L
	• Blood pressure
	  – <140/90 mmHg in all women
	  – <130/80 mm hg in women with complications
	• Lipids
	  – Cholesterol: No treatment target needed
	  – Triglycerides: <10 mmol/L (886 mg/dL)
	• Hypoglycaemia management
	  – Hypoglycaemic awareness formally assessed
	  – Management of severe hypoglycaemia reviewed
	• Folic acid use: Minimum 4 mg daily
	• Complete microvascular complication screening
	  – Retinopathy screening
	  – Urinary albumin creatinine ratio
	  – Serum creatinine
	  – Neurological examination
		• Insulin: If on mixed insulin on entry to preconception care, then consider conversion to MDI or CSII
		• Adjust insulin and carbohydrate ratios to meet glycaemic targets
		• Metformin: Continue
		• All other non-insulin glycaemic therapy: Discontinue
		• Antihypertensive therapy: See 'hypertension' section below
		• Lipid therapy: See 'Dyslipidaemia' section below

(continued)

Table 10.1 (continued)

Condition	Treatment targets	Medication adjustment
Hyperthyroidism (thyrotoxicosis)	• Free thyroxine (T4) concentrations: At or just above the upper limit of normal • TSH concentrations: No specific treatment target • Standard folic acid replacement	• Convert from methimazole or carbimazole to propylthiouracil • Minimise dose of antithyroid therapy as much as possible while maintaining treatment targets • Avoid radioiodine therapy
Hypothyroidism (primary or subclinical)	• Free thyroxine (T4) concentrations: No specific treatment target • TSH concentrations – TSH 0.2–2.5 mIU/L • Standard folic acid replacement	• Adjust thyroid supplementation as needed to achieve treatment targets
Adrenal insufficiency	• Ensure steroid replacement is adequate • Ensure annual review with endocrinologist is ongoing • Prepare steroid management plan for labour • Standard folic acid replacement	• No adjustment needed
Polycystic ovarian syndrome	• Regular menses (if possible) • Screen for diabetes • Ensure blood pressure is normal • Standard folic acid replacement	• No specific adjustment needed • If on metformin, then this can continue
Hyperprolactinaemia	• Regular menses • If menses not regular, then target is normal prolactin concentrations • Screen for pituitary tumour – Consult with endocrinologist regarding need for pituitary imaging • Standard folic acid replacement	• Reduce dose of dopamine agonist (cabergoline, bromocriptine) as much as possible while maintaining normal menses OR normal prolactin concentrations

Hypertension	• Blood pressure at least <150/90 mmHg in all women
	• Blood pressure at least <140/80 mmHg in women with associated cardiovascular or renal disease
	• Blood pressure at least <130/80 mmHg in women with comorbid complicated diabetes
	• Standard folic acid replacement
		• Discontinue
		  – Angiotensin receptor blockers
		  – Angiotensin-converting enzyme inhibitors
		  – Potassium-sparing diuretics
		• Continue or convert treatment to
		  – Appropriate beta blockers
		  – Methyldopa
		  – Nifedipine or other calcium channel antagonists
		  – Thiazide diuretics
		  – Hydralazine

Table 10.1 (continued)

Condition	Treatment targets	Medication adjustment
Dyslipidaemia	• Cholesterol: No treatment target needed • Triglycerides: <10 mmol/L (886 mg/dL) • Standard folic acid replacement	• Discontinue statins • Triglyceride therapy: Discontinue unless severe hypertriglyceridemia present • In cases of severe hypertriglyceridemia or other lipid disorders, then seek specialist advice
Epilepsy and seizure disorders	• Minimise maternal seizure activity • Folic acid 4–5 mg daily	• Discontinue sodium valproate if possible • Rationalise anticonvulsant therapy to a one agent regimen if possible • Prefer lamotrigine, carbamazepine, and levetiracetam as anticonvulsant therapy

consideration when crafting treatment plans to make sure she has the resources and support she needs to act on that plan—regardless of pregnancy intention.

Close liaison with the primary specialist team is essential to provide good pre-conception care. Histories of previous poor responses to alterations in treatment, for example, will be invaluable in amending medical therapy in the preconception phase. Specific specialist support in the management of disease complications will often be needed. Therefore, preconception care clinics focused on a specific disease or condition (as is increasingly available for women with diabetes) that includes both preconception care and medical specialists is a model to consider. People living with chronic conditions deserve quality care, which includes access to providers who are willing and able to help women who wish to become mothers achieve that goal in a way that supports their health and that of their future child.

10.10 Recommendations for Practice

- Preconception care of chronic medical conditions should involve the teams who usually provide specialist care for the woman planning pregnancy.
- Treatment targets should be agreed in collaboration with the woman and her primary specialist team and with reference to the existing evidence base.
- Medication adjustment should be made following consultation with the woman's primary specialist team: this is especially important in the case of epilepsy and disorders treated with disease-modifying therapy.
- Managing chronic medical conditions in pregnancy adds additional stress and anxiety for the prospective parents: women and men should be reassured that with good preconception care, pregnancy outcomes are expected to approach that of the reference population in most cases.

References

ABCD-DTN-UK. Best Practice Guide: Continuous subcutaneous insulin infusion (CSII). A clinical guide for adult diabetes services. https://abcd.care/sites/abcd.care/files/BP_DTN_v13%20 FINAL.pdf. 2018.

ACOG Practice Bulletin No. 203. Chronic hypertension in pregnancy. Obstet Gynecol 2019;133(1):e26-e50.

Alexander EK, Pearce EN, Brent GA, Brown RS, Chen H, Dosiou C, et al. 2017 guidelines of the American Thyroid Association for the diagnosis and management of thyroid disease during pregnancy and the postpartum. Thyroid. 2017;27(3):315–89.

American Diabetes Association. Management of diabetes in pregnancy: standards of medical care in diabetes-2019. Diabetes Care. 2019;42(Suppl 1):S165–S72.

Aoki Y, Belin RM, Clickner R, Jeffries R, Phillips L, Mahaffey KR. Serum TSH and total T4 in the United States population and their association with participant characteristics: National Health and Nutrition Examination Survey (NHANES 1999–2002). Thyroid. 2007;17(12):1211–23.

Artama M, Auvinen A, Raudaskoski T, Isojarvi I, Isojarvi J. Antiepileptic drug use of women with epilepsy and congenital malformations in offspring. Neurology. 2005;64(11):1874–8.

Baumfeld Y, Novack L, Wiznitzer A, Sheiner E, Henkin Y, Sherf M, et al. Pre-conception dyslipidemia is associated with development of preeclampsia and gestational diabetes mellitus. PLoS One. 2015;10(10):e0139164.

Becerra JE, Khoury MJ, Cordero JF, Erickson JD. Diabetes mellitus during pregnancy and the risks for specific birth defects: a population-based case-control study. Pediatrics. 1990;85(1):1–9.

Berg CJ, Callaghan WM, Syverson C, Henderson Z. Pregnancy-related mortality in the United States, 1998 to 2005. Obstet Gynecol. 2010;116(6):1302–9.

Blumer I, Hadar E, Hadden DR, Jovanovic L, Mestman JH, Murad MH, et al. Diabetes and pregnancy: an endocrine society clinical practice guideline. J Clin Endocrinol Metab. 2013;98(11):4227–49.

Boyd JM, Mehta A, Murphy DJ. Fertility and pregnancy outcomes in men and women with cystic fibrosis in the United Kingdom. Hum Reprod. 2004;19(10):2238–43.

Bozdag G, Mumusoglu S, Zengin D, Karabulut E, Yildiz BO. The prevalence and phenotypic features of polycystic ovary syndrome: a systematic review and meta-analysis. Hum Reprod. 2016;31(12):2841–55.

Bramham K, Parnell B, Nelson-Piercy C, Seed PT, Poston L, Chappell LC. Chronic hypertension and pregnancy outcomes: systematic review and meta-analysis. BMJ. 2014;348:g2301.

Bromley R, Weston J, Adab N, Greenhalgh J, Sanniti A, McKay AJ, et al. Treatment for epilepsy in pregnancy: neurodevelopmental outcomes in the child. Cochrane Database Syst Rev. 2014;10:CD010236.

Buckley LM, Bullaboy CA, Leichtman L, Marquez M. Multiple congenital anomalies associated with weekly low-dose methotrexate treatment of the mother. Arthritis Rheum. 1997;40(5):971–3.

Callaway LK, O'Callaghan M, McIntyre HD. Obesity and the hypertensive disorders of pregnancy. Hypertens Pregnancy. 2009;28(4):473–93.

CDC 2016. Center for Disease Control US Medical Eligibility for Contraceptive Use.

Chaker L, Bianco AC, Jonklaas J, Peeters RP. Hypothyroidism. Lancet. 2017;390(10101):1550–62.

Chen L, Hu R. Thyroid autoimmunity and miscarriage: a meta-analysis. Clin Endocrinol. 2011;74(4):513–9.

Cheng EY, Goss CH, McKone EF, Galic V, Debley CK, Tonelli MR, et al. Aggressive prenatal care results in successful fetal outcomes in CF women. J Cyst Fibros. 2006;5(2):85–91.

Choudhary P, Rickels MR, Senior PA, Vantyghem M-C, Maffi P, Kay TW, et al. Evidence-informed clinical practice recommendations for treatment of type 1 diabetes complicated by problematic hypoglycemia. Diabetes Care. 2015;38(6):1016–29.

Creanga AA, Berg CJ, Syverson C, Seed K, Bruce FC, Callaghan WM. Pregnancy-related mortality in the United States, 2006–2010. Obstet Gynecol. 2015;125(1):5–12.

Creanga AA, Syverson C, Seed K, Callaghan WM. Pregnancy-related mortality in the United States, 2011–2013. Obstet Gynecol. 2017;130(2):366–73.

Curtis KM, Tepper NK, Jatlaoui TC, Berry-Bibee E, Horton LG, Zapata LB, et al. U.S. medical eligibility criteria for contraceptive use, 2016. MMWR Recommend Rep. 2016;65(3):1–103.

Damm P, Houshmand-Oeregaard A, Kelstrup L, Lauenborg J, Mathiesen ER, Clausen TD. Gestational diabetes mellitus and long-term consequences for mother and offspring: a view from Denmark. Diabetologia. 2016;59(7):1396–9.

Danchenko N, Satia JA, Anthony MS. Epidemiology of systemic lupus erythematosus: a comparison of worldwide disease burden. Lupus. 2006;15(5):308–18.

Davies MJ, D'Alessio DA, Fradkin J, Kernan WN, Mathieu C, Mingrone G, et al. Management of hyperglycemia in Type 2 diabetes, 2018. A consensus report by the American Diabetes Association (ADA) and the European Association for the Study of Diabetes (EASD). Diabetes Care. 2018a;41(12):2669–701.

Davies MJ, D'Alessio DA, Fradkin J, Kernan WN, Mathieu C, Mingrone G, et al. Management of hyperglycaemia in type 2 diabetes, 2018. A consensus report by the American Diabetes Association (ADA) and the European Association for the Study of Diabetes (EASD). Diabetologia. 2018b;61(12):2461–98.

De Groot L, Abalovich M, Alexander EK, Amino N, Barbour L, Cobin RH, et al. Management of thyroid dysfunction during pregnancy and postpartum: an Endocrine Society clinical practice guideline. J Clin Endocrinol Metab. 2012;97(8):2543–65.

De Leo S, Lee SY, Braverman LE. Hyperthyroidism. Lancet. 2016;388(10047):906–18.

Deputy NP, Kim SY, Conrey EJ, Bullard KM. Prevalence and changes in preexisting diabetes and gestational diabetes among women who had a live birth - United States, 2012–2016. MMWR Morb Mortal Wkly Rep. 2018;67(43):1201–7.

Dhillon-Smith RK, Middleton LJ, Sunner KK, Cheed V, Baker K, Farrell-Carver S, et al. Levothyroxine in women with thyroid peroxidase antibodies before conception. N Engl J Med. 2019;380:1316–25.

Diabetes Control and Complications Trial Research Group, Nathan DM, Genuth S, Lachin J, Cleary P, et al. The effect of intensive treatment of diabetes on the development and progression of long-term complications in insulin-dependent diabetes mellitus. N Engl J Med 1993;329(14):977–986.

Donovan LE, Cundy T. Does exposure to hyperglycaemia in utero increase the risk of obesity and diabetes in the offspring? A critical reappraisal. Diabet Med. 2015;32(3):295–304.

Dugowson CE, Koepsell TD, Voigt LF, Bley L, Nelson JL, Daling JR. Rheumatoid arthritis in women. Incidence rates in group health cooperative, Seattle, Washington, 1987–1989. Arthritis Rheum. 1991;34(12):1502–7.

Edenborough FP, Stableforth DE, Webb AK, Mackenzie WE, Smith DL. Outcome of pregnancy in women with cystic fibrosis. Thorax. 1995;50(2):170–4.

Edenborough FP, Borgo G, Knoop C, Lannefors L, Mackenzie WE, Madge S, et al. Guidelines for the management of pregnancy in women with cystic fibrosis. J Cyst Fibros. 2008;7(Suppl 1):S2–32.

Edey S, Moran N, Nashef L. SUDEP and epilepsy-related mortality in pregnancy. Epilepsia. 2014;55(7):e72–4.

Ehrmann DA, Barnes RB, Rosenfield RL, Cavaghan MK, Imperial J. Prevalence of impaired glucose tolerance and diabetes in women with polycystic ovary syndrome. Diabetes Care. 1999;22(1):141–6.

Feig DS, Donovan LE, Corcoy R, Murphy KE, Amiel SA, Hunt KF, et al. Continuous glucose monitoring in pregnant women with type 1 diabetes (CONCEPTT): a multicentre international randomised controlled trial. Lancet. 2017;390(10110):2347–59.

Fiest KM, Sauro KM, Wiebe S, Patten SB, Kwon CS, Dykeman J, et al. Prevalence and incidence of epilepsy: a systematic review and meta-analysis of international studies. Neurology. 2017;88(3):296–303.

Firoz T, Magee LA, MacDonell K, Payne BA, Gordon R, Vidler M, et al. Oral antihypertensive therapy for severe hypertension in pregnancy and postpartum: a systematic review. BJOG. 2014;121(10):1210–8; discussion 20

Fitton CA, Steiner MFC, Aucott L, Pell JP, Mackay DF, Fleming M, et al. In-utero exposure to antihypertensive medication and neonatal and child health outcomes: a systematic review. J Hypertens. 2017;35(11):2123–37.

Flint J, Panchal S, Hurrell A, van de Venne M, Gayed M, Schreiber K, et al. BSR and BHPR guideline on prescribing drugs in pregnancy and breastfeeding—Part II: analgesics and other drugs used in rheumatology practice. Rheumatology. 2016a;55(9):1698–702.

Flint J, Panchal S, Hurrell A, van de Venne M, Gayed M, Schreiber K, et al. BSR and BHPR guideline on prescribing drugs in pregnancy and breastfeeding—Part I: standard and biologic disease modifying anti-rheumatic drugs and corticosteroids. Rheumatology. 2016b;55(9):1693–7.

Forde R, Collin J, Brackenridge A, Charmley M, Hunt K, Forbes A. A qualitative study exploring the factors that influence the uptake of pre-pregnancy care among women with type 2 diabetes. Diabet Med. 2019. May 25 [Epub ahead of print]. PMID: 31127872.

Frangolias DD, Nakielna EM, Wilcox PG. Pregnancy and cystic fibrosis: a case-controlled study. Chest. 1997;111(4):963–9.

FSRH 2016. Faculty of Sexual and Reproductive Health UK Medical Eligibility Criteria for Contraceptive Use.

Gaede P, Vedel P, Larsen N, Jensen GV, Parving HH, Pedersen O. Multifactorial intervention and cardiovascular disease in patients with type 2 diabetes. N Engl J Med. 2003;348(5):383–93.

Gilljam M, Antoniou M, Shin J, Dupuis A, Corey M, Tullis DE. Pregnancy in cystic fibrosis. Fetal and maternal outcome. Chest. 2000;118(1):85–91.

Girault A, Blanc J, Gayet V, Goffinet F, Hubert D. Maternal and perinatal outcomes of pregnancies in women with cystic fibrosis—a single Centre case-control study. Respir Med. 2016;113:22–7.

Gold AE, MacLeod KM, Frier BM. Frequency of severe hypoglycemia in patients with type I diabetes with impaired awareness of hypoglycemia. Diabetes Care. 1994;17(7):697–703.

Goldenberg RL, McClure EM, Harrison MS, Miodovnik M. Diabetes during pregnancy in low- and middle-income countries. Am J Perinatol. 2016;33(13):1227–35.

Gotestam Skorpen C, Hoeltzenbein M, Tincani A, Fischer-Betz R, Elefant E, Chambers C, et al. The EULAR points to consider for use of antirheumatic drugs before pregnancy, and during pregnancy and lactation. Ann Rheum Dis. 2016;75(5):795–810.

Greenwood EA, Pasch LA, Cedars MI, Legro RS, Huddleston HG, Eunice Kennedy Shriver National Institute of Child Health and Human Development Reproductive Medicine Network. Association among depression, symptom experience, and quality of life in polycystic ovary syndrome. Am J Obstet Gynecol. 2018;219(3):279 e1–7.

Hamosh A, FitzSimmons SC, Macek M Jr, Knowles MR, Rosenstein BJ, Cutting GR. Comparison of the clinical manifestations of cystic fibrosis in black and white patients. J Pediatr. 1998;132(2):255–9.

Harden CL, Hopp J, Ting TY, Pennell PB, French JA, Hauser WA, et al. Practice parameter update: management issues for women with epilepsy—focus on pregnancy (an evidence-based review): obstetrical complications and change in seizure frequency: report of the Quality Standards Subcommittee and Therapeutics and Technology Assessment Subcommittee of the American Academy of Neurology and American Epilepsy Society. Neurology. 2009a;73(2):126–32.

Harden CL, Pennell PB, Koppel BS, Hovinga CA, Gidal B, Meador KJ, et al. Practice parameter update: management issues for women with epilepsy—focus on pregnancy (an evidence-based review): vitamin K, folic acid, blood levels, and breastfeeding: report of the Quality Standards Subcommittee and Therapeutics and Technology Assessment Subcommittee of the American Academy of Neurology and American Epilepsy Society. Neurology. 2009b;73(2):142–9.

Hayes DK, Fan AZ, Smith RA, Bombard JM. Trends in selected chronic conditions and behavioral risk factors among women of reproductive age, behavioral risk factor surveillance system, 2001–2009. Prev Chronic Dis. 2011;8(6):A120.

Heltshe SL, Godfrey EM, Josephy T, Aitken ML, Taylor-Cousar JL. Pregnancy among cystic fibrosis women in the era of CFTR modulators. J Cyst Fibros. 2017;16(6):687–94.

Hopkins D, Lawrence I, Mansell P, Thompson G, Amiel S, Campbell M, et al. Improved biomedical and psychological outcomes 1 year after structured education in flexible insulin therapy for people with type 1 diabetes: the U.K. DAFNE experience. Diabetes Care. 2012;35(8):1638–42.

IDF. International Diabetes Federation Diabetes Atlas. 8th ed. Brussels, Belgium; 2017. https://diabetesatlas.org

Jones JM, Lawson ML, Daneman D, Olmsted MP, Rodin G. Eating disorders in adolescent females with and without type 1 diabetes: cross sectional study. BMJ. 2000;320(7249):1563–6.

Kan C, Silva N, Golden SH, Rajala U, Timonen M, Stahl D, et al. A systematic review and meta-analysis of the association between depression and insulin resistance. Diabetes Care. 2013;36(2):480–9.

Kannel WB, Abbott RD. Incidence and prognosis of unrecognized myocardial infarction. An update on the Framingham study. N Engl J Med. 1984;311(18):1144–7.

Kappelman MD, Rifas-Shiman SL, Kleinman K, Ollendorf D, Bousvaros A, Grand RJ, et al. The prevalence and geographic distribution of Crohn's disease and ulcerative colitis in the United States. Clin Gastroenterol Hepatol. 2007;5(12):1424–9.

Karalis DG, Hill AN, Clifton S, Wild RA. The risks of statin use in pregnancy: a systematic review. J Clin Lipidol. 2016;10(5):1081–90.

Kelso AaWA. On behalf of the MBBRACE-UK Neurological Disorders Chapter Writing Group. Learning from neurological complications. In: Knight MKS, Brocklehurst J, Nelson J, Shakespeare J, Kurincuk JJ, editors. Oxford: National Perinatal Epidemiology Unit, University of Oxford; 2014.

Lamont T, Cousins D, Hillson R, Bischler A, Terblanche M. Safer administration of insulin: summary of a safety report from the National Patient Safety Agency. BMJ. 2010;341:c5269.

Lau EM, Barnes DJ, Moriarty C, Ogle R, Dentice R, Civitico J, et al. Pregnancy outcomes in the current era of cystic fibrosis care: a 15-year experience. Aust N Z J Obstet Gynaecol. 2011;51(3):220–4.

Laz TH, Rahman M, Berenson AB. Trends in serum lipids and hypertension prevalence among non-pregnant reproductive-age women: United States National Health and Nutrition Examination Survey 1999-2008. Matern Child Health J. 2013;17(8):1424–31.

Lindsay JR, Nieman LK. The hypothalamic-pituitary-adrenal axis in pregnancy: challenges in disease detection and treatment. Endocr Rev. 2005;26(6):775–99.

Luewan S, Chakkabut P, Tongsong T. Outcomes of pregnancy complicated with hyperthyroidism: a cohort study. Arch Gynecol Obstet. 2011;283(2):243–7.

Magee LA, Group CS, von Dadelszen P, Singer J, Lee T, Rey E, et al. Do labetalol and methyldopa have different effects on pregnancy outcome? Analysis of data from the Control of Hypertension in Pregnancy Study (CHIPS) trial. BJOG. 2016;123(7):1143–51.

Mahadevan U, Robinson C, Bernasko N, Boland B, Chambers C, Dubinsky M, et al. Inflammatory bowel disease in pregnancy clinical care pathway: a report from the American Gastroenterological Association IBD parenthood project working group. Gastroenterology. 2019;156(5):1508–24.

Mannucci E, Rotella F, Ricca V, Moretti S, Placidi GF, Rotella CM. Eating disorders in patients with type 1 diabetes: a meta-analysis. J Endocrinol Investig. 2005;28(5):417–9.

Mawhinney E, Craig J, Morrow J, Russell A, Smithson WH, Parsons L, et al. Levetiracetam in pregnancy: results from the UK and Ireland epilepsy and pregnancy registers. Neurology. 2013;80(4):400–5.

Meador K, Reynolds MW, Crean S, Fahrbach K, Probst C. Pregnancy outcomes in women with epilepsy: a systematic review and meta-analysis of published pregnancy registries and cohorts. Epilepsy Res. 2008;81(1):1–13.

Mendelson MM, Lyass A, O'Donnell CJ, D'Agostino RB Sr, Levy D. Association of Maternal Prepregnancy Dyslipidemia with Adult Offspring Dyslipidemia in excess of anthropometric, lifestyle, and genetic factors in the Framingham Heart Study. JAMA Cardiol. 2016;1(1):26–35.

Molodecky NA, Soon IS, Rabi DM, Ghali WA, Ferris M, Chernoff G, et al. Increasing incidence and prevalence of the inflammatory bowel diseases with time, based on systematic review. Gastroenterology. 2012;142(1):46–54 e42; quiz e30

Moran A, Dunitz J, Nathan B, Saeed A, Holme B, Thomas W. Cystic fibrosis-related diabetes: current trends in prevalence, incidence, and mortality. Diabetes Care. 2009;32(9):1626–31.

Moussa HN, Hosseini Nasab S, Haidar ZA, Blackwell SC, Sibai BM. Folic acid supplementation: what is new? Fetal, obstetric, long-term benefits and risks. Future Sci OA. 2016;2(2):FSO116.

Narendranathan M, Sandler RS, Suchindran CM, Savitz DA. Male infertility in inflammatory bowel disease. J Clin Gastroenterol. 1989;11(4):403–6.

Nathan DM, Cleary PA, Backlund JY, Genuth SM, Lachin JM, Orchard TJ, et al. Intensive diabetes treatment and cardiovascular disease in patients with type 1 diabetes. N Engl J Med. 2005;353(25):2643–53.

Negro R, Mangieri T, Coppola L, Presicce G, Casavola EC, Gismondi R, et al. Levothyroxine treatment in thyroid peroxidase antibody-positive women undergoing assisted reproduction technologies: a prospective study. Hum Reprod. 2005;20(6):1529–33.

Negro R, Formoso G, Mangieri T, Pezzarossa A, Dazzi D, Hassan H. Levothyroxine treatment in euthyroid pregnant women with autoimmune thyroid disease: effects on obstetrical complications. J Clin Endocrinol Metab. 2006;91(7):2587–91.

Ng SC, Shi HY, Hamidi N, Underwood FE, Tang W, Benchimol EI, et al. Worldwide incidence and prevalence of inflammatory bowel disease in the 21st century: a systematic review of population-based studies. Lancet. 2018;390(10114):2769–78.

Nguyen GC, Seow CH, Maxwell C, Huang V, Leung Y, Jones J, et al. The Toronto consensus statements for the Management of Inflammatory Bowel Disease in pregnancy. Gastroenterology. 2016;150(3):734–57. e1.

NHS_Digital. National Pregnancy in Diabetes Audit Report, 2016. 2017. https://digital.nhs.uk/data-and-information/publications/statistical/national-pregnancy-in-diabetes-audit/national-pregnancy-in-diabetes-annual-report-2016

NICE. Continuous subcutaneous insulin infusion for the treatment of diabetes mellitus. Technology appraisal guidance. TA151. 2008.

NICE. Hypertension and pregnancy: diagnosis and management. 2011. https://www.nice.org.uk/guidance/cg107/chapter/1-Guidance#management-of-pregnancy-with-chronic-hypertension

NICE. Diabetes in pregnancy: management from preconception to the postnatal period. NICE guideline. NG3. 2015a.

NICE. Type 2 diabetes in adults: management. NICE Guideline NG28. www.nice.org.uk/guidance/ng28. 2015b, updated May 2017.

Norgard B, Hundborg HH, Jacobsen BA, Nielsen GL, Fonager K. Disease activity in pregnant women with Crohn's disease and birth outcomes: a regional Danish cohort study. Am J Gastroenterol. 2007;102(9):1947–54.

Ostensen M, Khamashta M, Lockshin M, Parke A, Brucato A, Carp H, et al. Anti-inflammatory and immunosuppressive drugs and reproduction. Arthritis Res Ther. 2006;8(3):209.

Ostensen M, Andreoli L, Brucato A, Cetin I, Chambers C, Clowse ME, et al. State of the art: reproduction and pregnancy in rheumatic diseases. Autoimmun Rev. 2015;14(5):376–86.

Patel EM, Swamy GK, Heine RP, Kuller JA, James AH, Grotegut CA. Medical and obstetric complications among pregnant women with cystic fibrosis. Am J Obstet Gynecol. 2015;212(1):98 e1–9.

Pedersen-Bjergaard U, Pramming S, Heller SR, Wallace TM, Rasmussen ÅK, Jørgensen HV, et al. Severe hypoglycaemia in 1076 adult patients with type 1 diabetes: influence of risk markers and selection. Diabetes Metab Res Rev. 2004;20(6):479–86.

Qin JZ, Pang LH, Li MJ, Fan XJ, Huang RD, Chen HY. Obstetric complications in women with polycystic ovary syndrome: a systematic review and meta-analysis. Reprod Biol Endocrinol RB&E. 2013;11:56.

Reynaud Q, Poupon-Bourdy S, Rabilloud M, Al Mufti L, Rousset Jablonski C, Lemonnier L, et al. Pregnancy outcome in women with cystic fibrosis-related diabetes. Acta Obstet Gynecol Scand. 2017;96(10):1223–7.

Shekhar S, Gupta N, Kirubakaran R, Pareek P. Oral nifedipine versus intravenous labetalol for severe hypertension during pregnancy: a systematic review and meta-analysis. BJOG. 2016;123(1):40–7.

Sibai BM. Chronic hypertension in pregnancy. Obstet Gynecol. 2002;100(2):369–77.

Soto-Pedre E, Newey PJ, Bevan JS, Greig N, Leese GP. The epidemiology of hyperprolactinaemia over 20 years in the Tayside region of Scotland: the Prolactin Epidemiology, Audit and Research Study (PROLEARS). Clin Endocrinol. 2017;86(1):60–7.

Sueblinvong V, Whittaker LA. Fertility and pregnancy: common concerns of the aging cystic fibrosis population. Clin Chest Med. 2007;28(2):433–43.

Taylor PN, Minassian C, Rehman A, Iqbal A, Draman MS, Hamilton W, et al. TSH levels and risk of miscarriage in women on long-term levothyroxine: a community-based study. J Clin Endocrinol Metab. 2014;99(10):3895–902.

Thangaratinam S, Tan A, Knox E, Kilby MD, Franklyn J, Coomarasamy A. Association between thyroid autoantibodies and miscarriage and preterm birth: meta-analysis of evidence. BMJ. 2011;342:d2616.

Thorogood M, Seed M, De Mott K, Guideline Development Group. Management of fertility in women with familial hypercholesterolaemia: summary of NICE guidance. BJOG. 2009;116(4):478–9.

Thorpe-Beeston JG, Madge S, Gyi K, Hodson M, Bilton D. The outcome of pregnancies in women with cystic fibrosis—single Centre experience 1998–2011. BJOG. 2013;120(3):354–61.

Tomson T, Battino D, Bonizzoni E, Craig J, Lindhout D, Sabers A, et al. Dose-dependent risk of malformations with antiepileptic drugs: an analysis of data from the EURAP epilepsy and pregnancy registry. Lancet Neurol. 2011;10(7):609–17.

Tunceli K, Bradley CJ, Nerenz D, Williams LK, Pladevall M, Elston LJ. The impact of diabetes on employment and work productivity. Diabetes Care. 2005;28(11):2662–7.

UK Prospective Diabetes Study (UKPDS) Group. Intensive blood-glucose control with sulphonylureas or insulin compared with conventional treatment and risk of complications in patients with type 2 diabetes (UKPDS 33). Lancet. 1998;352(9131):837–53.

Uramoto KM, Michet CJ Jr, Thumboo J, Sunku J, O'Fallon WM, Gabriel SE. Trends in the incidence and mortality of systemic lupus erythematosus, 1950–1992. Arthritis Rheum. 1999;42(1):46–50.

Van Assche G, Dignass A, Reinisch W, van der Woude CJ, Sturm A, De Vos M, et al. The second European evidence-based consensus on the diagnosis and management of Crohn's disease: special situations. J Crohns Colitis. 2010;4(1):63–101.

Vanderpump MP, Tunbridge WM, French JM, Appleton D, Bates D, Clark F, et al. The incidence of thyroid disorders in the community: a twenty-year follow-up of the Whickham survey. Clin Endocrinol. 1995;43(1):55–68.

Viale L, Allotey J, Cheong-See F, Arroyo-Manzano D, McCorry D, Bagary M, et al. Epilepsy in pregnancy and reproductive outcomes: a systematic review and meta-analysis. Lancet. 2015;386(10006):1845–52.

Voinescu PE, Pennell PB. Delivery of a personalized treatment approach to women with epilepsy. Semin Neurol. 2017;37(6):611–23.

Waljee A, Waljee J, Morris AM, Higgins PD. Threefold increased risk of infertility: a meta-analysis of infertility after ileal pouch anal anastomosis in ulcerative colitis. Gut. 2006;55(11):1575–80.

Wang H, Gao H, Chi H, Zeng L, Xiao W, Wang Y, et al. Effect of levothyroxine on miscarriage among women with Normal thyroid function and thyroid autoimmunity undergoing in vitro fertilization and embryo transfer: a randomized clinical trial. JAMA. 2017;318(22):2190–8.

Weindling AM. The confidential enquiry into maternal and child health (CEMACH). Arch Dis Child. 2003;88(12):1034–7.

WHO. Medical eligibility criteria for contraceptive use. 2015.

Wild S, Roglic G, Green A, Sicree R, King H. Global prevalence of diabetes: estimates for the year 2000 and projections for 2030. Diabetes Care. 2004;27(5):1047–53.

Wilson AM, Boyle AJ, Fox P. Management of ischaemic heart disease in women of child-bearing age. Intern Med J. 2004;34(12):694–7.

Wu FC, Aitken RJ, Ferguson A. Inflammatory bowel disease and male infertility: effects of sul-fasalazine and 5-aminosalicylic acid on sperm-fertilizing capacity and reactive oxygen species generation. Fertil Steril. 1989;52(5):842–5.

Yakoob MY, Bateman BT, Ho E, Hernandez-Diaz S, Franklin JM, Goodman JE, et al. The risk of congenital malformations associated with exposure to beta-blockers early in pregnancy: a meta-analysis. Hypertension. 2013;62(2):375–81.

Yamamoto JM, Hughes DJF, Evans ML, Karunakaran V, Clark JDA, Morrish NJ, et al. Community-based pre-pregnancy care programme improves pregnancy preparation in women with preges-tational diabetes. Diabetologia. 2018;61(7):1528–37.

Yoder SR, Thornburg LL, Bisognano JD. Hypertension in pregnancy and women of childbearing age. Am J Med. 2009;122(10):890–5.

Yuen KC, Chong LE, Koch CA. Adrenal insufficiency in pregnancy: challenging issues in diagno-sis and management. Endocrine. 2013;44(2):283–92.

Infectious Diseases

Dean V. Coonrod and Celeste V. Bailey

Infectious diseases play an important role in the lives of young adults, influencing their health and that of future children. Infections impact a number of important reproductive outcomes, including fertility, miscarriage and spontaneous abortion, fetal, newborn, delivery, and obstetric outcomes including low birthweight and preterm birth. Many different infectious agent types, including bacteria, parasites, and viruses, may influence birth outcomes as well as overall health. This chapter will focus on traditional infectious disease interventions in clinical care, such as treatment with appropriate anti-infective agents or prevention with immunizations. However, it is important to note that many infectious diseases include an element of environmental contribution and while not a focus of this discussion, the profound impact of public health interventions in mitigating infectious disease cannot be understated.

This chapter will purposefully not include breastfeeding, although this is an important intervention that has a connection with infectious disease. Likewise, the chapter will not focus on infections such as asymptomatic bacteriuria and screening for group B *Streptococcus* infection as they are addressed during pregnancy. Certain infectious conditions have previously been targeted for preconception care, but recent research suggested they are better addressed during pregnancy. For example, immunization for *pertussis* infection is now recommended during each pregnancy to promote optimal passive immunization and protection of the newborn. This chapter is meant to provide a general overview of key infections that should be addressed to support optimal health outcomes for young adults and their future children.

D. V. Coonrod (✉)
Department of Obstetrics and Gynecology, Valleywise Health / District Medical Group, Creighton University School of Medicine Regional Campus, Omaha, NE, USA

University of Arizona College of Medicine, Phoenix, AZ, USA
e-mail: dean_coonrod@dmgaz.org

C. V. Bailey
Obstetrics and Gynecology, Creighton University School of Medicine Regional Campus, Phoenix, USA
e-mail: Celeste.Bailey@valleywisehealth.org

© Springer Nature Switzerland AG 2020
J. Shawe et al. (eds.), *Preconception Health and Care: A Life Course Approach*,
https://doi.org/10.1007/978-3-030-31753-9_11

11.1 HIV and AIDS

The human immunodeficiency virus (HIV) is a virus that attacks the host immune system, causing acute and chronic infections (World Health Organization 2019h). It is transmitted through exchange of bodily fluids including semen, vaginal secretions, blood, and breastmilk (World Health Organization 2019h). At risk populations include individuals with a history of sexually transmitted infections; engaging in unprotected anal or vaginal sex; sharing needles while using intravenous drugs; and working in a healthcare setting (World Health Organization 2019h). Serodiscordant couples or non-monogamous couples are also at significant risk of seroconversion or acquired HIV infection (Centers for Disease Control and Prevention: US Public Health Service 2018). Research has shown that early detection of HIV leads to decreased transmission. The risk of vertical transmission in childbirth is related to antepartum viral load. Thus, early antiretoriviral therapy is a mainstay of prevention. (Committee Opinion No. 752 2018).

In 2017, an estimated 1.8 million people were infected with HIV with 36.9 million people worldwide living with HIV. The burden of disease is heavier in lower-income countries and lower-income areas of wealthy countries (UNAIDS 2018). Of those new infections, 180,000 were children, most of whom live in sub-Saharan Africa and were infected by vertical transmission (Centers for Disease Control and Prevention 2016a). An estimated 80% of HIV-seropositive pregnant woman worldwide had access to antiretrovirals to prevent vertical transmission (UNAIDS 2018).

A number of preconception strategies have been developed to decrease the risk of acquisition and vertical transmission. HIV testing should be done for anyone at risk. Partners should also be encouraged to get tested and counseled on safer sex practices. Healthcare providers need to discuss reproductive life planning with all women. For women with HIV positive male partners or in non-monogamous relationships, pre-exposure prophylaxis (PrEP) is encouraged. Men should be involved in reproductive goal planning and should be encouraged to participate in testing and safer sex/conception practices (Centers for Disease Control and Prevention: US Public Health Service 2018; AIDSinfo 2019). Open communication and disclosure of results between patient and partner should be encouraged by the care provider (World Health Organization 2019h; AIDSinfo 2019). Women with HIV of reproductive age should be on antiretroviral therapy. Serodiscordant couples will likely benefit from PrEP and HIV testing every 3 months, and they should be counseled to expect changes to their medical care during pregnancy. For example, medications may need to change depending on trimester and teratogenicity. For example, the use of dolutegravir is not recommended at less than 14 weeks and prior to conception due to risk of neural tube defects (AIDSinfo 2018). Furthermore, HIV-positive women are at increased risk of having a fetus with neural tube defects and should be encouraged to take a multivitamin with 400mcg folic acid (AIDSinfo 2019).

11.1.1 Recommendations for Practice

Given that the earlier antiretroviral treatment is started, the lower the risk of transmission, all women should be offered testing for HIV prior to pregnancy. Women and their partners should discuss reproductive life planning goals with providers. For serodiscordant couples, PrEP should be considered to reduce risk of seroconversion. Men and women in serodiscordant sexual relationships should get frequently tested and viral loads checked to ensure efficacy of the antiretroviral regimen. Shared decision-making regarding choice of antiretroviral medication is always important, but particularly prior to conception for some medications. All women, especially those that are HIV positive, should be on a multivitamin with folic acid. All people at risk for HIV infection should have access to testing and care.

11.2 Malaria

The sequelae of malaria infection can become a chronic challenge for all young adults and infection should be proactively prevented, screened for, and treated. Malaria in pregnancy significantly increases maternal and neonatal morbidity and mortality, largely due to risk of profound maternal anemia and low birth weight. The malaria parasite replicates in the placenta and placental parasitemia can cause low birth weight (World Health Organization 2017a). Complications of malaria infection in pregnancy include maternal and fetal anemia, spontaneous abortion, premature delivery, low birth weight, and congenital infection (Centers for Disease Control and Prevention 2019a).

In 2017 there were 435, 000 deaths from malaria. The disease is a significant burden on low-income countries. Most cases are concentrated in sub-Saharan Africa and India (World Health Organization 2018a). While mortality has decreased from 607,000 (2010) to 435,000 in 2017, there is an appreciable stagnation in preventing mortality (World Health Organization 2018a). It is estimated that one in four women in sub-Saharan Africa has evidence of placental malaria infection at birth (Desai et al. 2007).

Strategies for preconception prevention of malaria are similar to those employed for prevention outside of pregnancy. However, women trying to get pregnant in malaria endemic areas should be cautioned about the potential risks to fetus with doxycycline and atovaquone/proguanil. The teratogenicity of tetracyclines has been appreciated in the literature but not specifically doxycycline. Given this lack of evidence, there are certain cases where adjunct therapy with doxycycline may outweigh risk of teratogenicity (Cross et al. 2015).

The World Health Organization (WHO) recommends the use of long-lasting insecticidal nets (LLINs), intermittent preventive treatment in pregnancy (IPTp) with sulfadoxine-pyrimethamine (SP) as part of antenatal care services, and expediency in diagnosis and treatment of infection (World Health Organization 2017a).

11.2.1 Recommendations for Practice

Prevention of malaria infection is encouraged through environmental maintenance: management of mosquito breeding grounds, use of bed nets, use of insect repellent, and limiting activity at night (World Health Organization 2019a). Providers should discuss risks of travel to malaria-endemic areas with anyone of reproductive age. Women may consider use of reliable contraception to prevent conception while at risk for malaria exposure. In high-risk regions (sub-Saharan Africa), discuss with women opportunities to prevent acquisition of malaria in pregnancy using intermittent preventive treatment with sulfadoxine-pyrimethamine (IPTp-SP) (World Health Organization 2013).

11.3 Tuberculosis (TB)

Tuberculosis is primarily a pulmonary disease that can disseminate and cause further complications due to infection by *Mycobacterium tuberculosis* (Loto and Awowole 2012). Disseminated disease is more likely in the setting of HIV co-infection (Loto and Awowole 2012). TB outranks HIV/AIDS worldwide as a cause of death and is considered one of the top ten causes of mortality with 1.3 million deaths in 2017 in HIV-negative individuals and 300,000 more in those HIV positive (World Health Organization 2018b). Of the ten million individuals with TB disease, 3.2 are women and 1.0 million are children (World Health Organization 2018b). In addition to active TB, 25% of the world's population is affected with latent TB (World Health Organization 2018b).

Women of reproductive age suffer the greatest disease burden in areas of high prevalence (Marais et al. 2010), and TB is known to lead to tubal factor infertility (Namavar Jahromi et al. 2001). In pregnancy, TB leads to premature birth, low birth weight, growth restriction, fetal death, and rare instances of congenital TB (Loto and Awowole 2012; Marais et al. 2010). Infants of mothers with TB, especially those with maternal HIV, are at risk for TB and increased risk of mortality (Marais et al. 2010).

Screening and treatment before pregnancy is vital to avoid the risks of drugs that might pose a risk to the fetus such as streptomycin, pyrazinamide, and other second-line antituberculosis drugs (Marais et al. 2010). This means that counseling about birth control would be important in those of childbearing age.

In populations where latent TB treatment is the target, screening and treatment before pregnancy. This will avoid delays in treatment due to the risk of hepatotoxicity induced by isoniazid in pregnancy. The WHO prioritizes HIV-positive pregnant women for latent TB testing and treatment (Marais et al. 2010). The risk of hepatotoxicity induced by isoniazid in pregnancy can lead to complicated and delayed treatment plans (Marais et al. 2010). Focusing screening efforts in the preconception period for populations where latent TB treatment is the priority may lead to less complicated treatment decisions.

11.3.1 Recommendations for Practice

TB screening and treatment is best undertaken prior to pregnancy to avoid pregnancy complications associated with the disease and to simplify treatment decision-making around medication choice.

11.4 Listeria

Listeriosis is a serious foodborne illness caused by *Listeria monocytogenes* which causes noninvasive and invasive forms of the illness. Pregnant women are at a 20 times higher risk for listeriosis than other healthy adults. Further, they are at a higher risk for invasive disease, which includes sepsis and meningitis. Clinical course of this invasive form is complicated by a variable incubation period between a few days to 3 months. Pregnant women are at further risk of miscarriage, stillbirth, and preterm birth. Transplacental transmission can cause neonatal sepsis and meningitis which occur through transplacental transmission to the fetus (Marais et al. 2010).

Listeriosis is uncommon with about 0.1–10 cases per million. However, if invasive disease occurs, the mortality rate is high, about 20–30% (Marais et al. 2010), and the CDC estimates that listeriosis is the third leading cause of foodborne-related death in the United States (Centers for Disease Control and Prevention 2016b). Outbreaks attributed to specific foods are known to occur (World Health Organization 2007). Return to baseline infection rates result once the food causing the outbreak is identified and removed from circulation (World Health Organization 2007).

Food safety for the population is key since it includes reproductive-age women (World Health Organization 2007). This includes good hygiene practices and microbial testing strategies in the food supply (World Health Organization 2007). The long incubation period of invasive disease means that preconception exposures can lead to spontaneous abortion or severe disease in the mother during early pregnancy. Lifestyle changes to reduce risk of exposure are encouraged for women at risk of pregnancy or planning a pregnancy. These practices should be continued during the pregnancy (World Health Organization 2018c). Goals to prevent and treat infection are focused on vaccination and immune response to *L. monocytogenes* might represent future strategies (Clark et al. 2014).

11.4.1 Recommendations for Practice

At a preventive visit, during the preconception and the pregnancy period it can be discussed with women to avoid unpasteurized dairy products, deli/ready-to-eat meats, and cold-smoked seafood that pose a risk, i.e., smoked salmon. These foods should be cooked/heated to a steaming temperature (Ross et al. 2006). Storage and shelf-life instructions should be followed (World Health Organization 2018c). Educational materials about this can be found at the WHO (World Health Organization 2018d) and CDC web sites with the latter including specific education about exposures more common in certain subgroups (e.g., queso fresco—unpasteurized cheese among Latinos) and other high-risk foods such as raw sprouts and melons (Centers for Disease Control and Prevention 2016b).

11.5 Periodontal Disease

Periodontal disease is an inflammatory response to bacterial accumulation around the teeth (Amar and Kim 2008; Jiang et al. 2013). Pre-existing periodontal infection has been associated with risk of preterm labor, low birth weight, and preeclampsia (Daalderop et al. 2018). The mechanism is thought to be related to the chronic inflammatory state that a periodontal infection incites (Amar and Kim 2008; Crowther et al. 2005). It is also well-accepted that many women with periodontal disease fall within a more vulnerable patient population because good health literacy and adequate finances are needed to understand the importance of and to dedicate time to dental health.

It is estimated that 40% of pregnant women in the United States have periodontal disease in pregnancy (Committee Opinion No. 569 2017). Globally the prevalence of severe periodontitis in adults is estimated at 10%. The high prevalence of periodontal disease worldwide and its suspected influence on birth outcomes has made it a global health priority (Daalderop et al. 2018).

Women should be encouraged to seek out dental healthcare for their own health and well-being. Women may be more receptive to dental care if they are planning a pregnancy and made aware of the protection it could confer. Treatment of periodontal disease during pregnancy has not been shown to impact outcomes of preterm birth, low birth weight, or preeclampsia (Daalderop et al. 2018). However, providers should consider that this could be related to the already existing inflammatory response ongoing in the body. Dental disease treated in the preconception period has been theorized to be more directly beneficial (Xiong et al. 2011); although data is lacking, there is at least one planned randomized trial to test this in place (Jiang et al. 2013). Worldwide the disparity in adequate oral health continues to grow as people have less access to fluoride alongside heavy marketing of sugars, alcohol, and tobacco (World Health Organization 2018e). The American College of Obstetricians and Gynecologists (ACOG) oral health guidance should be discussed with all patients including those in the preconception window. They may be advised that they can have dental care at any time during pregnancy and care providers should create relationships with local dentists to provide care for underserved populations (Committee Opinion No. 569 2017).

11.5.1 Recommendations for Practice

Dental care should be discussed prior to pregnancy as the opportunity arises with an emphasis on good dental care, including attention to periodontal care. Patients can be told that pregnancy is not a reason to defer dental care. It is possible that there may be an advantage to treating periodontal disease prior pregnancy.

11.6 Sexually Transmitted Infections: Syphilis, Chlamydia, Gonorrhea, HPV, Hepatitis B and C, and HSV

11.6.1 Chlamydia

Infection with *Chlamydia trachomatis* remains the most prevalent sexually transmitted infection (STI) since 1994. Chlamydia infection can have profound impact on the future health of women, men, and offspring. Short-term sequelae of chlamydia infection include pelvic inflammatory disease (PID), epididymitis, and increased risk of infection with HIV. Long-term sequelae include infertility and chronic pelvic pain (Centers for Disease Control and Prevention 2018a). Genital chlamydia infection in pregnancy can have severe impacts on the neonate. Neonatal chlamydia infection may cause ophthalmia neonatorum or pneumonitis. There is also an increased risk of postpartum endometritis in genital chlamydia infection (Lingman et al. 2017).

The at-risk population includes women and men under the age of 25 years old and those older than 25 with multiple sexual partners, new sexual partners, or a history of sexually transmitted infections. Globally, criminalized and marginalized groups bear the burden of infection rates—people who inject drugs, sex workers, transgender people, men who have sex with men (MSM), and internally displaced and low-income individuals (World Health Organization 2019b). In the United States, chlamydia infection disproportionately affects blacks when compared to all other race/ethnicity groups (Centers for Disease Control and Prevention 2018a). The CDC reported over 1.7 million cases of chlamydia in the United States in 2017 with increasing rates over the last 4 years (Centers for Disease Control and Prevention 2018a). There is a similar picture worldwide with an estimated 131 million new cases of chlamydia annually (World Health Organization 2016a).

The focus in the preconception period should be on screening for chlamydia and evaluation of sexual behavior of patient and their partner(s) that may increase risk of infection (Committee Opinion No. 762 2002). Care providers should provide nonjudgmental inquiry into patients' sexual behavior and preferences to gather accurate assessment of risk (Committee Opinion No. 706 2017). The WHO recognizes that the best strategy to approach eradication of chlamydia is not yet defined

(World Health Organization 2016a). Current global prevention strategies focus on access to health information, condoms, and testing/treatment (World Health Organization 2016a).

11.6.1.1 Recommendations for Practice

Screening for chlamydia is an important aspect of preventive healthcare. There is some evidence to suggest that screening for chlamydia can reduce the risk of PID (Low et al. 2016). Screening should be done for any at-risk population, men and women younger than 25, and anyone with multiple sexual partners or new partner(s) (Centers for Disease Control and Prevention 2018a).

11.6.2 Gonorrhea

Infection with the organism, *Neisseria gonorrhoeae*, most commonly presents as a mucopurulent cervicitis in women or urethritis in men. It is transmitted through sexual contact. Infections can often be asymptomatic, making diagnosis and early treatment difficult (World Health Organization 2016b). Untreated infections can lead to pelvic inflammatory disease, ectopic pregnancy, and infertility in women and men. In neonates, vertical transmission of gonorrhea can cause neonatal conjunctivitis. Similar to chlamydia infections, gonococcal infections can also increase risk of HIV transmission (World Health Organization 2016b; World Health Organization 2019c).

Worldwide, there were an estimated 86.9 million new infections in 2016 (World Health Organization 2019b). In the United States, there are approximately 820,000 new infections annually, according to 2015 statistics (Centers for Disease Control and Prevention 2015a). Treatment-resistant gonorrhea infections are a rising concern. The WHO estimates 70% of countries participating in surveillance report antimicrobial resistance to *Neisseria gonorrhea* (World Health Organization 2016a). The most important component to prevention is annual screening and testing in those age 25 and under who are sexually active with new or multiple partners (World Health Organization 2016a; Committee Opinion No. 762 2002; Centers for Disease Control and Prevention 2015a).

11.6.2.1 Recommendations for Practice

Patient education is integral to prevention and treatment of sexually transmitted infections. Practitioners should utilize clinic visits as a nonjudgmental space to evaluate and encourage safe sex practices that decrease risk of sexually transmitted infections. Worldwide, healthcare providers need to offer nondiscriminatory and comprehensive testing and treatment for men and women at risk for or newly diagnosed with a STI (World Health Organization 2019b). Women who are at risk, as described above, should be offered sexually transmitted infection screening (World Health Organization 2016a; Committee Opinion No. 762 2002). In-clinic testing should be done for any woman with complaints consistent with possible gonococcal infection (Centers for Disease Control and Prevention 2015a). The risk of future infertility and chronic sequelae from sexually transmitted infections should also be emphasized (World Health Organization 2016a).

11.6.3 Syphilis

Syphilis is caused by the spirochete, *Treponema pallidum*, and is transmitted through sexual contact, vertical transmission in childbirth, and transplacental or intravenous drug use (Tsimis and Sheffield 2017). Syphilis infection presents in three stages. Primary syphilis is characterized by a painless, nontender, ulcerated lesion called a chancre. Often, because these are painless chancres, they may go unnoticed and syphilis is not often diagnosed in the primary stage (Tsimis and Sheffield 2017). The secondary stage is defined by infection of any organ system with the spirochete and can occur 4–10 years after initial infection. Patients may present with constitutional symptoms and maculopapular rash of palms and soles (Centers for Disease Control and Prevention 2019b). Finally, tertiary syphilis is characterized by local granulomatous lesions, called gumma, cardiovascular complications, and neurosyphilis. The tertiary stage is less commonly found in reproductive-aged women because of strong screening efforts in this population and long latency period (Tsimis and Sheffield 2017).

The early 2000s saw many successes in identification and treatment of disease, but since 2013 there has been a worldwide increase in the incidence of syphilis (Tsimis and Sheffield 2017; American College of Obstetricians and Gynecologists 2017). Populations at risk are men who have sex with men (MSM), individuals engaged in substance use or prostitution, communities of low socioeconomic status, and marginalized groups such as African-Americans and Hispanics in the United States (Tsimis and Sheffield 2017; World Health Organization 2019d). Data from 2017 demonstrates a dramatic correlation between recreational drug use and increased cases of syphilis in men who have sex with women (MSW) and in women (Centers for Disease Control and Prevention 2019b). Further, there is an increased risk of HIV transmission in patients with syphilis (Tsimis and Sheffield 2017). Maternal syphilis infection is an important cause of stillbirth and any woman with a stillbirth should be tested for the disease per ACOG guidelines. Clinical manifestation of congenital syphilis is extensive and includes nephrotic syndrome, deafness, or hepatosplenomegaly (Center for Disease Control and Prevention 2018).

The incidence of syphilis has been increasing (Tsimis and Sheffield 2017; World Health Organization 2019d)—globally, maternal syphilis infection causes 300,000 fetal and neonatal deaths a year (World Health Organization 2019a). The CDC estimates a 76% increase in number of syphilis cases in the United States over the last 6 years (Centers for Disease Control and Prevention 2019c). Further, the incidence of congenital syphilis has increased 43% from 2016 to 2017 (Centers for Disease Control and Prevention 2017). These changes represent a global challenge in preconception and peripartum care.

There is a need for increased screening in at-risk populations but also for care providers re-education on the importance of screening (Committee Opinion No. 569 2017). As the rates of syphilis had declined significantly after the 1990s, provider emphasis on screening did too (American College of Obstetricians and Gynecologists 2017). It is well accepted that strides in syphilis elimination were made with increased screening and access to treatment. The preconception period is a valuable opportunity for syphilis screening and education on safe sex practices.

11.6.3.1 Recommendations for Practice

The decentralization of testing and treatment centers has led to many successes in identification and treatment of syphilis in the developing world (World Health Organization 2019d). This model should be applied throughout low-resource settings with high syphilis prevalence. The increase in syphilis infection in MSW and women demonstrates a lack of population health perspective in prevention efforts. It is an important reminder to screen not only women in preconception period but encourage their partners to get screened as well.

11.6.4 Human Papilloma Virus (HPV)

The human papilloma virus (HPV) is a collection of over 120 different viruses that are associated with anogenital cancers and are transmitted through sexual contact (Immunization for Women 2015). In the United States, 66% of cervical cancer cases are attributed to HPV 16 and 18 and 90% of genital warts caused by HPV 6 and 11 (Human Papillomavirus Vaccination 2017). There is emerging evidence to support an association between HPV infection and risk of preterm birth and preeclampsia (Lawton et al. 2018; McDonnold et al. 2014).

The human papillomavirus is the most commonly transmitted sexual infection and causes the majority of cervical cancers (Immunization for Women 2015; Human Papillomavirus Vaccination 2017). Worldwide, there are an estimated 530,000 cervical cancer cases each year. There are 264,000 cases of cervical cancer deaths per year, contributing a significant burden of disability-adjusted life years (DALYs) globally (Global, Regional, and Cancer 2018). In the United States, there are an estimated 4000 deaths a year from cervical cancer (Immunization for Women 2015).

New data suggests that prior receipt of the quadrivalent HPV vaccine is protective against preterm birth (Lawton et al. 2018). The confirmation of this outcome with larger population studies would demonstrate an important public health opportunity globally.

11.6.4.1 Recommendations for Practice

- Routine screening for HPV infection and cervical cell dysplasia along with routine vaccination starting at 11–12 years old for young women and men (Immunization for Women 2015).
- Men should be vaccinated in the following cases: younger than age 21, men who have sex with men through age 26, transgender men through age 26, and men with immunocompromised conditions (CDC).

- Any patient who has not been vaccinated age 26 or younger should be offered the HPV vaccination (Human Papillomavirus Vaccination 2017).
- The WHO recommends HPV vaccination programs that educate individuals about cervical cancer while providing the vaccine (World Health Organization 2019a).

11.6.5 Hepatitis B

The hepatitis B virus (HBV) is an enveloped DNA virus that infects the liver and can eventually lead to liver cancer, liver failure, and death (World Health Organization 2015; American College of Obstetricians and Gynecologists 2007). The virus is transmitted through percutaneous or mucosal exposure and can survive up to 7 days outside of host on environmental surfaces (Schillie et al. 2018). Adults resolve the majority of infections (85%), but about 10% become chronically infected (American College of Obstetricians and Gynecologists 2007). HBV infection also puts people at risk of hepatitis D virus superinfection which has a significantly higher morbidity (70% develop cirrhosis) and mortality (25%). Populations most at risk are individuals who inject drugs, have multiple sexual partners, or have sexual partners with these risk-taking behaviors (American College of Obstetricians and Gynecologists 2007). Vertical transmission is the largest cause of chronic HBV infection worldwide; neonates and children under age 5 with HBV are much more likely to have chronic HBV compared to adults that get infected (World Health Organization 2015; American College of Obstetricians and Gynecologists 2007). Fortunately, infection is preventable with the hepatitis B vaccination, and the WHO and CDC recommend vaccination of children with the three-part series starting at birth (World Health Organization 2015; Schillie et al. 2018). For women with known HBV infection at time of birth, infants are given the vaccination and immunoglobulin to prevent chronic infection. Given the opportunity for prevention, the preconception period is an important time for action; the vaccination is also safe to be given in pregnancy (American College of Obstetricians and Gynecologists 2007).

There are an estimated 257 million individuals living with chronic HBV infection worldwide (World Health Organization 2017b). The CDC and WHO report gaps in diagnosis. Vertical transmission of HBV occurs in about 10–20% of women who are HBV positive. The risk of vertical transmission increases dramatically with concurrent hepatitis E virus (HEV) infection to 85–95% without neonatal prophylaxis.

The WHO encourages prevention of HBV infection through vaccination of nonpregnant and at-risk pregnant women as a priority action for countries (World Health Organization 2019b). Hepatitis B screening is a routine part of the prenatal visit. ACOG encourages screening tests to be labeled as "prenatal" so that they are done expeditiously and increase the chance of appropriate prophylaxis/treatment of vertical transmission (American College of Obstetricians and Gynecologists 2007). In serodiscordant couples, vaccination is highly encouraged (World Health Organization 2019b). If partner status is unknown, testing is encouraged (World Health Organization 2019b).

11.6.5.1 Recommendations for Practice

- It is well-accepted that the three-step HepB vaccination series should be started at birth (World Health Organization 2019b; American College of Obstetricians and Gynecologists 2007; Schillie et al. 2018).
- Anticipatory guidance for women with known HBV infection includes plan to start antiviral therapy with Tenofovir at 28 to 32 weeks of gestational age if they have high hepatitis B viral loads (Schillie et al. 2018). In this setting, neonates would still get HepB vaccination and HBIG within 12 hours of postpartum (Schillie et al. 2018).
- Screening for women at risk of HBV infection can lead to early treatment and better control of viral loads improving their well-being.
- Harm reduction intervention programs for people who inject drugs are a critical component of preventing HBV transmission (World Health Organization 2017b).

11.6.6 Hepatitis C

Infection in women with hepatitis C can lead to vertical infection to the infant (Lanini et al. 2016). Unlike hepatitis B, vertical transmission contributes less to the overall burden of disease for this condition, but it is a leading cause of childhood infection (Lanini et al. 2016). More common risk factors than vertical transmission include injection drug use, transfusions, and therapeutic injections given in unsafe conditions; the latter two are more important in developing countries (Lanini et al. 2016). Tattooing, scarification, and genital cutting have also been identified as contributing factors (Lanini et al. 2016). Important co-factors that contribute to complications include HIV and alcohol use (Lanini et al. 2016). Heterosexual sexual transmission is not a major contributor to disease acquisition; sexual transmission in men who have sex with men (MSM) who are HIV positive has been identified to contribute to outbreaks (Lanini et al. 2016).

It is estimated that 100 million are affected globally with about 700,000 deaths annually due to liver-related conditions (Lanini et al. 2016). Vertical transmission occurs in about 6% of newborns with HIV-negative mothers and 11% of those HIV positive (Benova et al. 2014).

With the appearance of antiretroviral therapies, screening for risk factors for hepatitis C with laboratory testing of those with risk factors is a strategy for control where access to therapy is available and affordable (World Health Organization 2018f). Direct-acting antiviral (DAA) therapies have limited information about use in pregnancy such that they are not recommended in pregnancy (World Health Organization 2018f). Ribavirin has been associated with fetal malformations such that contraception with two methods is recommended to be used during treatment and for 6 months after treatment (World Health Organization 2018f). Screening reproductive-age women and treatment prior to pregnancy can be a strategy to prevent vertical transmission (World Health Organization 2017c) and might represent a benefit over screening in pregnancy with post-pregnancy treatment (Hughes et al. 2017).

11.6.6.1 Recommendations for Practice

If screening for hepatitis C risk factors is recommended in primary care or pregnancy, it may be reasonable to do so as part of preconception care with a goal of prevention of maternal child transmission.

11.6.7 Herpes Simplex Virus (HSV)

Herpes simplex virus (HSV) is one of the most common sexually transmitted infections (Centers for Disease Control and Prevention 2017). It is transmitted through direct contact when the mucosa or opened skin is exposed. Traditionally, it was thought that only HSV-2 causes genital lesions, but there has been an emergence of HSV-1-specific genital lesions (American College of Obstetricians and Gynecologists 2002). After initial infection it can take almost 2 weeks before any noticeable inflammation or lesion occurs on the host's skin. Individuals affected then have recurrence of these lesions that can be painful and very irritating and can expose neonates to vertical transmission (American College of Obstetricians and Gynecologists 2002). An underlying herpes infection can also increase risk of transmission of HIV (World Health Organization 2019a). A primary lesion has a significantly higher viral load and is therefore more concerning for neonatal transmission in labor. There is no cure for herpes infection, only antiviral suppression therapy (Centers for Disease Control and Prevention 2017). Neonatal herpes manifests as disseminated disease, central nervous system disease, or mucosal surface infections. It is most commonly caused by HSV-1, and long-term sequelae are present in approximately 20% of neonatal HSV cases (American College of Obstetricians and Gynecologists 2002).

Globally, an estimated 412 million people are infected with HSV-2 (World Health Organization 2019a); the estimated prevalence of HSV-2 ranges from about 20% (Eastern Mediterranean) to 80% (Africa). In the United States, approximately 50 million individuals are infected with HSV-2; the strain most commonly attributed to genital herpes.

Vaccination for herpes virus has entered clinical trials (World Health Organization 2019b); this represents a promising preconception strategy. At this time, there is only treatment and prevention for outbreaks, but a method for prevention of initial infection would transform outcomes. Encouraging partners of known seronegative women seeking preconception counseling to get tested is an approach in prevention of seroconversion. This is especially important given the increased risk of vertical transmission with primary lesions. It is important for serodiscordant couples to use a barrier method when sexually active in pregnancy and to avoid any sexual intercourse in the third trimester. The risk of seroconversion and possibility of neonatal morbidity is high (American College of Obstetricians and Gynecologists 2002). At this time, however, there are no US recommendations to screen women for HSV serostatus (Centers for Disease Control and Prevention 2015b).

11.6.7.1 Recommendations for Practice

Some studies have suggested that a strategy for the prevention of infection includes encouraging partner testing for known seronegative women (Delaney et al. 2012). At present time, recommendations for practice are focused on viral suppression at 36 weeks for pregnant women with known herpes simplex infection. Avoiding sexual intercourse in serodiscordant couples during third trimester and consistent use of barrier contraception in first and second trimesters can assist with reducing the burden of disease (American College of Obstetricians and Gynecologists 2002).

11.7 Vaccine Preventable Diseases

11.7.1 Influenza

In a typical seasonal epidemic year, it is estimated that 5–15% of the population are affected worldwide (Nunes and Madhi 2018) leading to 300,000–650,000 deaths (Iuliano et al. 2018). Much of the burden is among those older than 65 or under age 1 (Nunes and Madhi 2018). Influenza infection is caused by a respiratory virus which can circulate in seasonal/epidemic form and pandemic forms (Epidemiology and Prevention of Vaccine-Preventable Diseases 2015a). Acute respiratory infection occurs with cases worsening and leading to death due to severe disease or secondary infection (Epidemiology and Prevention of Vaccine-Preventable Diseases 2015a). Those more prone to complications or worse disease include pregnant women and newborns (Epidemiology and Prevention of Vaccine-Preventable Diseases 2015a). Pregnant women have risks of complications similar to other groups deemed to be high risk (Epidemiology and Prevention of Vaccine-Preventable Diseases 2015a). Newborns have a greater risk due to undeveloped immune responses (Nunes and Madhi 2018). Vaccination in children is not recommended until age 6 months or more (Epidemiology and Prevention of Vaccine-Preventable Diseases 2015a) meaning that passive immunization is an important means of protection (Centers for Disease Control and Prevention 2018b).

In the United States, it is recommended that all individuals older than 6 months be vaccinated yearly for the influenza subtypes most likely to be in circulation (Epidemiology and Prevention of Vaccine-Preventable Diseases 2015a). This includes reproductive aged women and, if not yet vaccinated, pregnant women (Epidemiology and Prevention of Vaccine-Preventable Diseases 2015a; National Health Service 2019). In the United Kingdom, women free of chronic disease are recommended to be vaccinated only if pregnant (National Health Service 2019). These strategies lead to fewer complications for the woman in pregnancy and the newborn in the first few months of life, through passive immunization (Nunes and Madhi 2018; Epidemiology and Prevention of Vaccine-Preventable Diseases 2015a; American College of Obstetricians and Gynecologists 2018).

11.7.1.1 Recommendations for Practice

Reproductive-aged women should be advised to obtain the annual influenza vaccine or educated about the importance of the vaccine in pregnancy. Such vaccination provides benefit to both the pregnant mother and her newborn.

11.7.2 Varicella/Chickenpox

Prevention of congenital infection is the principal concern for consideration in preconception care for herpes zoster virus infection. This virus can cause both chickenpox and varicella zoster infection. In pregnancy, the former may be more serious for maternal health (varicella pneumonia) and rarely can be a concern for transmission if delivery occurs during acute infection (Gardella and Brown 2007). Congenital infection is characterized by scarred skin lesions, limb paresis or hypoplasia, optic lesion, and microcephaly (Gardella and Brown 2007).

Natural infection in childhood is quite likely and leads to protective immunity in the childbearing years, with 90% of adults showing immunity (Gardella and Brown 2007). Congenital varicella occurs in 0.4–2% of fetuses whose mother was primarily infected, i.e., chickenpox not varicella zoster which is a secondary infection (Gardella and Brown 2007).

A strategy of immunizing in childhood or prior to pregnancy is employed in the United States with the CDC citing a 90% decline in incidence, hospitalization, deaths, and infants (Centers for Disease Control and Prevention 2018b). Currently the United Kingdom does not recommend childhood vaccination citing concerns with a shift to more adult chickenpox and varicella zoster, further citing that natural immunity to childhood chickenpox leads to more protective immunity (National Health Service 2016). The WHO recommends countries with a high burden of VZV infection consider childhood vaccination so long as a goal of >80% coverage can be met, as lower levels risk shifting the burden to older age individuals and increased morbidity and mortality (World Health Organization 2014).

11.7.2.1 Recommendations for Practice

Screen for immunity at a preconception care visit with either a reliable history or documentation of vaccination. In a negative history of chickenpox, VZV antibodies can be assessed to document immunity. In the absence of immunity, a vaccine series might be recommended prior to pregnancy. It is considered contraindicated in pregnancy since it is a live attenuated vaccine (World Health Organization 2014).

11.7.3 Rubella

The rubella virus is transmitted through droplet exposure from infected persons (World Health Organization 2016c). Rubella infection is characterized by a prodromal maculopapular rash and subsequent low-grade fever, malaise, lymphadenopathy, upper respiratory symptoms, and arthralgias. Some infections may be subclinical (Bhise and Dhib-Jalbut 2014). Typically, rubella infections in an otherwise healthy adult are self-limited. Rubella infection in pregnancy, however, can cause fetal death, spontaneous abortion, or preterm delivery. Further, infection in pregnancy can lead to congenital rubella syndrome (CRS). The constellation of outcomes from CRS includes cataracts, deafness, cardiac defects, and intellectual developmental delay (IDD). Later manifestations of disease include diabetes mellitus or progressive encephalopathy diagnosed in childhood (Bhise and Dhib-Jalbut 2014).

Prior to the rubella vaccine, 4 in every 1000 live births were born with CRS (World Health Organization 2016c). In 2004, endemic transmission of rubella in the United States was determined to have ended (Centers for Disease Control and Prevention 2019d). Globally, there remains a significant burden of disease from rubella (Bhise and Dhib-Jalbut 2014), and it is the leading cause of vaccine-preventable birth defects (World Health Organization 2019e).

Vaccination is the key to prevention. Any child or adult without a contraindication should receive vaccination against rubella (MMR or MMRV) (World Health Organization 2016c; Centers for Disease Control and Prevention 2019d). Women need to understand risks associated with rubella infection in pregnancy and counseled on the risks of transmission in areas where prevalence remains high.

11.7.3.1 Recommendations for Practice

Women of childbearing age should be vaccinated for rubella. It is a live vaccine, however, and there is a theoretical risk of CRS if vaccination given in pregnancy. It is recommended that after getting vaccinated, women wait 4 weeks before becoming pregnant (World Health Organization 2016c; Centers for Disease Control and Prevention 2019d) and contraceptive counseling is important.

11.7.4 Tetanus

Tetanus occurs after wound infection by *Clostridium tetani* spores that are widespread in soil (Epidemiology and Prevention of Vaccine-Preventable Diseases 2015b). In hypoxic wounds, or closed-off wounds, it leads to development of a neurotoxin which can be highly fatal. The neurotoxin causes trismus (lockjaw) and muscle rigidity including respiratory muscles (Epidemiology and Prevention of Vaccine-Preventable Diseases 2015b). This is dangerous for all people regardless of childbearing intentions. Neonates can acquire this when the umbilical stump is cut with instruments contaminated with the spores. Neonatal tetanus has high case fatality (Epidemiology and Prevention of Vaccine-Preventable Diseases 2015b; World Health Organization 2019f). This mortal condition most often occurs in areas with poor hygiene at delivery and where tetanus toxoid coverage is low (Epidemiology and Prevention of Vaccine-Preventable Diseases 2015b; World Health Organization 2019f).

Globally 30,848 newborns died of tetanus in 2017 (World Health Organization 2019f). As of March 2018, 13 countries have not achieved the goal of elimination of maternal neonatal tetanus (World Health Organization 2019f).

Clinicians should ensure that women of reproductive age, including pregnant women, are vaccinated with the tetanus toxoid. This is through six doses of tetanus containing vaccine in childhood (three as infants and three more before adolescence) to allow for immunity to be robust in the reproductive years (World Health Organization 2019g; Thwaites et al. 2014).

11.7.4.1 Recommendations for Practice

In areas with high rates of neonatal tetanus, target special efforts to women of reproductive age and during pregnancy and promote hygienic childbirth practices (World Health Organization 2019g; Thwaites et al. 2014). Sustainability of immunity can be achieved through routine vaccination, booster administration, and maintaining hygienic childbirth practices (World Health Organization 2019g; Thwaites et al. 2014).

11.8 Prevention of Congenital Infections

11.8.1 Toxoplasmosis

Maternal infection with the protozoan parasite *Toxoplasma gondii* can cause congenital toxoplasmosis which may lead to significant morbidity to the fetus and newborn. Congenital toxoplasmosis may cause intellectual developmental delay, blindness, and epilepsy (Preventing Congenital Toxoplasmosis 2000). Typically, infection does not occur if a woman is infected prior to conception but can transmit across the placenta if she is infected after conception (Preventing Congenital Toxoplasmosis 2000). Exposure to the parasite occurs through eating or handling undercooked, contaminated meat or shellfish, drinking unpasteurized goat's milk or contaminated water, handling cat litter, or through contaminated soil (Centers for Disease Control and Prevention 2018c).

The exact burden of disease is difficult to estimate given that many immunocompetent individuals are asymptomatic. It is estimated that the highest burden of disease from congenital toxoplasmosis (CT) is in South America, and the highest incidence is in parts of Africa and the Middle East (Torgerson and Mastroiacovo 2013). The MMWR estimates 400–4000 cases of CT per year in the United States, but these statistics are from 2000 (Preventing Congenital Toxoplasmosis 2000).

Prevention of exposure is the goal of preconception strategies. This includes avoiding undercooked meats, making sure to wash fruits and vegetables, diligent handwashing before handling food, wearing gloves when working with soil, and avoiding contact with cat feces (Preventing Congenital Toxoplasmosis 2000; World Health Organization 2018g).

11.8.1.1   Recommendations for Practice

Prevention strategies should be reinforced at a preconception visit. Education in the preconception period has been associated with decreased infections (Ross et al. 2006; Breugelmans et al. 2005). Further, prepregnancy patient education can include information on opportunities for testing and treatment during pregnancy should a concern for fetal infection arise (World Health Organization 2018g).

11.8.2 Cytomegalovirus (CMV)

CMV infection is of greatest concern for the fetus as disease in adults is almost always mild and/or asymptomatic. It is the most common congenital infection (Practice Bulletin No. 151 2015). This herpes virus causes findings such as hearing loss, non-immune hydrops, growth restriction, myocarditis, petechiae, jaundice, and hepatosplenomegaly in the affected fetus (Practice Bulletin No. 151 2015). This can occur with either primary or secondary infection. Severe disease is possible with either form although much more likely with primary disease (Practice Bulletin No. 151 2015). Secondary infection leads to congenital hearing loss as its more serious consequence (Practice Bulletin No. 151 2015). As with adults, most infants are asymptomatic at birth (Practice Bulletin No. 151 2015).

CMV has been estimated to affect 0.2–2% of neonates (Practice Bulletin No. 151 2015); in developing countries 1–5% of births are affected (Manicklal et al. 2013). HIV infected newborns are at a three- to fivefold higher risk of infection (Manicklal et al. 2013).

A vaccine would prove beneficial for reducing the burden of disease of this virus with a number in development; this has been a long-term goal with few breakthroughs to date (Schleiss 2016). In the absence of a vaccine, prevention to avoid child-to-adult transmission has been recommended as a strategy to reduce congenital infection. As the virus is found in urine and saliva, efforts might include handwashing after feeding and changing diapers and avoiding saliva by not sharing of utensils and cups or when kissing young children. A subgroup at high risk, those seronegative working in day care, has had some data indicating targeted education would be a promising approach (Adler et al. 1996). Despite this, serologic screening is not recommended in or before pregnancy by organizations in the United States or the United Kingdom (Practice Bulletin No. 151 2015; NICE Guidance: Pregnancy 2019). Further since implementing educational recommendations might be burdensome and their efficacy has not been definitely demonstrated, these preventive actions have not been endorsed (Practice Bulletin No. 151 2015).

11.8.3 Recommendations for Practice

At this time, no special recommendations for CMV should be undertaken in the preconception time period. Those working in day care may choose to follow the preventive measures (handwashing after feeding and diaper changes; avoid sharing saliva when kissing children and avoid sharing utensils and cups); however, these appear to represent good general hygiene measures. Serologic testing to find those at risk for primary disease is not recommended.

11.9 Zika Virus

Zika virus infection in adults occurs because of mosquito bites or sexual transmission. In utero and perinatal transmission can cause congenital Zika syndrome: microcephaly, thinning of the cerebral cortices, ocular findings of macular scarring and localized retinal pigmentary mottling, contractures, and hypertonia (Moore et al. 2017). Both men and women can be infected; usually it causes mild disease in the affected adult—maculopapular rash, fever, and conjunctivitis that sometimes can be difficult to distinguish from other infections. Much of the concern with this infection has to do with congenital infection as these neurologically affected infected children can be a burden for the family and society (Satterfield-Nash et al. 2017).

Congenital Zika occurs in 5–10% of those with Zika infection that has been confirmed, with risks higher in the first trimester (8–15%) than the second or third (4–5%) (Reynolds et al. 2017) (Shapiro-Mendoza et al. 2017). The presence of symptoms does not appear to be predictive of congenital infection (Shapiro-Mendoza et al. 2017). In the United States, cases were rare before 2015 when an outbreak in the Americas and Puerto Rico led to travel-associated Zika—it declined in 2017 with no reported cases in 2018 or 2019 (Centers for Disease Control and Prevention 2019e). The outbreak in Brazil and Columbia was felt to be due to large number of vectors (principally *A. aegypti*) and low immunity in the population (Pan American Health Organization 2017). Its subsequent fall has returned to a more a more endemic pattern of transmission (Pan American Health Organization 2017).

Approaches to preconception care depend on whether travel is planned to Zika endemic areas or if ongoing exposure within the area is occurring. Current maps are updated by the CDC (https://wwwnc.cdc.gov/travel/page/zika-travel-information).

The CDC gives advice for reproductive-age men and women for those who travel, plan to conceive, or could conceive in areas with Zika transmission: Avoid mosquito bites by *A. aegypti* and other mosquitos with repellant, skin covering, screens, and use of air conditioning if available and avoid home standing water (Polen et al. 2018). If one gets sick with Zika, prevent spread by following the above measures since it is in the blood at high levels in the first week of symptoms (Centers for Disease Control and Prevention 2019f). If males or both partners travel to areas at high risk, the advice is to abstain from sex or use condoms for 3 months after symptoms or last exposure (Polen et al. 2018). If women only travel or are affected, 2 months of abstinence or condom use are recommended (Polen et al. 2018). If a male partner is exposed or has symptoms and the partner is pregnant, abstain from sex or use condoms during the entire pregnancy. The advice is longer for males because the virus survives longer in sperm (Polen et al. 2018). For those living in areas with ongoing exposure, weigh risks and benefits with timing and avoid exposure. If either partner is known to have symptomatic infection or infected, follow the above guidelines for abstinence or condom use (Polen et al. 2018). Sample scripts for counseling have been provided by the CDC for this scenario and the ones above (Centers for Disease Control and Prevention 2019g). These include information on family planning and contraception with reproductive life planning.

11.9.1 Recommendations for Practice

Zika infection is an area with emerging data and changes in epidemiology that might guide changing practice so consulting the CDC or WHO would be a prudent strategy: https://www.cdc.gov/zika/index.html; https://www.who.int/emergencies/diseases/zika/en/. This is also an area in which preconception immunization would be an important strategy should one be developed or approved (Poland et al. 2018).

11.10 Emerging Issues

- It is believed that infectious diseases cause a significant portion of preterm births. The medical community currently lacks the ability to identify and treat these infections early enough to prevent the effect on the pregnancy. For this reason, the preconception period might prove to be an important time for prevention and treatment of potential causes of preterm birth.
- We are still learning about early changes to the human system that may be associated with preterm birth, such as the role of various microbiomes or HPV infection.
- Alteration in the vaginal microbiome has been associated with preterm birth (Elovitz et al. 2019). Further, data suggests that subclinical infection may have an onset many weeks prior to any preterm labor (Parry and Strauss 1998) indicating that early pregnancy or preconceptual interventions to restore a vaginal microbiome could be an important part of preconception care.
- A large cohort found HPV vaccination prior to pregnancy was associated with lower rates of preterm birth (Lawton et al. 2018). HPV, however, has not been an infectious agent associated with preterm birth.
- Maternal sepsis is a critical issue for maternal mortality that we are only starting to understand. The role of preconception care in prevention of maternal sepsis is unclear.

11.11 Conclusion

Adequate preventive care in the preconception period can have a significant impact on maternal and neonatal outcomes. Infectious diseases play an important role in the preconception period—global and national data is important for creating a cause for action. Specifically, education on preventable diseases such as listeria and the role of vaccination when available for cases like hepatitis B is essential. This chapter outlined the management of chronic diseases like HIV and hepatitis C for those desiring pregnancy, noting the role of the partner in preventing seroconversion for these chronic diseases cannot be underestimated. There are a number of emerging issues such as the association of HPV infection and preterm birth which may add to the list of considerations of preconception management of infectious disease to improve maternal and pregnancy outcomes.

References

Adler SP, Finney JW, Manganello AM, Best AM. Prevention of child-to-mother transmission of cytomegalovirus by changing behaviors: a randomized controlled trial. Pediatr Infect Dis J. 1996;15(3):240–6. https://doi.org/10.1097/00006454-199603000-00013.

AIDSinfo. Panel on treatment of pregnant women with HIV infection and prevention of perinatal transmission. recommendations for the use of antiretroviral drugs in pregnant women with HIV infection and interventions to reduce perinatal HIV transmission in the United States. 2018. https://aidsinfo.nih.gov/e-news. Accessed 27 Apr 2019.

AIDSinfo. Preconception Counseling and Care for Women of Childbearing Age Living with HIV. 2019. https://aidsinfo.nih.gov/guidelines/html/3/perinatal/152/overview. Accessed 25 Apr 2019.

Amar J, Kim S. Periodontal disease and systemic conditions: a bidirectional relationship. Odontol PMC. 2008;94(1):10–21.

American College of Obstetricians and Gynecologists. Practice Bulletin No. 82: herpes in pregnancy. 2002;108(82):1–15.

American College of Obstetricians and Gynecologists. Practice Bulletin No. 86: viral hepatitis in pregnancy. 2007;86.

American College of Obstetricians and Gynecologists. Clinical practice: syphilis resurgence reminds us of the importance of STD screening and treatment during prenatal Caree. 2017. https://www.acog.org/About-ACOG/ACOG-Departments/ACOG-Rounds/May-2017/Syphilis-Resurgence?IsMobileSet=false. Accessed 5 June 2019.

American College of Obstetricians and Gynecologists. Committee Opinion No. 732: influenza vaccination during pregnancy. 2018;131(4):e109–e114. https://doi.org/10.1097/AOG.0000000000002588.

Benova L, Mohamoud YA, Calvert C, Abu-Raddad LJ. Vertical transmission of hepatitis C virus: systematic review and meta-analysis. Clin Infect Dis. 2014;59(6):765–73.

Bhise V, Dhib-Jalbut S. Rubella virus. Encycl Neurol Sci. 2014;76–8. https://doi.org/10.1016/B978-0-12-385157-4.00387-0.

Breugelmans M, Naessens A, Foulon W. Prevention of toxoplasmosis during pregnancy—an epidemiologic survey over 22 consecutive years. J Perinat Med. 2005;32(3):211–4. https://doi.org/10.1515/JPM.2004.039.

Center for Disease Control and Prevention. Syphilis (*Treponema pallidum*) 2018 case definition. 2018. https://wwwn.cdc.gov/nndss/conditions/syphilis/case-definition/2018/. Accessed 6 May 2019.

Centers for Disease Control and Prevention. Gonococcal infections. 2015a. https://www.cdc.gov/std/tg2015/gonorrhea.htm. Accessed 13 June 2019.

Centers for Disease Control and Prevention. Genital HSV infections. 2015b. https://www.cdc.gov/std/tg2015/herpes.htm. Accessed 13 June 2019.

Centers for Disease Control and Prevention. Today's HIV/AIDS epidemic the scope and impact of HIV in the United States. 2016a. https://www.cdc.gov/hiv/default.html. Accessed 27 May 2019.

Centers for Disease Control and Prevention. Listeria (listeriosis): people at risk—pregnant women and newborns. 2016b. https://www.cdc.gov/listeria/risk-groups/pregnant-women.html. Accessed 5 Mar 2019.

Centers for Disease Control and Prevention. Sexually transmitted disease surveillance. 2017. https://www.cdc.gov/std/stats. Accessed 5 June 2019.

Centers for Disease Control and Prevention. Sexually transmitted disease surveillance 2017: Chlamydia. 2018a. https://wwwcdcgov/std/stats17/chlamydiahtm#ref5. Accessed 27 May 2019.

Centers for Disease Control and Prevention. Chickenpox (varicella): for healthcare professionals. 2018b. https://www.cdc.gov/chickenpox/hcp/index.html?CDC_AA_refVal=https%3A%2F%2Fwww.cdc.gov%2Fchickenpox%2Fhcp%2Fimmunity.html. Accessed 5 Mar 2019.

Centers for Disease Control and Prevention. Toxoplasmosis. 2018c. https://www.cdc.gov/parasites/toxoplasmosis/index.html. Accessed 6 May 2019.

Centers for Disease Control and Prevention. Treatment of malaria (guidelines for clinicians). 2019a. http://www.cdc.gov/malaria/resources/pdf/treatmenttable.pdf. Accessed 5 May 2019.

Centers for Disease Control and Prevention. Syphilis surveillance supplement 2013–2017. 2019b. https://www.cdc.gov/std/stats17/syphilis2017/default.htm. Accessed 5 June 2019.

Centers for Disease Control and Prevention. National STD Infographic. 2019c. https://www.cdc.gov/std/products/infographics.htm. Accessed 5 June 2019.

Centers for Disease Control and Prevention. Vaccines and preventable diseases—routine measles, mumps, and rubella vaccination. 2019d. https://www.cdc.gov/vaccines/vpd/mmr/hcp/recommendations.html. Accessed 7 May 2019.

Centers for Disease Control and Prevention. Zika virus: statistics and maps. 2019e. https://www.cdc.gov/zika/reporting/index.html. Accessed 8 Sept 2019.

Centers for Disease Control and Prevention. Counseling travelers on zika virus risks. 2019f. https://www.cdc.gov/pregnancy/zika/materials/documents/travelcounseling-fs.pdf. Accessed 9 Sept 2019.

Centers for Disease Control and Prevention. Preconception counseling for men and women living in areas with ongoing spread of zika virus who are interested in conceiving. 2019g. https://www.cdc.gov/pregnancy/zika/testing-follow-up/documents/Preconception-Counseling.pdf. Accessed 9 Sept 2019.

Centers for Disease Control and Prevention: US Public Health Service. Preexposure Prophylaxis for the Prevention of HIV Infection in the United State—2017 Update Clinical Practice Guideline. 2018. https://www.cdc.gov/hiv/pdf/risk/prep/cdc-hiv-prep-guidelines-2017.pdf. Accessed 4 Aug 2019.

Clark DR, Chaturvedi V, Kinder JM, Jiang TT, Xin L, Ertelt JM, et al. Perinatal *Listeria monocytogenes* susceptibility despite preconceptual priming and maintenance of pathogen-specific CD8+T cells during pregnancy. Cell Mol Immunol. 2014;11(6):595–605. https://doi.org/10.1038/cmi.2014.84.

Committee Opinion No. 569. Oral health care during pregnancy and through the lifespan. Am Coll Obstet Gynecol. 2017;569

Committee Opinion No. 706. Sexual health. Am Coll Obstet Gynecol. 2017;706

Committee Opinion No. 752. Prenatal and perinatal human immunodeficiency virus testing. Am Coll Obstet Gynecol. 2018;132:e138–42.

Committee Opinion No. 762. Prepregnancy counseling. Am Coll Obstet Gynecol. 2002;98(2):357–64.

Cross R, Ling C, Day NPJ, McGready R, Paris DH. Revisiting doxycycline in pregnancy and early childhood—time to rebuild its reputation? Expert Opin Drug Saf. 2015;15(3):367–82. https://doi.org/10.1517/14740338.2016.1133584.

Crowther CA, Thomas N, Middleton P, Chua M-C, Esposito M. Treating periodontal disease for preventing preterm birth in pregnant women. Cochrane Database Syst Rev. 2005;6 https://doi.org/10.1002/14651858.cd005297.

Daalderop LA, Wieland BV, Tomsin K, Reyes L, Kramer BW, Vanterpool SF, et al. Periodontal disease and pregnancy outcomes: overview of systematic reviews. JDR Clin Transl Res. 2018;3(1):10–27.

Delaney S, Gardella C, Daruthayan C, Saracino M, Drolette L, Corey L, et al. A prospective cohort study of partner testing for herpes simplex virus and sexual behavior during pregnancy. J Infect Dis. 2012;206(4):486–94.

Desai M, ter Kuile FO, Nosten F, McGready R, Asamoa K, Brabin B, Newman RD. Epidemiology and burden of malaria in pregnancy. Lancet Infect Dis. 2007;7(2):93–104.

Elovitz MA, Gajer P, Riis V, Brown AG, Humphrys MS, Holm JB, et al. Cervicovaginal microbiota and local immune response modulate the risk of spontaneous preterm delivery. Nat Commun. 2019;10(1):1305. https://doi.org/10.1038/s41467-019-09285-9.

Epidemiology and Prevention of Vaccine-Preventable Diseases. Influenza virus. In: Hamborsky J, Kroger A WS, editors. Washington, DC: Public Health Foundation; 2015a. p. 187–207.

Epidemiology and Prevention of Vaccine-Preventable Diseases. Tetanus. In: Hamborsky J, Kroger A WS, editors. Washington, DC: Public Health Foundation; 2015b.

Gardella C, Brown ZA. Managing varicella zoster infection in pregnancy. Cleve Clin J Med. 2007;74(4):290–6. https://doi.org/10.3949/ccjm.74.4.290.

Global, Regional and National Cancer. Incidence, mortality, years of life lost, years lived with disability, and disability-adjusted life-years for 29 Cancer groups, 1990 to 2016: a systematic analysis for the global burden of disease study. JAMA Oncol. 2018;4(11):1553–68.

Hughes BL, Page CM, Kuller JA. Hepatitis C in pregnancy: screening, treatment, and management. Am J Obstet Gynecol. 2017;217(5):B2–12.

Human Papillomavirus Vaccination. Obstet Gynecol. 2017;129(6):1155–6. https://doi.org/10.1097/AOG.0000000000002111.

Immunization for Women. About human papillomavirus. 2015. http://immunizationforwomen.org/providers/diseases-vaccines/hpv/about-hpv.php. Accessed 6 June 2019.

Iuliano AD, Roguski KM, Chang HH, Muscatello DJ, Palekar R, Tempia S, et al. Estimates of global seasonal influenza-associated respiratory mortality: a modelling study. Lancet. 2018;391(10127):1285–300.

Jiang H, Xiong X, Su Y, Zhang Y, Wu H, Jiang Z, et al. A randomized controlled trial of pre-conception treatment for periodontal disease to improve periodontal status during pregnancy and birth outcomes. BMC Pregnancy Childbirth. 2013;13:228. https://doi.org/10.1186/1471-2393-13-228.

Lanini S, Easterbrook PJ, Zumla A, Ippolito G. Hepatitis C: global epidemiology and strategies for control. Clin Microbiol Infect. 2016;22(10):833–8.

Lawton B, Howe AS, Turner N, Filoche S, Slatter T, Devenish C, et al. Association of prior HPV vaccination with reduced preterm birth: a population based study. Vaccine. 2018;36(1):134–40.

Lingman GK, Bengtsson K, Cluver C, Eriksson DO, Novikova N. Interventions for treating genital Chlamydia trachomatis infection in pregnancy. Cochrane Database Syst Rev. 2017;9 https://doi.org/10.1002/14651858.cd010485.pub2.

Loto OM, Awowole I. Tuberculosis in pregnancy: a review. J Pregnancy. 2012;2012:1. https://doi.org/10.1155/2012/379271.

Low N, Redmond S, Uuskula A, van Bergen J, Ward H, Andersen B, et al. Screening for genital chlamydia infection. Cochrane Rev. 2016;12:2–5. https://doi.org/10.1002/14651858.CD010866.

Manicklal S, Emery VC, Lazzarotto T, Boppana SB, Gupta RK. The "silent" global burden of congenital cytomegalovirus. Clin Microbiol Rev. 2013;26(1):86–102. https://doi.org/10.1128/cmr.00062-12.

Marais BJ, Gupta A, Starke JR, El Sony A. Tuberculosis in women and children. Lancet. 2010;375(9731):2057–9. https://doi.org/10.1016/S0140-6736(10)60579-X.

McDonnold M, Dunn H, Hester A, Pacheco LD, Hankins GDV, Saade GR, et al. High risk human papillomavirus at entry to prenatal care and risk of preeclampsia. Am J Obstet Gynecol. 2014;210(2):138.e1–5.

Moore CA, Staples JE, Dobyns WB, Pessoa A, Ventura CV, Fonseca EB d, et al. Characterizing the pattern of anomalies in congenital Zika syndrome for pediatric clinicians. JAMA Pediatr. 2017;171(3):288–95. https://doi.org/10.1001/jamapediatrics.2016.3982.

Namavar Jahromi B, Parsanezhad ME, Ghane-Shirazi R. Female genital tuberculosis and infertility. Int J Gynaecol Obstet. 2001;75(3):269–72. https://doi.org/10.1016/s0020-7292(01)00494-5.

National Health Service. Why aren't children in the UK vaccinated against chickenpox? 2016. https://www.nhs.uk/common-health-questions/childrens-health/why-are-children-in-the-uk-not-vaccinated-against-chickenpox. Accessed Mar 5 2019.

National Health Service. Flu vaccine overview. 2019. https://www.nhs.uk/about-us/about-the-nhs-website. Accessed 8 Sep 2019.

NICE Guidance: Pregnancy. 2019. https://www.nice.org.uk/donotdo/the-available-evidence-does-not-support-routine-cytomegalovirus-screening-in-pregnant-women-and-it-should-not-be-offered. Accessed 6 Oct 2019.

Nunes MC, Madhi SA. Prevention of influenza-related illness in young infants by maternal vaccination during pregnancy. F1000Research. 2018;7:122. https://doi.org/10.12688/f1000research.12473.1.

Pan American Health Organization. Zika virus: an epidemiological update. 2017. https://www.paho.org/hq/index.php?option=com_content&view=article&id=11599:regional-zika-epidemiological-update-americas&Itemid=41691&lang=en. Accessed 8 Sept 2019.

Parry S, Strauss J. Premature rupture of the fetal membranes. N Engl J Med. 1998;338:663–70. https://doi.org/10.1038/s41467-019-09285-9.

Poland GA, Kennedy RB, Ovsyannikova IG, Palacios R, Ho PL, Kalil J. Development of vaccines against Zika virus. Lancet Infect Dis. 2018;18(7):e211–9. https://doi.org/10.1016/S1473-3099(18)30063-X.

Polen KD, Gilboa SM, Hills S, Oduyebo T, Kohl KS, Brooks JT, et al. Update: interim guidance for preconception counseling and prevention of sexual transmission of zika virus for men with possible zika virus exposure. Morb Mortal Wkly Rep. 2018;67(31):868–71. https://doi.org/10.15585/mmwr.mm6731e2.

Practice Bulletin No. 151 Cytomegalovirus, parvovirus B19, varicella zoster, and toxoplasmosis in pregnancy. Am Coll Obstet Gynecol 2015;125(6):1510–1525. https://doi.org/10.1097/01.AOG.0000466430.19823.53.

Preventing Congenital Toxoplasmosis. Morb Mortal Wkly Rep. 2000. https://www.cdc.gov/mmwr/preview/mmwrhtml/rr4902a5.htm. Accessed 6 May 2019.

Reynolds MR, Jones AM, Petersen EE, Lee EH, Rice ME, Bingham A, et al. Vital signs: update on zika virus-associated birth defects and evaluation of all U.S. infants with congenital zika virus exposure. Morb Mortal Wkly Rep. 2017;66(13):366–73. https://doi.org/10.15585/mmwr.mm6613e1.

Ross DS, Jones JL, Lynch MF. Toxoplasmosis, cytomegalovirus, listeriosis, and preconception care. Matern Child Health J. 2006;10(S1):189–93. https://doi.org/10.1007/s10995-006-0092-0.

Satterfield-Nash A, Kotzky K, Allen J, Bertolli J, Moore CA, Pereira IO, et al. Health and development at age 19–24 months of 19 children who were born with microcephaly and laboratory evidence of congenital zika virus infection during the 2015 zika virus outbreak. Morb Mortal Wkly Rep. 2017;66(49):1347–51. https://doi.org/10.15585/mmwr.mm6649a2.

Schillie S, Vellozzi C, Reingold A. Prevention of hepatitis B virus infection in the United States: recommendations of the advisory committee on immunization practices. Morb Mortal Wkly Rep. 2018;67:455.

Schleiss MR. Cytomegalovirus vaccines under clinical development. J Virus Erad. 2016;2(4):198–207.

Shapiro-Mendoza CK, Rice ME, Galang RR, Fulton AC, VanMaldeghem K, Prado MV, et al. Pregnancy outcomes after maternal zika virus infection during pregnancy. Morb Mortal Wkly Rep. 2017;66(23):615–21. https://doi.org/10.15585/mmwr.mm6623e1.

Thwaites CL, Beeching NJ, Newton CR. Maternal and neonatal tetanus. Lancet. 2014;385(9965):362–70. https://doi.org/10.1016/s0140-6736(14)60236-1.

Torgerson PR, Mastroiacovo P. The global burden of congenital toxoplasmosis: a systematic review. 2013;91:501–508. https://doi.org/10.2471/BLT.12.111732.

Tsimis ME, Sheffield JS. Update on syphilis and pregnancy. Birth Defects Res. 2017;109(5):347–52. https://doi.org/10.1002/bdra.23562.

UNAIDS. Fact sheet—World Aids Day. 2018. https://www.unaids.org/en/resources/fact-sheet. Accessed 27 May 2019.

World Health Organization. Guidelines on the application of general principles of food hygiene to the control of *Listeria monocytogenes* in foods. 2007. http://www.fao.org/input/download/standards/10740/CXG_061e.pdf. Accessed 5 Mar 2019.

World Health Organization. WHO policy brief for the Implementation of Intermittent Preventive Treatment of Malaria in Pregnancy Using Sulfadoxine-Pyrimethamine (IPTp-SP). 2013 (rev. 2014). http://www.who.int/malaria/publications/atoz/iptp-sp-updated-policy-brief-24jan2014.pdf?ua=1. Accessed 5 May 2019.

World Health Organization. Varicella and herpes zoster vaccines. 2014;89(25):265–87. http://www.who.int/wer/2014/wer8925.pdf?ua=1. Accessed 8 Sept 2019.

World Health Organization. Guidelines for the prevention, care and treatment of persons with chronic hepatitis B infection. 2015. Licence:CC BY-NC-SA 3.0 IGO.

World Health Organization. Sexually transmitted infections. 2016a. Licence: CC BY-NC-SA 3.0 IGO.

World Health Organization. Guidelines for the treatment of *Neisseria gonorrhoeae*. 2016b;50. Licence: CC BY-NC-SA 3.0 IGO.

World Health Organization. Immunization, vaccines, biologicals: rubella. 2016c. https://www.who.int/immunization/diseases/rubella/en. Accessed June 13 2019.

World Health Organization. Malaria in pregnant women. 2017a. https://www.who.int/malaria/areas/high_risk_groups/pregnancy/en/. Accessed 5 May 2019.

World Health Organization. Global hepatitis report, 2017. 2017b. Licence: CC BY-NC-SA 3.0 IGO.

World Health Organization. Guidelines on hepatitis B and C testing. 2017c. p. 1–170. Licence: CC BY-NC-SA 3.0 IGO.

World Health Organization. World malaria report. 2018a. Licence :CC BY-NC-SA 3.0 IGO.

World Health Organization. Global Health Tuberculosis Report. 2018b. Licence: CC BY-NC-SA 3.0 IGO.

World Health Organization. Listeriosis Fact Sheet. 2018c. www.who.int/mediacentre/factsheets/listeriosis/en. Accessed 5 Apr 2019.

World Health Organization. Listeriosis. 2018d. https://www.who.int/ith/diseases/listeriosis/en. Accessed 5 Apr 2019.

World Health Organization. Oral health. 2018e. https://www.who.int/news-room/fact-sheets/detail/oral-health. Accessed 31 Aug 2019.

World Health Organization. Guidelines for the care and treatment of persons diagnosed with chronic hepatitis C virus infection. 2018f. Licence: CC BY-NC-SA 3.0 IGO.

World Health Organization. Toxoplasmosis infection resources for health professionals. 2018g. https://www.cdc.gov/parasites/toxoplasmosis/health_professionals/index.html. Accessed 5 May 2019.

World Health Organization. World malaria report. 2019a. Licence: CC BY-NC-SA 3.0 IGO.

World Health Organization. Progress report on HIV, viral hepatitis and sexually transmitted infections. Accountability for the global health sector strategies. 2019b. Licence: CC BY-NC-SA 3.0 IGO.

World Health Organization. Sexually transmitted infections: key facts. 2019c. https://www.who.int/news-room/fact-sheets/detail/sexually-transmitted-infections-(stis). Accessed 27 May 2019.

World Health Organization. Disease watch focus: syphilis. 2019d. https://www.who.int/tdr/publications/disease_watch/syphilis/en/. Accessed 5 June 2019.

World Health Organization. Rubella. 2019e. https://www.who.int/en/news-room/fact-sheets/detail/rubella. Accessed 13 June 2019.

World Health Organization. Maternal and neonatal tetanus elimination (MNTE). 2019f. https://www.who.int/immunization/diseases/MNTE_initiative/en. Accessed 8 Sept 2019.

World Health Organization. Protecting all against tetanus: guide to sustaining maternal and neonatal tetanus elimination and broadening tetanus protection for all populations. 2019g. Licence: CC BY-NCSA 3.0 IGO.

World Health Organization. HIV/AIDS. 2019h. https://www.who.int/news-room/fact-sheets/detail/hiv-aids. Accessed 12 June 2019.

Xiong X, Buekens P, Goldenberg RL, Offenbacher S, Qian X. Optimal timing of periodontal disease treatment for prevention of adverse pregnancy outcomes: before or during pregnancy? Am J Obstet Gynecol. 2011;205(2):111.e1–6. https://doi.org/10.1016/j.ajog.2011.03.017.

Environment and Occupation

12

A. N. Rosman, Ch. Schaefer, and T. Brand

12.1 Introduction

A growing number of women have paid jobs before and during pregnancy. Thus, increasingly more women are potentially exposed to occupational hazards by working with organic solvents, pollutants, toxins, or contaminated water. Working in these areas can lead to adverse effects on the health of young women as well as on pregnancy outcomes and their health in later life (Garlantézac et al. 2009; Snijder et al. 2012; Robledo et al. 2015).

There has been an increase in waste products of (bio-)chemical industries and man-made waste due to a higher standard of living with an increased use of chemically processed products like disposable materials or the use of preservatives and pesticides. This ends up in the food chain or in surface water. Therefore, the environment is polluted with toxicants easily entering the human body and exposing (germ) cells to potential endocrine disrupting processes which can harm the reproductive systems and perinatal outcomes on short and long term.

The aim of this chapter is to provide information about work-related risks and the consequences of environmental pollutants on preconceptional health and

A. N. Rosman (✉)
Department of Health Care Studies, Rotterdam University of Applied Sciences, EK, Rotterdam, The Netherlands

Perined, Perinatal Registry Netherlands, BL, Utrecht, The Netherlands
e-mail: a.n.rosman@hr.nl

C. Schaefer
Department of Pharmacology and Embryotoxocology, Charité-University of Berlin, Berlin, Germany

T. Brand
Amsterdam University Medical Center, Coronel Institute of Occupational Health, AZ, Amsterdam, The Netherlands

© Springer Nature Switzerland AG 2020
J. Shawe et al. (eds.), *Preconception Health and Care: A Life Course Approach*,
https://doi.org/10.1007/978-3-030-31753-9_12

early pregnancy. Most will be described from the perspectives of women but men will not be forgotten.

There are three periods of time for consideration around exposure to toxins: (a) planning a pregnancy and exposure, (b) exposure during an unplanned pregnancy, and (c) exposure considered the cause in a case of an adverse outcome (e.g., delivery or a child with a birth defect). Providers should be careful to prevent unjustified anxiety or feelings of guilt, so any risk should be carefully weighed and specified regarding its likelihood of occurrence. Even significant results should be carefully interpreted on clinical relevance before sharing them with people potentially exposed to harm for themselves and future offspring. Likewise, communities have the right to know about pollutants in their homes and environments in order to advocate for themselves and families.

12.2 Occupation

The employment rate of women has increased over the last 15 years. In the European Union the percentage of women with a paid job increased from 59% in 2004 to 67% in 2017 (Statistics Netherlands, Eurostat 2019). Also, outside the European Union an increase of working women is visible. For example, the percentage of employed women in the United States rose from 33% in 1950 toward 57% in 2015 (US Department of Labour 2017). In Africa the percentage of employed women in 2016 was 55% (African Statistics n.d.).

The average age that men and women start to work is between 20 and 30 years. This is also the period men and women start to plan a (first) pregnancy. This means that potential risks for adverse pregnancy outcomes or adverse effects in later life need to be eliminated or to be made as small as possible. Therefore, it is important that men and women are aware of potential occupational risks in the preconception period. But this awareness is not only important for women and men, the surrounding area as well as health-care professionals need to be informed about occupational risks, occupational hazards, and environmental risks, especially in the preconceptional period (O'Brien et al. 2018; Kotelchuck and Lu 2017; Stephenson et al. 2018).

12.3 Environment

Environmental pollutants can be divided into three specific groups: (a) soil pollutants (e.g., heavy metals, pesticides or herbicides, organic chemicals, oils, and tars), (b) air pollutants (e.g., carbon monoxide, particulate matter, ozone, sulfur dioxide, lead), and (c) water pollutants (e.g., mercury, nitrates, fecal coliform, and bacterial pollution). Environmental pollutants are a worldwide problem. They are hidden players in reproductive health. Clinicians, scientists, and communities need to understand the impact of environmental pollutants on current and future generations.

This chapter focuses on occupational risks, occupational hazards, environmental pollutants (air, soil, heat), toxins, and contaminated water. The authors discuss definitions, impact on the health of both women and men regarding future pregnancies, and the implications for preconception care. All information on risks exposures in pregnancy are read in three different situations: (a) planning a pregnancy and exposure, (b) exposure happened during an (unplanned) pregnancy, and (c) exposure considered the cause in a case of an adverse outcome (e.g., delivery or a child with a birth defect).

12.4 Definitions

Occupational hazards can cause injuries or ailments resulting from the work one does or from the environment in which one works. It concerns both short-term and long-term risks associated with the workplace environment. Occupational hazards can increase the possibility of disabilities, illnesses, or even the death of the employee. Occupational hazards in the preconceptional period can harm the oocyte and sperm with consequent problems with the conception, the development of the embryo and fetus, and even to a disordered development in later life (Sheiner et al. 2003; Figà-Talamanca 2006).

Environmental pollutants are defined as the contamination of the physical and biological components of the earth/atmosphere system to such an extent that normal environmental processes are adversely affected. Pollutants can be naturally occurring substances or energies (e.g., fog, mist, ozone, ash, soot, salt spray, sulfur dioxide), but they are considered contaminants when in excess of nature levels. Environmental pollutants are significantly associated with reduced fertility in men and women as well as with reproductive disorders in women (Chiang et al. 2017).

Toxins are defined as naturally organic poisons. Toxins can and do affect every part of the body. Toxins can also make changes within cells and affect the DNA. Some effects of toxins are irreversible. Damaged DNA can cause spontaneous abortions, preterm birth, congenital malformations, or syndromes of the offspring (Pizzorno 2018).

Contaminated water or water pollution is defined as water that is physically changed or has the presence of certain chemicals or microbes. Water and soil pollution are two of the main categories within environmental pollution. Contaminated water is a concerning major global problem as the chemicals or microbes can alter multiple physiologic processes and, in case of endocrine disruptors, can interfere with many facets of hormone activity including reproductive hormones (Rashtian et al. 2019).

Fetal pregnancy outcomes are defined as congenital malformations, spontaneous abortion, low birth weight, intra-uterine growth restriction, small for gestational age, preterm delivery (birth before 37 weeks gestation), and perinatal death.

12.5 Occupational Hazards

Occupational hazards can cause an injury or ailment resulting from the work one does or from the environment in which one works. It concerns both short term as long-term risks associated with the workplace environment. Occupational hazards can increase the possibility of disabilities, illness, or even the death of the employee. Occupational hazards in the preconceptional period can harm the oocyte and sperm with consequent problems with the conception, the development of the embryo and fetus, and even to a disordered development in later life. But occupational hazards can also cause metabolic diseases like diabetes and cardiovascular diseases, affect mental health, affect the thyroid axis, and affect the respiratory tract and the digestive system.

An in-depth review of Figà-Talamanca et al. revealed that in the past decades knowledge about associations between occupational hazards and reproductive outcomes has significantly increased. Initially, the research focused primarily on the fetus, but after realizing that occupational hazards could affect reproductive hormones, menstrual cycle, and fertility, the focus shifted toward the impact on reproduction health of men and women (Figà-Talamanca 2006).

12.6 Chemical Agents in the Workplace Affecting Reproductive Health: Heavy Metals

Chemical agents include heavy metals, solvents, and pesticides. Heavy metals like lead, mercury, nickel, and manganese have been known to be toxic for many years. Lead is known to damage the general health of lead workers slowly. The body accumulates lead and excretion is very difficult. The first signs of lead poisoning are not very specific (nausea, vomiting, headache). In the second stage of lead poisoning, anemia occurs and nerve and kidney damage as well. Failure to recognize lead poisoning in time can lead to death.

In the first part of the nineteenth century, it became clear that exposure to high levels of lead was associated with recurrent abortions and immature deliveries. Men who were exposed to high levels of lead seemed to be less fertile by having a reduced amount of sperm and more abnormal sperm. For women, no adverse effects of working with lead on fertility was found. However, female workers with lead need to be very careful as exposure to lead during pregnancy can damage the fetus permanently. Lead damages the fetal blood production and the central nervous system (Yun et al. 2015; Hu et al. 2006).

Regarding the adverse effects of working with lead and the adverse effects on the reproductive health of men, they are advised to protect themselves carefully to minimize the contamination with lead. Women are advised not to work with lead or lead components at least 3 months before planning a pregnancy. In some countries like the Netherlands, laws inhibit fertile women to work with lead during pregnancy and breastfeeding (Dutch Law on Lead Exposure 1988).

Mercury is also a heavy metal causing problems with fertility, menstrual disorders, delayed conception, and adverse pregnancy outcomes. Mercury can be divided into organic mercury and nonorganic mercury. The WHO distinguishes elemental mercury and inorganic mercury compounds (WHO 2019). Elemental mercury can easily enter the body by inhalation. In the 2003 report of the WHO, the committee reported that several studies have been conducted on the effect of occupational exposure to mercury vapor on spontaneous abortions, which are consistently negative. Several other studies focused on male fertility but none could find correlations between exposure to elemental mercury and (in)fertility. Some older studies on females exposed to elemental mercury vapor in the workplace found increased time to pregnancies and spontaneous abortions; however, the results of these studies should be carefully interpreted due to methodological issues. Rowland et al. reported that the fecundity of female dental assistants was at higher risk for abovementioned adverse effects (Rowland et al. 1994). If preparing more than 30 amalgam fillings per week, the fecundity rate was 63% (95% CI 42–95) of that of unexposed controls, although dental assistants with lower mercury exposure were more fertile than the referents. Figà-Talamica et al. and Lindbolm et al. reported that increasing mercury levels in blood could affect the endocrine systems, which could explain menstrual disorders and hormonal fertility problems (Figà-Talamanca 2006; Lindbohm et al. 2007).

The volatility of inorganic mercury compounds is low. This form of mercury can enter the body by the gastrointestinal tract or by skin contact. The WHO 2003 report reported that no valid information was available on the reproductive toxicity of inorganic mercury compounds in humans.

12.7   Chemical Agents in the Workplace Affecting Reproductive Health: Solvents

Solvents can be seen as one family, sometimes with different effects depending on the specific solvent. Many studies revealed associations between exposure to solvents and time to pregnancy, spontaneous abortion, and congenital malformations of offspring among exposed men and women (Taskinen et al. 1989; Logman et al. 2005; Snijder et al. 2012). Snijder et al. reviewed nine studies for the association between occupational exposure to solvents and time to pregnancy (TTP) (Snijder et al. 2012). Time to pregnancy was defined as the time it takes to become pregnant after actively trying to conceive and is used as an indicator for the fertility of a couple. Chemicals that influence the TTP are also suspect to influence subsequent pregnancies and adverse pregnancy outcomes. The review of Snijder et al. included four studies (Taskinen et al. 1989; Sallmén et al. 1995; Wennborg et al. 2001; Sallmen et al. 1998) on women working with solvents and concluded that the fecundability ratios ranged from 0.44 to 1.09 for different solvents if compared to women not working with solvents (Sallmén et al. 1995; Taskinen et al. 1989; Wennborg et al. 2001). Fecundability was defined as the chance of conception leading to a live birth per menstrual cycle given unprotected intercourse. The four studies focused on specific groups, e.g., a sub-study in a previous study on spontaneous abortions, shoe workers, female woodworkers exposed to formaldehyde, and female personnel in biomedical laboratories in Sweden. Five studies (Eskenazi et al. 1991; Sallmen et al. 1998; Kolstad et al. 2000; Luderer et al. 2004; Hooiveld et al. 2006) were conducted among men working with solvents (Eskenazi et al. 1991; Sallmen et al. 1998; Kolstad et al. 2000; Luderer et al. 2004; Hooiveld et al. 2006). In these five studies the fecundability ratio ranged from 0.52 to 1.09 if compared to men not working with solvents. The review of Snijder et al. included in total 49 studies of different occupational risks and time to pregnancy. The review by Snijder et al. suggested publication bias, whereby smaller studies with a decreased FR were more likely to be published since almost no small studies published negative findings.

A meta-analysis performed by Logman et al. to assess the risks of spontaneous abortions and major malformations after paternal exposure to organic solvents concluded that paternal exposure was associated with an increased risk for neural tube defects, but not for spontaneous abortions (Logman et al. 2005). One possible explanation for the higher incidence of major malformations could be a direct impact of solvents on sperm DNA, producing mutations or chromosomal abnormalities. A limitation of the study of Logman is that response bias and/or recall bias could not be excluded. Some of the included studies were interview based, and parents of children with adverse outcomes are more likely to search for an explanation, while parents of healthy children could lack such a motivation. The review of Logman also met problems with the assessment of exposure to organic solvents. An actual exposure, duration, and timing are difficult to quantify which made that the interpretation of associations should be done carefully. Another possible explanation according to Olshan et al. was that there could be indirect effects by transmission of agents to the mother through seminal fluid or maternal exposure through the male partner (skin to skin contact, sneezing) (Olshan et al. 1991). Olshan et al. advised already in the early 1990s of the past century, pending good epidemiological research, to avoid working with chemicals in the preconceptional period and early pregnancy by taking adequate preventive measures for both men and women (Olshan et al. 1991). But this study also met some limitations whereby the results of the study must be viewed with caution. The study was limited to live-born children, and the variables available from the birth certificates were limited. Paternal occupation could be misclassified which could influence the associations between occupation and birth defect. For example, in some cases paternal occupation was classified at birth and not in the preconception phase which could differ from the occupation at birth.

Rosofsky et al. published the results of a Danish cohort study: "Exposure to multiple chemicals in a cohort reproductive-aged Danish women" (Rosofsky et al. 2017). Aim of the study was to examine the extent of chemical exposure during their reproductive ages to identify potential risks for exposure in utero and fetal susceptibility as a lot of chemical biomarkers can pass the placental barrier. Concentration of chemicals in a one single spot blood and urine samples at one point in time of 73 women aged 18–40 years was measured in the preconception phase. To ensure that concentration was measured in the preconception period, only women who stopped contraceptives because they were planning a pregnancy were eligible for the study. In blood or urine samples, an average of 95 different chemical biomarkers could be identified, of which some are known to disrupt endocrine processes. Another Finnish study found an increased risk, however not significant, for reduced fertility among primiparous women with higher exposure to toluene, aromatic and aliphatic hydrocarbons. For those who were exposed (shoe factories, dry-cleaning shops, and metal industry), the probability to conceive was reduced by half compared to those who were not exposed (Sallmén et al. 1995).

Another group, comprised largely of women, who is exposed to occupational risks on a daily basis, are hairdressers and cosmetologists. Hair shampooing, dyeing hair, performing hair curling treatments, cleaning nails with acetone, and applying cremes to the facial skin and other beauty treatments are moments when hairdressers and cosmetologists could be exposed to chemical substances if personal protective measures are not sufficient or not applied. Reproductive disorders for some of those exposures are described by Rylander et al. (2002) and Rylander and Källén (2005). On the other hand, there are also studies published which could not confirm adverse effects for reproductive disorders by occupational exposure of hairdressers and cosmetologists (Hougaard et al. 2006; Gallichio et al. 2010). Driven by conflicting results of studies under hairdressers and cosmetologists, Kim et al. included 19 studies in a meta-analysis to explore the occupational risks for hairdressers and cosmetologists (Kim et al. 2016). Chemical exposure is mentioned as the most hazardous risks for hairdressers and cosmetologists. Toluene in nail polish, nitrosamines in hair dye, and phthalates in both hair dye and in nail polish are some chemical substances which adversely interfere with fertility. The meta-analysis revealed that hairdressers and cosmetologists had a significant increased risk of infertility and preterm delivery. All studies reported a high potential for recall bias which should be considered by interpreting the results.

12.8 Chemical Agents in the Workplace Affecting Reproductive Health: Pesticides

Pesticides include a group of agents used as insecticides, fungicides, herbicides, and rodenticides. Pesticides are studied for many years and are associated with reduced fertility, spontaneous abortions, and congenital malformations. Pesticides are known as endocrine disrupting chemicals. They can influence the hypothalamus, pituitary, ovary, uterus, fertility, and reproductive senescence. Pesticides can be divided into organophosphates, organochlorines, carbamates, pyrethroids, and triazines. Well-known pesticides include DDT (dichlorodiphenyltrichloroethane) and malathion.

There is limited evidence available in human research, but research in rats showed that exposure during adulthood (females) to a small amount of pesticides increases significantly the gonadotropin-releasing hormone (GnRH) mRNA levels in GT1–7 cells (Gore 2011). The carbamate molinate suppresses LH pulse frequency, leading to delayed ovulation (Stoker et al. 2005). Atrazine both activated the release of pituitary hormones (Fraites et al. 2009) and inhibited LH release from the pituitary (Fraites et al. 2009; Foradori et al. 2011; Goldman et al. 2013).

The same applies for the impact on ovaries and the uterus. Research in animal studies showed that pesticides lower the weight of the ovaries, follicle growth, and oocyte viability (Borgeest et al. 2002; Tiemann 2008). Most pesticides affect the hormonal release by the oocyte. DDT is associated with decreased progesterone levels and a shorter luteal phase (Windham et al. 2005). Other pesticides inhibit the production of estradiol, testosterone, androstenedione, and progesterone. Some pesticides are associated with a decreased uterine weight or endometrial hyperplasia.

More evidence in human studies is known over the impact of pesticides on fertility. Exposure to organochlorine pesticides is associated with a prolonged time to pregnancy (Chevrier et al. 2013). A study of female Danish greenhouse workers who worked with spraying pesticides without sufficient protecting measures showed a significant reduction in fecundity and a prolonged time to pregnancy (Abell et al. 2000). This was also shown for health-care nurses who worked ≥1 h a week with high-level disinfectants if prepared without sufficient protective materials (gloves, masks) (Gaskins et al. 2017). The use of adequate protective materials attenuated the effects of high-level disinfectants with 9% for respiratory protection and 69% for the use of gloves compared to women who were never exposed to high-level disinfectants.

It has become evident that occupational exposure to pesticides damages the testicular functions, impacting male fertility (Bonde 2010; Mima et al. 2018). The spermatogenesis is very vulnerable for toxicological hazards by the continuously ongoing large number of cell divisions. Specific substances, for example, dibromochloropropane or epichlorohydrin, affect cells of the male reproductive tissues. Occupational exposure might reduce the sperm quality e.g. sperm density and motility, inhibition of spermatogenesis, reduction of testis weights, reduction of sperm counts, motility, viability and density, inducing sperm DNA damage, and increasing abnormal sperm morphology. DDT and its metabolites could have estrogenic effects on males (Mima et al. 2018; Mehrpour et al. 2014).

A study of fruit growers in the Netherlands revealed a prolonged time for conception after a seasonal exposure to pesticides of male workers (De Cock et al. 1994; Bretveld et al. 2008a). Bretveld et al. (2008a) found that male greenhouse workers were less fecund when trying to conceive their first pregnancy compared to a control group who was not occupationally exposed to pesticides (Bretveld et al. 2008a). However, in another study of Bretveld et al. (2008b) the conclusion was that primigravidous couples had a slightly elevated risk of prolonged TTP and an increased risk of spontaneous abortion among female greenhouse workers (Bretveld et al. 2008b). Among partners of male greenhouse workers, a decreased risk of preterm birth was found.

On the contrary, other researchers assume that working with pesticides has more impact on fetal growth and development. A review of Goodman et al. (2014) focused on spontaneous abortions and fetal outcomes like birth defects, birth weight, preterm birth, small for gestational age, and a small head circumference (Goodman et al. 2014). The results of this review showed associations between specific use of atrazine and birth defects, but results were limited as in many studies, it was unclear how they corrected for confounders such as maternal age or smoking. The Generation R study of Snijder et al. (2012) revealed a significant association between occupational exposure to pesticides and phthalate exposure and a decreased placental weight (Snijder et al. 2012). This study revealed negative effects on fetal growth (fetal head circumference, fetal weight, and fetal length) if the mother was occupationally exposed to polycyclic aromatic hydrocarbons, phthalates, or alkylphenolic compounds.

Pesticides have been used in modern agriculture for many years. Although there are growing concerns about the impact of pesticides on human health and fertility, eliminating pesticides is still far away. Therefore, it is important to prevent pesticide accidents. Pesticide hazards can occur everywhere but are more likely to happen in developing countries with poor standards of the workplace or by the lack of safety rules and protection measures, especially if they interfere with production quota. Being aware of the adverse effects of working with pesticides without sufficient and adequate protection should be a point of attention for every employer and employee. Preventing actions like offering and an obliged use of personal equipment tools like glasses, mask, boots, coveralls, and gloves can limit the adverse effects on human fertility and the early pregnancy. This is important as major malformations occur in the early pregnancy (Fig. 12.1). Ashiru and

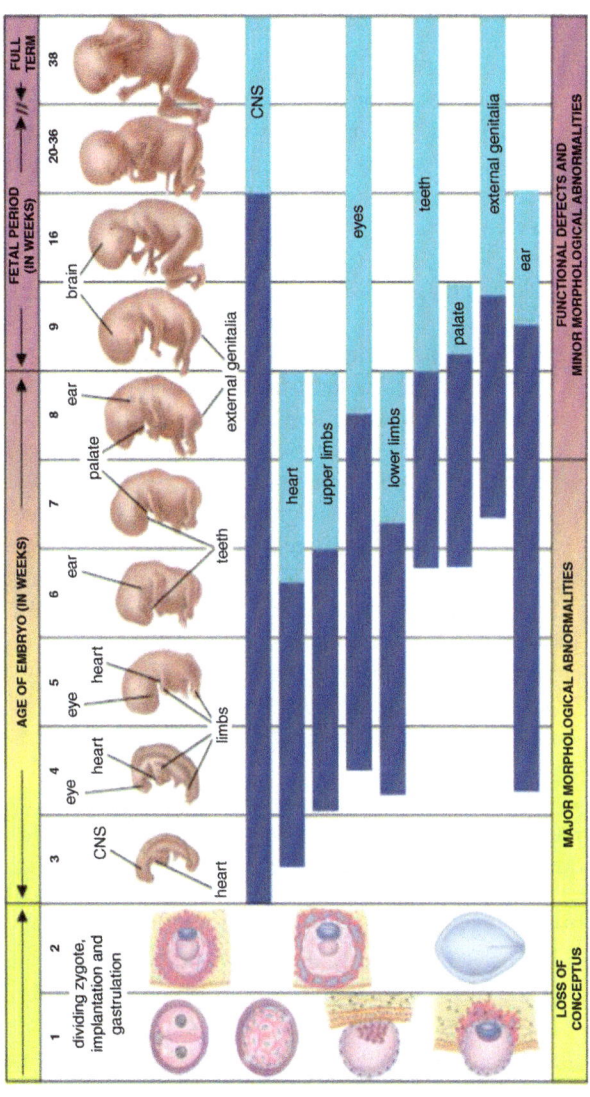

Fig. 12.1 Embryological development and periods of susceptibility. *Source*: Fetal development over time, demonstrating the effects of teratogens on organogenesis. (Retrieved from http://www.slideshare.net/SDRTL/fetal-development-10766134)

Odusanya (2009) showed that employees who were well protected did not suffer from adverse effects on fertility and adverse fetal pregnancy outcomes (Ashiru and Odusanya 2009).

12.9 Prevention and Protection

Next to personal protecting measures (not only for working with pesticides but for all exposures to chemicals in the working place), training of employees and creating awareness of work-related risks and protecting laws are opportunities to prevent adverse effects on fertility and the health of future generations. Training should include the importance of personal hygiene, proper use of protecting materials, and the associations between unprotected work and adverse effects on human fertility and pregnancy outcomes.

In the Netherlands, and likely all western countries, there are guidelines, decrees, and regulations regarding the protection of parents-to-be. The Dutch Occupational Health and Safety Decree and the Occupational Health and Safety Regulation state that the following strategy can be adopted when supporting couples who want to have children or pregnant women who have been exposed to chemical agents at work. There must be no exposure to substances with a direct genotoxic mechanism of action around the time of conception, during pregnancy, or during breastfeeding. These include all mutagens and a significant proportion of carcinogenic substances. This is because it is not possible to determine a safe exposure level for these compounds. It may be possible to determine a safe exposure level for substances which have been identified as potentially harmful to the unborn child or infant but which definitely do not have a genotoxic mechanism of action. However, this requires a high level of expertise which not every occupational health and safety officer can automatically be presumed to possess. If, however, it proves impossible to establish a safe exposure level, then the precautionary principle will apply: i.e., avoid all exposure.

If the reprotoxic effect has been taken into account when setting the statutory limit value for the substance in question, then women may work with this substance during pregnancy and breastfeeding providing it can be shown that the statutory limit value is not exceeded. It should be borne in mind here that the statutory limit value may be out of date. An occupational health and safety specialist should, in any case, carefully consult the Health Council advisory reports about the substances in question.

If insufficient data are available about the possible reprotoxic properties of a substance and/or if there is uncertainty about the safety of the actual exposure level (and absorption through the skin is considered possible), then the precautionary principle should be applied. In other words, the advice must be avoid exposure (Ten Kate et al. 2007). Occupational health workers could contribute to healthy working circumstances by screening working places and the risks for employees (Brand et al. 2009). Finally, there is a responsibility for government and governmental agencies to create laws that guarantee a safe working environment for their inhabitants in order to minimize risks for the health of their labor force and future generations. There is a need to demand for mother/parental protection laws and a strict application and the control of their application.

12.10 Recommendations

- An occupational health worker can conduct workplace screenings and assess the working conditions of both women and men in order to eliminate risks.
- Protecting measures like gloves, boots, glasses, coveralls, and respirators but also training about work-related risks should be provided to all workers who are exposed to occupational risks.
- Governments can have an impact on healthy generations by formulating protecting laws regarding to work with endocrine-disrupting chemicals like heavy metals, solvents, and pesticides.

12.11 Environmental Toxins

Environmental toxins are defined as any organic or inorganic substances, compounds, agents in the environment that are potentially harmful to human health. Environmental toxins include a large number of hazardous chemicals and physical and biological substances such as pesticides, industrial toxic substances, heavy metals, radioactive materials, as well as various forms of energy (e.g., noise, radiation, heat). These pollutants may be inhaled, absorbed through skin and mucous membranes, or ingested. The impact of chemicals and biological substances are discussed later.

Many environmental toxins are everywhere, at home, in the workplace, and in the community via air, water, soil, and food. Women are exposed increasingly to a variety of toxins in the workplace and environment. A growing concern has been raised about the consequences of adverse effects of environmental toxins on the reproductive system, germ cells, fertility, and fetal development. Various substances in the environment are related to oxidative stress and infertility. Factors like an increased use of cosmetics containing heavy metals and phthalates, further industrialization of nations, drinking contaminated water which is poisoned by pesticides as well as using food additives and preservatives, daily contact with household cleaning reagents, and an increased exposure to waves of mobile phones can directly or indirectly cause deleterious effects on fertility or on a developing fetus (Pizzorno 2018).

Phthalates are chemical substances that are used as plasticizers in plastic. They are found in packaging for food, detergents, lubricating oils, and cosmetic products like shampoos, lotions, and soap. Phthalates enter the body through food, skin, or the respiratory tract and can inhibit the production of sperm and damage the DNA. Sulfur dioxide (E-220) is used as a preservative in, among other things, dried fruits, potato products, fruit sauce and syrup, wine, fruit desserts, lemonade syrup, and seasoned sauces.

Timing, intensity, and cumulation of the exposure to environmental toxins will determine the impact of the effects on the reproduction systems. Infertility or a decreased fertility caused by environmental toxins originate by endocrine disruption, damage to the female reproductive systems, and damage to the male reproductive systems.

Endocrine disruption is mainly responsible for a loss of blood-sugar control resulting in diabetes or metabolic syndrome and in obesity (men) and polycystic ovary syndrome (PCOS) in women. Aforementioned diseases and syndromes are associated with lower fertility. Women with PCOS have increased risks for developing gestational diabetes (OR 2.9), pregnancy-induced hypertension, pre-eclampsia, preterm birth, NICU admission of their offspring, and perinatal mortality (Pizzorno 2018).

Multiple studies in humans suggest a negative impact of environmental toxins on male fertility, especially the semen quality (concentration, mobility, and morphology). The etiology is still under research but decreased sperm mobility may be due to mitochondrial dysfunction from the loss of intracellular ATP and increased reactive oxygen species (ROS) generation. An increased generation of ROS can damage cell structures including DNA. Exposure of spermatozoa to oxidative stress is a major causative agent of male infertility. Oxidative stress occurs when the amount of ROS exceeds the natural antioxidant capacity of the body. ROS are produced by spermatozoa and leucocytes in semen. Due to ROS, the mobility of sperm decreases as also the capability to bind to the zona pellucida and to fertilize the egg. Immature spermatozoa produce more ROS than mature spermatozoa. The male body has developed different strategies to protect sperm against oxidative stress. The sperm and semen have enzymes and antioxidants to protect against ROS. Most important enzyme antioxidants are SOD (superoxide dismutase), catalase, and GPX (glutathione peroxidase). Antioxidants in semen protect sperm against oxidative stress after ejaculation. During the spermatogenesis and preservation in the testicles, the sperm is not protected. During these phases sperm is extra sensitive for environmental toxins or endocrine-disrupting chemicals like phthalates (Guz et al. 2013; Wright et al. 2014).

12.12 Environmental Toxins: Ionizing and Non-ionizing Radiation and Heat

In modern society men and women are frequently exposed to different types of radiation which comes from sources like laptops, mobile phones, microwaves, and occupational equipment. Radiation can be divided into two groups depending on the energy of the radiated particles: ionizing and non-ionizing radiation.

12.12.1 Non-ionizing Radiation

Non-ionizing radiation is defined by electromagnetic fields (EMFs) that do not have enough energy to release electrons (non-ionizing) but enlarge the movements of electrons. EMFs are divided into four classes of frequencies: (Garlantézac et al.

2009) extremely low frequencies with frequencies below 300 HZ (military equipment); (Snijder et al. 2012) intermediate frequencies ranging from 300 Hz to 10 MHz (television, computer monitors, industrial cables); (Robledo et al. 2015) hyper frequencies ranging from 10 MHz to 3000 GHz (mobile phones, radio); and (Statistics Netherlands, Eurostat 2019) static EMFs that have zero frequency (MRI) (Marci et al. 2018).

For females, most research studies on the effects of non-ionizing radiation on human reproduction are animal studies with mice. These studies reveal that non-ionizing radiation is associated with an inhibition of ovulations, reduction of the total number of corpora lutea, a reduction of the development of antral follicles and to extend the lifetime of free radicals increasing oxidative stress resulting in damaging the DNA. Antral follicles are follicles which contain mature oocytes, waiting for a hormonal release. Non-ionizing radiation during pregnancy is associated with a higher abortion rate and increased number of congenital malformations (Marci et al. 2018).

Non-ionizing radiation affects the spermatogenesis and male fertility. Figure 12.2 shows how non-ionizing radiation affects the Leydig cells, which are responsible for the production of testosterone and the Sertoli cells and seminiferous tubules. Damaging the Leydig and Sertoli cells and the tubuli alters the spermatogenesis, hence resulting in a decreased sperm count, sperm motility, sperm morphology, sperm viability, and antioxidants.

An additional problem with the use of non-ionizing devices is the heat flux they generate during use. This heat doesn't have to interfere with fertility, but if men store their mobile phones in their pants or work with a laptop on their lap, heat is nearby the scrotum. Thermal mapping of the skin and testicles during the use of heat flux devices was researched by Safari et al. on human models (Safari et al. 2017). The research revealed that the temperature in the scrotum and abdomen increased but did not exceed the IEEE Standard for Safety Levels with Respect to Humans (2005). The effect on pregnant women was not studied.

12.12.2 Ionizing Radiation

Ionizing radiation is much more harmful to human reproductive systems as it damages directly or indirectly the cell's DNA. Sources of ionizing radiation can be found in natural sources as well as in artificial sources. Natural ionizing radiation sources, specific γ-rays, are the sun, uranium in the earth, and cosmic radiation. Artificial sources of ionizing radiation can be found in medical care and in radioactive waste. The effects of ionizing radiation can be divided into two types: (Garlantézac et al. 2009) deterministic effects which are dose dependent and (Snijder et al. 2012) stochastic effects which are the result of symmetrical translocation during cell replication. Deterministic effects only occur if the radiation exceeds the threshold and cause a functional impairment of tissues or organs like reduced fertility which is related to ovarian dysfunction. Stochastic effects occur when the dose of radiation exceeds. There is a linear association between the dose of radiation and stochastic effects. It is known that high dose levels of cosmic radiation cause

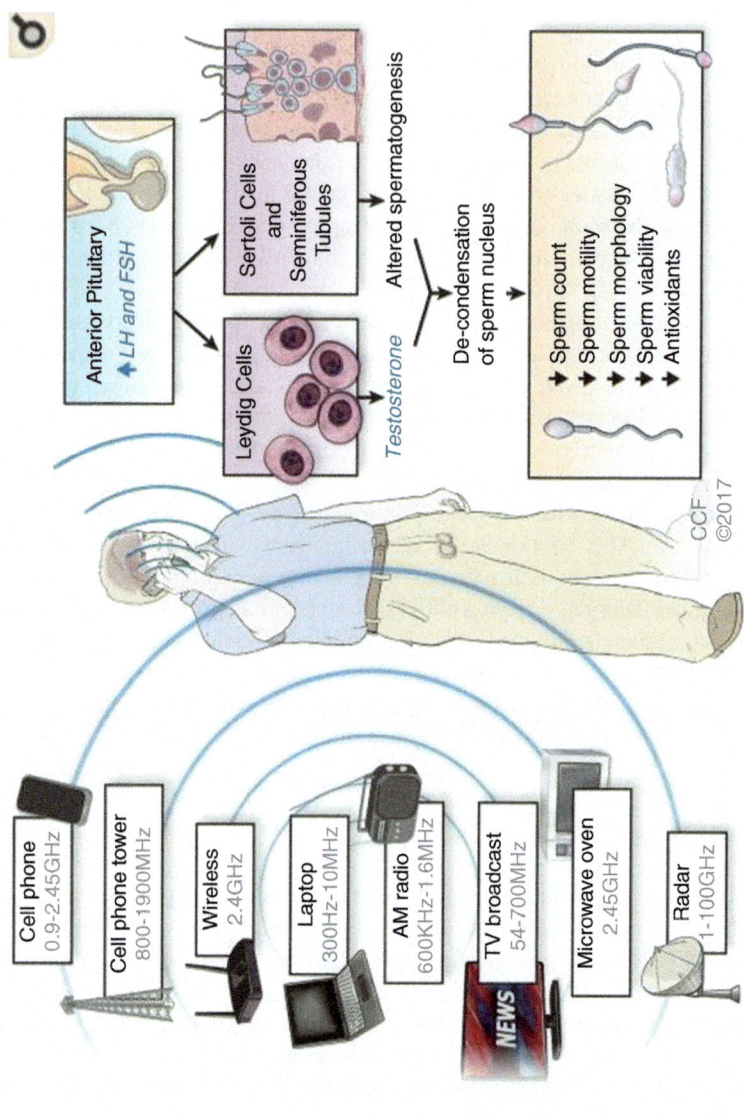

Fig. 12.2 Diagrammatic representation of various sources of EMF exposure effect on the brain and testicular organ and deleterious outcome. (Retrieved on April 18th, 2019 from: Kesari et al. Radiations and male fertility. Reproductive Biology and Endocrinology. 2018 16:118. https://doi.org/10.1186/s12958-018-0431-1) (Kesari et al. 2018)

damage to cells (skin cancer) and DNA and oxidative stress. Oxidative stress is (as earlier stated) associated with a reduced fertility for both men and women.

Ionizing radiation is used commonly in health care (X-rays diagnostics, radiotherapy). With an increasing number of humans affected by cancers, radiotherapy is becoming more and more the first treatment options. Cancers of the reproductive systems are representing one third of all the cancers affecting a young group of humans ≤45 years (cancer of the female reproductive system 9%, cancer of the male reproductive system 11%, cancer of the endocrine system 11%). Several cancers require intensive radiotherapy like cervical cancer, endometrium cancer, and bladder or rectal cancer. The impact of radiation on the reproductive capacity depends on the type, dose, and duration of the treatment. Pelvic irradiation affects the ovary and the uterus. Cranial irradiation for brain tumors can affect the hypothalamic-pituitary-gonadal axis. It is unknown to what extent damage by radiation is irreversible.

During radiotherapy not only the affected tissues are radiated, also healthy tissues will be exposed to radiation. Regarding the ovaries, radiotherapy can damage the follicle growth as the aim of radiation is to stop cell development. A reduced growth of follicles inhibit female's fecundity. The younger a woman is exposed to radiotherapy in the pelvic, the greater the damage is on the ovarian function and the greater (and irreversible) the effect is on females fertility (Safari et al. 2017). For males, the most sensible organ for radiation are the testicles. The germinal epithelium and the spermatogonia are more sensitive to radiation than other cells (Kesari et al. 2018).

12.12.3 Environmental Toxins: Contaminated Water, Soil and Air Pollution, and Extreme Heat

Environmental toxins like contaminated water and air and soil pollution are an increasing global problem for human fertility. Water and soil pollutants represent two categories of environmental pollution. Most water and soil pollutants are often man-made pollution: household waste, manufacturing waste, agricultural waste by the use of fertilizers by farmers, oil spill, and radioactive waste. Once in local waters, the pollution can expand to rivers, sea, and oceans threatening life in and around the water which interferes directly and indirectly with human life. Polluted water and soil can cause acute toxicity but can also alter the human genes by damaging the cell DNA.

Water and soil pollution is a global problem as water and soil pass borders, so hazards in one country can easily be spread to surrounding countries. One of the most found substances in water and soil pollution is bisphenol A (BPA). BPA is a chemical structure which was widely used, and toxic effects of BPA are proven but dose dependent. BPA can be found in toilet papers, plastic bottles, paint, and toys but also in medical devices, cell phones, and printer ink. BPA is easily spread in the environment by human-made waste, for example, throwing away plastic bottles in nature and the plastic ocean soup. Free coming toxins are easily picked up by microorganisms, algae, and plants which are then taken up by plants and larger animals (fish) and eventually humans. Humans are also contaminated with BPA through eating prepackaged or canned food, drinking out of plastic bottles, working with printed documents, and medical devices, and the use of mobile phones. BPA has endocrine disruption properties and influences both the female and male reproduction. Studies under infertile women showed that BPA was associated with a lower number of oocytes, fewer mature oocytes, lower serum E2 levels, and a trend for having lower blastocysts formation (Ehrlich et al. 2012; Bloom et al. 2011).

BPA affects the endocrine-reproductive function in men. De Nisio and Foresta (2019) published in Reproductive Biology (2019) a clear schematic overview of pathways of BPA and other environmental toxins like phthalates to disrupt endocrine functions within male fertility. There is sufficient evidence that soil pollutants like BPA impair males' fertility by a reduced quality of sperm (concentration, mobility, and morphology).

In Europe but also in the United States and Canada, the use of BPA is limited by law since 2010 due to its toxic effects on the general and reproductive health (EFSA, European Food and Safety Authority 2011). Canada was the first country to declare bisphenol A toxic (Canadian Environmental Protection Act 1999).

12.12.4   Air Pollution

Whether air pollution affects female infertility is under discussion. A systematic review of Conforti et al. (2018) focused on air pollution and female infertility due to conflicting results of earlier published results and an increasing exposure to air pollutants (Conforti et al. 2018). Increasing industrial development of nations, subsequent more emission of potential harmful gasses, and more traffic in cities are major concerns for air pollution which is not only specific for developed countries but also for the developing countries. Air pollution can be divided into four categories: (Garlantézac et al. 2009) gaseous pollutants, (Snijder et al. 2012) organic compounds, (Robledo et al. 2015) heavy metals, and (Statistics Netherlands, Eurostat 2019) particulate matter. Gaseous pollutants are, for example, carbon monoxide (CO) and nitrogen oxide (NO). Examples of organic compounds are dung and fertilizers. Air pollution by heavy metals occurs by soot of traffic and industries. Particulate matter is a cause of smog.

Air pollutants enter the body by inhalation. Therefore, most common diseases caused by air pollutants are in the respiratory tract, but some air pollutants seem to have adverse effects on female fertility by endocrine-disrupting processes. Some air pollutants influence the estrogen, antiestrogen, and antiandrogenic processes, and some interfere with the function of the thyroid axis causing an increased risk of obesity, metabolic disorders, and diabetes. These diseases are directly linked to a reduced fertility of both men and women.

Perin et al. studied short-term exposure to air pollutants in the preconception period of women undergoing fertility treatments for male infertility. The study was a retrospective cohort study of 400 first IVF/ET cycles of women exposed to ambient particulate matter during the follicular phase. Particulate matter was classified in quartiles from low to high. Perin et al. found an increased risk for miscarriages for women in the highest quartile compared to women from the first to third quartile (Perin et al. 2010). Others could not identify adverse effects on female reproductivity (Salma et al. 2013).

Nieuwenhuijsen et al. studied the impact of particulate matter and the fecundability ratio. He found a significant decrease in the female fertility ratio with traffic-related air pollution, in particular by particulate matter, specific PM_{coarse} (Nieuwenhuijsen et al. 2013). PM_{coarse} are the larger particles of particulate matter with a diagram >10 μm. Lafuente et al. performed a systematic review for air pollution and semen quality (Lafuente et al. 2016). Although reduced semen quality was found, the results must be interpreted carefully by the lack of homogeneity of included studies and the lack of a clear standardizing of air pollution (Lafuente et al. 2016).

12.12.5 Air Pollution and Extreme Heat

With global climate change, the world will encounter more environmental hazards. Next to ambient air pollution outdoors, people will have to adapt their lifestyle to more periods of extreme heat and changing indoor circumstances. Air pollution spread by air conditioning is an example of potential indoor air pollution. Although data are lacking about the impact of extreme heat on the preconception health of young men and women, it is plausible that extreme heat affects vulnerable people, for example, women with cardiovascular diseases or metabolic diseases. During extreme heat, the mortality and morbidity rates increase. Coping with extreme heat is a physical strain which can lead to a disruption of metabolic processes. Once metabolic processes are disrupted, the endocrine system can also become disrupted which can have an impact on the reproductive system (Barreca et al. 2016, 2018; Hansen 2009; Ellison et al. 2005). Therefore, it is important to control the indoor climates of houses and office buildings in order to minimize indoor air pollution and to make the adverse effects of air pollution on fertility as small as possible.

12.13 Prevention and Protecting

Environmental toxins are everywhere and at any time and thereby a global issue. Prevention and protection against environmental toxins can be divided in three categories: (Garlantézac et al. 2009) personal prevention and protection, (Snijder et al. 2012) national prevention and protection, and (Robledo et al. 2015) global prevention and protection.

12.14 Recommendations

Men and women should be advised to protect themselves as much as possible from exposure to environmental toxins, particularly if they are planning to become pregnant. Risk assessment of the environment after a reproductive problem such as habitual abortions should be one of the first focuses for a physician, obstetrician, or midwife. Information about environmental toxins and potential risks for fertility problems, general health problems, and adverse pregnancy outcomes should be easily accessible for men and women contemplating a pregnancy.

12.15 The Role of Health-Care Professionals, Government, Governmental Agencies, and Academic Centers

Health-care professionals like midwives, obstetricians, pediatricians, general practitioners, and occupational physicians have regular contact with young men and women. Many of these men and women are working and therefore at risk for occupational hazards. In daily life men and women are exposed to possible harmful environmental hazards. Therefore, it is important that health-care professionals are aware of their role regarding informing and possibly protecting young men and women for occupational and environmental hazards.

Sutton et al. published an article about this topic in the American Journal of Obstetrics and Gynecology (AJOG (Sutton et al. 2012)). Sutton et al. stated that preconception and prenatal exposure to environmental chemicals are of particular importance because they may have a profound and lasting impact on health across the life course. The importance of the preconception period was previously brought to attention by David Barker. Barker described that the origin of health and diseases have their origin in the preconception period of human life (Barker 1995). Nowadays the theory of Barker is known as the Barker hypothesis or as the DOHad (Developmental Origin of Health and Diseases). Prevention activities spread by health-care professionals, especially of reproductive health-care professionals, are of great importance to protect a new generation against occupational and environmental hazards. Therefore, these professionals must ring the clock in communities but also in the political arena to underline the importance of prevention and protection. Sutton et al. described that pediatricians are focused on environmental hazards for a long time. They screen their patients (and their parents) on potential harmful exposure to environmental hazards searching for explanations of diseases of children. The American Academy of Pediatrics had an environmental committee and wrote a textbook for clinicians about hazardous environmental factors (Sutton et al. 2012).

Workplace assessment for occupational hazards and environmental hazards is a specialty of occupational health workers. In the Netherlands, every employee has access to an occupational health worker. They can be consulted without permission of their employer and are familial with laws and regulations on working with chemical substances and exposure to harmful environmental factors. The occupational health worker can alert someone to potential danger and also provide education about preventing exposure (Brand et al. 2009). Raynal et al. wrote a letter to plead for legislation for the mandatory provision of occupational health services either by the state or by employers (Raynal et al. 2019). Lack of these services can harm the labor force because they are denied from early detection of harmful risks. This type of care should be available to workers globally.

But what do general physicians and reproductive health-care professionals like obstetricians, midwives, and even pediatricians need to know and need to ask? What questions are the right questions to screen on occupational or environmental risks in the workplace? Gerritsen et al. stated that first it is important to understand the reciprocal relation between work and health as a basis for why and how to screen for occupational and environmental risks (Gerritsen et al. 2013). If knowledge and understanding is sufficient, physicians and reproductive health-care professionals must be able to take a work and context history. A context history should not only include questions about work but also the living environment and conditions. If knowledge regarding work-related factors of health-care professionals is not sufficient, professionals should point out men and women, preferably in the preconception period but certainly in the early pregnancy, on the possibility of screening the workplace environment to an occupational physician or a safety committee or union or other configuration.

Exposure to hazardous environmental factors does not only harm working young men and women; damage can continue for generations. This knowledge, revealed by research by academic centers, is not only important for reproductive health-care professionals but should also be shared with governments and governmental agencies who have an obligation to inform their citizens about how to cope with (avoidable) risks like occupational and environmental hazards. They also have a responsibility to act to protect citizens of all ages from dangerous exposures. Steegers et al. highlight that to maximize the chance for a healthy pregnancy, couples should be screened in the preconception period on environmental and occupational risks (Steegers et al. 2016). This should not only be addressed to reproductive health-care professionals but also to public health professionals.

References

Abell A, Juul S, Bonde JPE. Time to pregnancy among female greenhouse workers. Scand J Work Environ Health. 2000;26:131–6.

African Statistics. n.d. https://www.africaneconomicoutlook.org/statistics/. Accessed 10 Jan 2020.

Ashiru OA, Odusanya OO. Fertility and occupational hazards: review of the literature. Afr J Reprod Health. 2009;13:159–65.

Barker DJP. Intrauterine programming of adult disease. Mol Med Today. 1995;1(9):418–23.

Barreca A, Clay K, Greenstone M, Deschenes O, Shapiro J. Adapting to climate change: the remarkable decline in the U.S. temperature-mortality relationship over the 20th century. J Polit Econ. 2016;124:105–59.

Barreca A, Deschenes O, Guldi M. Maybe next month? Temperature shocks and dynamic adjustments in birth rates. Demography. 2018;55(4):1269–93.

Bloom MS, Vom Saal FA, Kom D, Taylor JA, Lamb JD, Fujimoto VY. Serum unconjugated bisphenol A concentrations in men may influence embryo quality indicators during in vitro fertilization. Environ Toxicol Pharmacol. 2011;32(2):319–23.

Bonde JP. Male reproductive organs are at risk from environmental hazards. Asian J Androl. 2010;12:152–6.

Borgeest C, Greenfeld C, Tomic D, Flaws JA. The effects of endocrine disrupting chemicals on the ovary. Front Biosci. 2002;7:1941–8.

Brand T, van Haperen VW, van Vliet-Lachotzki EH, Steegers EA. Preconceptual care should include looking at the effect of working conditions on pregnancy. Ned Tijdschr Geneeskund. 2009;153:A363 [Article in Dutch].

Bretveld R, Kik S, Hooiveld M, van Rooij I, Zielhuis G, Roeleveld N. Time-to-pregnancy among male greenhouse workers. Occup Environ Med. 2008a;65:185–90.

Bretveld RW, Hooiveld M, Zielhuis GA, Pellegrino A, van Rooij JA, Roeleveld N. Reproductive disorders among male and female greenhouse workers. Reprod Toxicol. 2008b;25:107–14.

Canadian Environmental Protection Act. Canada Gazette Part II. 1999. Order adding a toxic substance to schedule 1 to the Canadian Environmental Protection Act, 1999. 2010-10-13.

Chevrier C, Warembourg C, Gaudreau E, Monfort C, Le Blanc A, Guldner L, Cordier S. Organochlorine pesticides, polychlorinated biphenyls, seafood consumption, and time to pregnancy. Epidemiology. 2013;24:251–60.

Chiang C, Mahalingam S, Flaws JA. Environmental contaminants affecting fertility and somatic health. Semin Reprod Med. 2017;35:241–9.

Conforti A, Mascia M, Cioffi G, De Angelis C, Coppola G, De Rosa P, Pivonello R, Alviggi C, De Placido G. Air pollution and female fertility: a systematic review of literature. Reprod Biol Endocrinol. 2018;16(1):117.

De Cock J, Westveer K, Heederik D, te Velde E, van Kooij R. Time to pregnancy and occupational exposure to pesticides in fruit growers in the Netherlands. Occup Environ Med. 1994;51:639.

De Nisio A, Foresta C. Water and soil pollution as determinant of water and food quality/ contamination and its impact on male fertility. Reprod Biol Endocrinol. 2019;6(1):4.

Dutch Law on Lead Exposure. 1988. https://wetten.overheid.nl/BWBR0022918/2007-12-02. Accessed 5 Apr 2019.

EFSA, European Food and Safety Authority. Bisphenol A. 2011. Retrieved from https://www.efsa.europa.eu/en/topics/topic/bisphenol. Accessed 6 Apr 2019.

Ehrlich S, Williams PL, Missmer SA, Flaws JA, Ye X, Calafat AM, Petrozza JC, Wright D, Hauser R. Urinary bisphenol A concentrations and early reproductive health outcomes among women undergoing IVF. Hum Reprod. 2012;17(12):3583–92.

Ellison PT, Valeggia CR, Sherry DS. Human birth seasonality. In: Brockman DK, van Schaik CP, editors. Seasonality in primates: studies of living and extinct human and non-human primates. Cambridge: Cambridge University Press; 2005. p. 379–400.

Eskenazi B, Fenster L, Hudes M, Wyrobek AJ, Katz DF, Gerson J, Rempel DM. A study of the effect of perchloroethylene exposure on the reproductive outcomes of wives of dry-cleaning workers. Am J Ind Med. 1991;20(5):593–600.

Figà-Talamanca I. Occupational risk factors and reproductive health of women. Occup Med. 2006;56:521–31.

Foradori CD, Hinds LR, Quihuis AM, Lacagnina AF, Breckenridge CB, Handa RJ. The differential effect of atrazine on luteinizing hormone release in adrenalectomized adult female Wistar rats. Biol Reprod. 2011;85:684–9.

Fraites MJP, Cooper RL, Buckalew A, Jayaraman S, Mills L, Laws SC. Characterization of the hypothalamic-pituitary-adrenal axis response to Atrazine and metabolites in the female rat. Toxicol Sci. 2009;112:88–99.

Gallichio L, Miller SR, Green T, Zacur H, Flaws JA. Health outcomes of children born to cosmetologists compared to children of women in other occupations. Reprod Toxicol. 2010;29:361–5.

Garlantézac R, Monfort C, Rouget F, Cordier S. Maternal occupational exposure to solvents and congenital malformations: a prospective study in the general population. Occup Environ Med. 2009;66:456–63.

Gaskins AJ, Chavarro JE, Rich-Edwards JW, Missmer SA, Laden F, Henn SA, Lawson CC. Occupational use of high-level disinfectants and fecundity among nurses. Scand J Work Environ Health. 2017;43:171–80.

Gerritsen JC, Smits PB, Brand T. Every physician should know how to take an occupational history: the importance of teaching occupational medicine in medical school. 2013;157(14):A5787 [Article in Dutch].

Goldman JM, Davis LK, Murr AS, Cooper RL. Atrazine-induced elevation or attenuation of the LH surge in the ovariectomized, estrogen-primed female rat: role of adrenal progesterone. Reproduction. 2013;145:305–14.

Goodman M, Mandel JS, DeSesso JM, Scialli AR. Atrazine and pregnancy outcomes: a systematic review of epidemiologic evidence. Birth Defects Res B Dev Reprod Toxicol. 2014;10:215–36.

Gore AC. Environmental toxicant effects on neuroendocrine function. Endocrine. 2011;14:235–46.

Guz J, Gackowski D, Foksinski M, Rozalski R, Zarakowska E, Siomek A, Szpila A, Kotzbach M, Kotzbach R, Olinski R. Comparison of oxidative stress/ DNA damage in semen and blood of fertile and infertile men. PLoS One. 2013;8(7):e68490.

Hansen PJ. Effects of heat stress on mammalian reproduction. Philos Trans Roy Soc B Biol Sci. 2009;364:3341–50.

Hooiveld M, Haveman W, Roskes K, Bretveld R, Burstyn I, Roeleveld N. Adverse reproductive outcomes among male painters with occupational exposure to organic solvents. Occup Environ Med. 2006;63(8):538–44.

Hougaard KS, Hannerz H, Bonde JP, Feveille H, Burr H. The risk of infertility among hairdressers. Five-year follow-up of female hairdressers in a Danish national registry. Hum Reprod. 2006;12:3122–6.

Hu H, Téllez-Rojo MM, Bellinger D, Smith D, Ettinger AS, Lamadrid-Figueroa H, Schwartz J, Schnaas L, Mercado-Garcia A, Hernández-Avila M. Fetal lead exposure at each stage of pregnancy as a predictor of infant mental development. Environ Health Perspect. 2006;114:1730–5.

Kesari KK, Agarwal A, Henkel R. Radiations and male fertility. Reprod Biol Endocrinol. 2018;16(1):118.

Kim D, Kang MY, Choi S, Park J, Lee HJ, Kim EA. Reproductive disorders among cosmetologists and hairdressers: a meta- analysis. Int Arch Occup Environ Health. 2016;89:739–53.

Kolstad HA, Bisanti L, Roeleveld N, Baldi R, Bonde JP, Joffe M. Time to pregnancy among male workers of the reinforced plastics industry in Denmark, Italy and the Netherlands: ASCLEPIOS. Scand J Work Environ Health. 2000;26(4):353–8.

Kotelchuck M, Lu M. Father's role in preconception health. Matern Child Health J. 2017;21:2025–39.

Lafuente H, García-Blàquez N, Jacquemin B, Checa MA. Outdoor air pollution and sperm quality. Fertil Steril. 2016;106(4):880–96.

Lindbohm ML, Ylöstalo P, Sallmén M, Henriks-Eckerman ML, Nurminen T, Forss H, Taskinen H. Occupational exposure in dentistry and miscarriage. Occup Environ Med. 2007;64:127–33.

Logman JFS, de Vries LE, Hemels MEH, Khattak S, Einarson TR. Paternal organic solvents exposure and adverse pregnancy outcomes: a meta-analysis. Am J Ind Med. 2005;47:37–44.

Luderer U, Bushley A, Stover BD, Bremmer WJ, Faustman EM, Takaro TK, Checkoway H, Brodin CA. Effects of occupational solvent exposure on reproductive hormone concentrations and fecundability in men. Am J Ind Med. 2004;46(6):614–26.

Marci R, Mallozzi M, Di Benedetto L, Schimberni M, Mossa S, Soave I, Palombo S, Caserta D. Radiations and female fertility. Reprod Biol Endocrinol. 2018;16(1):112.

Mehrpour O, Karrari P, Zamani N, Tsatsakis AM, Abdollahi M. Occupational exposure to pesticides and consequences on male semen and fertility: a review. Toxicol Lett. 2014;15:146–56.

Mima M, Greenwald D, Ohlander S. Environmental toxins and male fertility. Curr Urol Rep. 2018;17:50.

Nieuwenhuijsen MJ, Dadvand P, Grellier J, Martinez D, Vrijheid M. Environmental risk factors of pregnancy outcomes: a summary of recent meta-analysis of epidemiological studies. Environ Health. 2013;12:6.

O'Brien AP, Hurley J, Linsley P, McNeil KA, Fletcher R, Aitken JR. Men's preconception health: a primary health-care viewpoint. Am J Men's Health. 2018;12:1575–81.

Olshan A, Teschke A, Baird P. Paternal occupation and congenital malformations in offspring. Am J Ind Med. 1991;20:447–75.

Perin PM, Sedrakyan S, Guiliani S, Da Sacco S, Carraro G, Shiri L, Lemley KV, Rosol M, Wu S, Atala A, Warburton D, De Filippo RE. Impact of short-term preconceptional exposure to particulate air pollution on treatment outcome in couples undergoing in vitro fertilization and embryo transfer (IVF/ET). J Assist Reprod Genet. 2010;27(7):371–82.

Pizzorno J. Environmental toxins and infertility. Integr Med. 2018;17:8–11.

Rashtian J, Chavkin DE, Merhi Z. Water and soil pollution as determinant of water and food quality/contamination and its impact on female fertility. Reprod Biol Endocrinol. 2019;13:5.

Raynal A, Hermanns R, Robson S, Weir M, Carry D. Everybody should have access to occupational health services. BMJ. 2019;364:k5220.

Robledo CA, Yeung E, Mendola P, Sundaram R, Maisog J, Sweeney AM, Boyd Barr D, Buck LG. Preconception maternal and paternal exposure to persistent organic pollutants and birth size: the LIFE study. Environ Health Perspect. 2015;1:88–94.

Rosofsky A, Janulewicz P, Thayer KA, McClean M, Wise LA, Calafat AM, Mikkelsen EM, Taylor KW, Hatch EE. Exposure to multiple chemicals in a cohort of reproductive-aged Danish women. Environ Res. 2017;154:73–85.

Rowland AS, Baird DD, Weinberg CR, Shore DL, Shy CM, Wilcox AJ. The effect of occupational exposure to mercury vapour on the fertility of female dental assistants. Occup Environ Med. 1994;51(1):28–34.

Rylander L, Källén B. Reproductive outcomes among hairdressers. Scand J Work Environ Health. 2005;31:212–7.

Rylander L, Axmon A, Torén K, Albin M. Reproductive outcome among female hairdressers. Occup Environ Med. 2002;59:517–22.

Safari M, Mosleminiya N, Abdolali A. Thermal mapping on male genital and skin tissues of laptop thermal sources and electromagnetic interaction. Bioelectromagnetics. 2017;38:550–8.

Sallmén M, Lindbohm ML, Kyyrönen P, Nykyri E, Anttila A, Taskinen H, Hemminki K. Reduced fertility among women exposed to organic solvents. Am J Ind Med. 1995;27:699–713.

Sallmen M, Lindbohm ML, Anttila A, Kyrrönen P, Taskinen H, Nykyri E, Hemminiki K. Time to pregnancy among the wives of men exposed to organic solvents. Occup Environ Med. 1998;55(1):24–30.

Salma R, Bottagisi S, Solansky I, Lepeule J, Giorgis-Allemand L, Sram R. Short-term impact of atmospheric pollution on fecundability. Epidemiology. 2013;24(6):871–9.

Sheiner EK, Sheiner E, Hammel RD, Potashnik G, Carel R. Effect of occupational exposure on male fertility: literature review. Ind Health. 2003;41:55–62.

Snijder CA, te Velde E, Roeleveld N, Burdorf A. Occupational exposure to chemical substances and time to pregnancy: a systematic review. Hum Reprod Update. 2012;3:284–300.

Statistics Netherlands, Eurostat. 2019. https://ec.europa.eu/eurostat. Accessed 5 Apr 2019

Steegers EA, Barker ME, Steegers-Theunissen RP, Williams MA. Societal valorisation of new knowledge to improve perinatal health: time to act. Paediatr Perinat Epidemiol. 2016;30(2):201–4.

Stephenson J, Heslehurst N, Hall J, Schoenaker DAJM, Hutchinson J, Cade JE, Poston L, Barret G, Crozier SR, Barker M, Kumaran K, Yajnik CS, Baird J, Mishra GD. Before the beginning: nutrition and lifestyle in the preconception period and its importance for future health. Lancet. 2018;5:1830–41.

Stoker TE, Perreault SD, Bremser K, Marshall RS, Murr A, Cooper RL. Acute exposure to molinate alters neuroendocrine control of ovulation in the rat. Toxicol Sci. 2005;1:38–48.

Sutton P, Woodruff TJ, Perron J, Stotland N, Conry JA, Miller MD, Giudice LC. Toxic environmental chemicals: the role of reproductive health professionals in preventing harmful exposures. Am J Obstet Gynecol. 2012;20(7):164–73.

Taskinen H, Antilla A, Lindbohm ML, Sallmen M, Hemminki K. Spontaneous abortions and congenital malformations among wives of men occupationally exposed to organic solvents. Scan J Work Environ Health. 1989;15:345–52.

Ten Kate LP, Assendelft WJJ, Brand T, Groeneveld PC, Hirasing RA, van Huis AM et al. Preconception care: a good beginning, chapter 4. 2007; 49–57.

Tiemann U. In vivo and in vitro effects of the organochlorine pesticides DDT, TCPM, methoxychlor, and lindane on the female reproductive tract of mammals: a review. Reprod Toxicol. 2008;25:316–26.

US Department of Labour. 2017.

Wennborg H, Bodin L, Vainio H, Axelsson G. Sovent use and time to pregnancy among female personnel in biomedical laboratories in Sweden. Occup Environ Med. 2001;62(1):43–55.

WHO. Elemental mercury and inorganic mercury compounds: human health aspects. https://www.who.int/ipcs/publications/cicad/en/cicad50.pdf. Accessed 13 May 2019.

Windham GC, Lee D, Mitchell P, Anderson M, Petreas M, Lasley B. Exposure to organochlorine compounds and effects on ovarian function. Epidemiology. 2005;16:182–90.

Wright C, Milne S, Leeson H. Sperm DNA damage caused by oxidative stress: modifiable clinical, lifestyle and nutritional factors in male infertility. Reprod Biomed Online. 2014;28:684–703.

Yun L, Zhang W, Qin K. Relationship among maternal blood lead, ALAD gene polymorphism and neonatal neurobehavioral development. Int J Clin Exp Pathol. 2015;8:7277–81.

Social Environment: Interpersonal Violence

13

Adja J. M. Waelput

13.1 Introduction

Social determinants of health, which can be protective or risk factors, influence the preconception period and therefore the health of future children and generations. These factors cover a wide range such as housing, working conditions, socio-economic status, exposure to noise or air pollution, safety, poverty, or interpersonal and sexual violence. Violence against women is experienced by millions of women and girls all around the world and can occur from prebirth to old age. Violence against women and girls is a fundamental violation of women's rights and is grounded in power inequalities, which are based on harmful and strict gender norms justifying male dominance and control over women.

Violence against women influences their physical and mental health, with long-lasting effects and even intergenerational effects. The violence can hinder them socially and economically, with a reduced ability to study, work, and care for themselves and their family. Their families and communities may suffer as well.

This chapter focuses on violence against women and how this influences the health and wellbeing of women, parents to be, and the next generation. The types of violence that women experience as well as the prevalence and impact will be discussed. This chapter will review the role of the health system in addressing violence and the comprehensive approach that is needed. By working together, communities, men and women, health, legal and social services, and professionals can

A. J. M. Waelput (✉)
Division of Obstetrics and Prenatal Medicine, Department of Obstetrics and Gynaecology, Erasmus Medical Centre Rotterdam, Rotterdam, The Netherlands
e-mail: a.waelput@erasmusmc.nl

© Springer Nature Switzerland AG 2020
J. Shawe et al. (eds.), *Preconception Health and Care: A Life Course Approach*,
https://doi.org/10.1007/978-3-030-31753-9_13

create awareness on the magnitude of violence and the lifelong effect of violence. Together they can introduce, link, and maintain programs for prevention and necessary services by healthcare professionals within the broader health systems and societal systems.

Women who have experienced violence often feel there is nowhere to turn to. Help and support might not be available, or the services might not be known or accessible. Pregnancy and the preconception period are windows of opportunity for detecting and addressing violence. For some women, these periods are the only ones in which they are in (regular) contact with healthcare professionals.

13.2   Violence Against Women and Girls

Violence against women and girls is a worldwide problem and can affect all women, in all stages of life. Globally, one in three women have experienced sexual or physical violence at least once in her life. One out of four children has a mother who has to deal with intimate partner violence. Experiencing violence at home influences health and wellbeing of children, both in the short and long term. Witnessing violence at home as a young child increases the risk of perpetrating or tolerating intimate partner violence (World Health Organization 2019).

13.2.1   Different Forms of Violence Against Women

According to the United Nations Declaration on the Elimination of Violence Against Women (United Nations General Assembly 1994), violence against women means '…any act of gender-based violence that results in, or is likely to result in, physical, sexual or psychological harm or suffering to women, including threats of such acts, coercion or arbitrary deprivation of liberty, whether occurring in public or in private life.' Violence against women has many different forms (World Health Organization 2013c):

- Physical and/or sexual violence by an intimate partner (intimate partner violence).
- Rape/sexual assault and other forms of sexual violence perpetrated by someone other than a partner such as friends, acquaintances, other family members, or utter strangers (non-partner sexual violence).
- Female genital mutilation (also known as female genital cutting or circumcision).
- Honour killing.
- Human trafficking.

Definitions of Different Forms of Violence Against Women (Raymond 2002; World Health Organization 2013c; IAWG 2019; OECD 2019)

Intimate partner violence	Self-reported experience of one or more acts of physical and/or sexual violence by a current or former partner (heterosexual or same-sex relationship) from the age of 15 years. This threshold is being used to distinguish between child sexual abuse (violence between 15–18 years) and violence against women and girls: • Physical violence: Being slapped or having something thrown at you that could hurt you; being pushed or shoved; being hit with a fist or something else that could hurt; being kicked, dragged, or beaten up; being choked or burnt on purpose; and/or being threatened with, or actually, having a gun, knife, or other weapon used on you. • Sexual violence: Being physically forced to have sexual intercourse when a person did not want to, having sexual intercourse because a person was afraid of what her partner might do, and/or being forced to do something sexual that a person found humiliating or degrading. It includes (attempted) rape, an act of non-consensual sexual intercourse, sexual abuse, and sexual exploitation.
Current partner violence	Being victim of (self-reported) partner violence of at least one act of physical or sexual violence within the past 12 months.
Perinatal intimate partner violence	Intimate partner violence in the year before conception, throughout pregnancy, during, and up to one year after giving birth.
Non-partner sexual violence	Experience of being forced to perform any sexual act that a person from the age of 15 did not want to by someone other than her husband/partner.
Female genital mutilation (FGM)	All procedures to the female genital organs for non-medical reasons such as partial or total removal of the external female genitalia or other injuries to the female genital.
Forced (early) marriage	The marriage of an individual against her or his will. The marriage is arranged and forced upon by parents, or others, for different reasons. The ones to be married off are not allowed or, if the are under 18, not old enough for informed consent to marry.
Psychological/ emotional violence	Systematic humiliation and belittling, degrading treatment, insulting, or making a woman feel bad about herself and threats to hurt her or her beloved ones and/or controlling behaviour such as isolation, ignoring her, monitoring what she does or who she meets, and controlling her access to healthcare, education, or the labour market.
Economic abuse	Denial of resources, services, and opportunities such as restricting access to financial means (even her own income), healthcare, education, or other resources with the purpose of controlling or subjugating a person. This might lead to poverty and hardship.
Honour killings	Murders in the name of honour.
Trafficking of women	Recruiting, transporting, harbouring, or receiving persons under threat or use of force or other types of coercion for purposes of exploiting individuals for prostitution, other types of sexual exploitation, forced labour or services, slavery or practices similar to slavery, servitude or the removal of organs.
Cyberbullying	The distribution of sexually explicit photos and videos to embarrass and shame the victim. Because of the difficulty in removing them, this abuse can have long-lasting consequences.

In case of a wide acceptance or justification of violence against women, it can be hard to change this attitude, behaviour, and practices. Nevertheless, attitudes on violence against women *are* changing. Surveys indicate that the acceptance of wife-beating is decreasing amongst women as well as men. Attitudes on female genital mutilation/cutting are changing as well, mainly in countries with a relatively low prevalence of female genital mutilation/cutting. In these countries the number of people, both women and men, who believe that the practice should end, is growing (U Nations - Affairs DoEaS 2015).

13.3 Violence against Women in Numbers

One in three women have experienced sexual or physical violence at least once in their lives. It is a worldwide problem and can affect all women, in all stages of life. Less than 40% seek help for their experience with violence. Less than 4% of women seeking help (i.e less than 2% of all women experiencing violence) seek help from the police (U Nations - Affairs DoEaS 2015).

Violence against women and girls can occur during any stage of the life cycle, from prebirth to old age. Through the life cycle, it has different forms: from female infanticide to abuse and neglect of older women, from genital mutilation of young girls to forced prostitution and trafficking, and from domestic violence to sexual harassment at work.

In general, violence peaks in the reproductive years. In Europe, the prevalence for both partner and non-partner violence women was highest amongst women aged 18 to 29 years and seems to decline with age (U Nations - Affairs DoEaS 2015). In comparison to other periods in the life course, the risk for physical forms of intimate partner abuse seems to be lower during pregnancy (Desmarais et al. 2014).

Most sexual violence against children takes place at home, or by someone close or known to them (UNICEF 2018). Experiencing sexual violence at school, or on the way to and from school, hampers girls in attending school (safely), both primary school and secondary school. In the USA, it is estimated that one in five women is sexually assaulted during college (Muehlenhard et al. 2017).

During pregnancy, childbirth, and the postpartum period, women can be confronted with disrespectful, neglectful, and abusive treatment by healthcare professionals. This violates their human rights as well as their rights to be free from discrimination and their rights to respectful care. This might influence the likelihood to seek and use reproductive and maternal healthcare services (World Health Organization 2014; Miller and Lalonde 2015).

Older women (i.e. over 60 years) may experience physical, sexual, or psychological abuse. Financial exploitation or neglect by intimate partners, family members, or caregivers might play a part in the violence against older women. This is especially the case for the ones having a mental or physical disease or living in a residence for elderly people.

13.3.1 Availability of Data on Violence Against Women

Despite the high prevalence of violence against women, data were scarce (U Nations - Affairs DoEaS 2015). Because only a small proportion of women turn to the police for help, violence against women is often under-reported. In addition to the prevailing norms on violence against women, the low number of female police officers might be one of the reasons for this under-reporting.

Since 1995, a more standardized way of collecting data and key indicators on violence against women has been implemented (World Health Organization 2005; U Nations - Affairs DoEaS 2015). These national surveys on violence against women are compiled by the United Nations Statistics Division (U Nations - Affairs DoEaS 2015).

Although the availability of data on violence against women has increased, under-reporting is still likely and may differ between and even within countries. This might be due to stigma and taboos on (raising) the subject and to the possible harmful social, physical, psychological, or legal consequences of disclosure of the act of violence.

The available data do not cover the whole spectrum of violence against women. Lack of standardization is still an obstacle in data collection, for example, on issues like emotional/psychological abuse (Hill et al. 2016) or disrespectful and abusive treatment in maternal healthcare (World Health Organization 2014). Data gaps are known for specific groups, such as elderly women who are often excluded from surveys due to their age or residency (no longer part of a household, but institutionalized) (World Health Organization 2013c; U Nations - Affairs DoEaS 2015).

Some data, such as data on 'honour' killings and trafficking, are limited to data on women and girls who have been detected by national authorities. Between 2012 and 2014 over 63,000 victims of trafficking were detected. About 71% of all victims are women (51%) and girls (20%), mostly for sexual exploitation. About 75% of all child trafficking victims are girls (UNODC 2016).

Data on topics which rely on self-reporting such as cyberbullying are scarce as well (OECD 2019). Across the OECD countries with available data, about 12% of girls aged 15 report having been cyberbullied at least once, compared to 8% for boys.

Violence by an intimate partner is the most reported and researched form of sexual or physical violence against women. It affects 30% of women worldwide

Case: Complementary Data Sources to Measure Violence Against Women in Canada (U Nations - Affairs DoEaS 2015)

Since 1962 Canada measures violence against women through police-reported administrative surveys. Since 1988 the survey includes data on the victim, the accused, the relationship between victim and accused, their sex and age, the location of the event, charge rates, etc. The survey is mandatory. Because of the common definitions across the counties, the data are nationally representative and enables comparisons over time and across regions. The main challenge is the victims' hesitation to report their case to the police. Therefore, this survey is complemented with data from victimization surveys. Over time the surveys have evolved to provide more insight in both violence against women and in spousal violence, for which women and men are targeted.

and accounts for 60–80% of all the experienced and reported violence in a lifetime. Abuse solely by someone other than an intimate partner is reported by less than one third of the women who reported violence. Data specific on physical violence against women in their lifetime varies between 7 and 77% and from 5 to 32% for sexual violence during lifetime, both irrespective of the perpetrator being a partner or not (U Nations - Affairs DoEaS 2015).

The 12-month prevalence of current partner violence has been researched in more depth, including the association with macro-level characteristics. Using data from 66 surveys from 44 countries, this study focused on the associations between macro-level measures of socio-economic development, women's status, gender inequality, and gender-related norms and the prevalence of current partner violence at a population level (Heise and Kotsadam 2015). In many high-income countries, less than 4% of the women aged 15–49 experienced current partner violence in the last 12 months. In some low-income countries, the prevalence was as high as 40%. Strikingly, in low-income countries, the lifetime prevalence and 12-month prevalence of intimate partner's violence are much alike. This might indicate it is hard to leave a violent relationship (U Nations - Affairs DoEaS 2015).

It is estimated that at least 200 million women and girls in 30 countries with representative data have undergone FMG, mostly before the age of 5. As a result of migration and refuge, women and girls with (risk on) FGM live across the globe (U Nations - Affairs DoEaS 2015). Overall, the prevalence in female genital mutilation in Africa is declining from 1 to 2 in 1985 to 1 in 3 recent years. The prevalence ranges from 1.4 to 89% (UNFPA 2019). However, the expected number of girls that have FGM will rise from 3,9 million in 2015 to 4,6 million in 2030. This rise is caused by the population growth amongst young girls in 25 countries with a high prevalence of FGM (UNFPA 2018).

The rates for FGM vary according to ethnicity, religion, urban or rural residence, economic status, age, education, and income. In general, reported levels of female genital mutilation are lower in urban areas, amongst younger women, in families with higher levels of household income, and amongst girls and women with higher educated mothers (U Nations - Affairs DoEaS 2015).

It is estimated that 650 million women and girls and 115 million men and boys living in the world were married before age 18. In the last decade, the global rate of child marriage has declined from 25 to 20% in women aged 20–24 years, especially amongst girls under age 15. In the early 1980s, one in three women were married in childhood (UNICEF 2018) and 1 in 30 boys were married before the age of 18. About 20% of these boys were younger than 15 at the moment of marriage (Murray Gáson et al. 2019).

Despite years of research on violence against women, data on the period from 1 year before conception and 1 year after childbirth tend to come from rather small studies, using different methodologies and including specific groups in specific settings such as women in maternity wards or shelters. It is assumed that under-reporting is widespread, due to stigma and taboos on (raising the) subject and to the possible harmful consequences of disclosure of the act of violence.

Population-based data on violence during pregnancy are scarce. Devries et al. used data from 19 countries. They showed that 2–13.5% of all women ever pregnant did experience intimate partner violence during their pregnancy (Devries et al. 2010). In an earlier study with data from 15 (other) countries, violence during pregnancy ranged from 1.2–27.6%. Half of these studies showed an estimated prevalence between 3.8 and 8.8% (García-Moreno et al. 2005). Based on a meta-analyses into domestic violence during pregnancy, James et al. concluded that 19.8% of pregnant women had to deal with domestic violence, which consisted of emotional abuse (28.4%), physical abuse (13.8%), and sexual abuse during pregnancy (8.0%) (James et al. 2013).

At the end of the 1990s, an American study was the first to differentiate between moment of physical violence before, during, and after pregnancy (Martin et al. 2001). In 2006–2007 a Canadian study on physical and sexual violence, by any perpetrator, differentiate any abuse before, during, or after pregnancy only or at any combination of these times. They interviewed 6,421 women 5–9 months after giving (live) birth; 791 women reported abuse. More than half of them were abused solely before pregnancy, nearly 5% at all three moments. About 30% of the women experienced abuse during pregnancy (solely or in combination with any other period). For nearly half of them, the abuse started during pregnancy (Daoud et al. 2012).

A Belgian study reported 14.3% interpersonal violence in the 12 months before pregnancy and 10.6% during pregnancy. Women reported 2.4% psychological, 1.1% sexual, and 12.8% physical abuse during pregnancy. Part of the women experienced violence both before and during pregnancy (Van Parys et al. 2014). A Swedish study into the prevalence of domestic violence during pregnancy and 1–1½ years postpartum showed an increase of domestic violence over time from 2.5% of domestic violence during pregnancy to 3.3% postpartum. All women who reported domestic violence at 1–1½ years postpartum had a history of violence (Finnbogadóttir and Dykes 2016).

Pregnancy seems to be a protective factor in intimate partner violence. Compared to the lifetime and past year period prevalence, the prevalence of intimate partner violence is lower during pregnancy. Between one third and two thirds of the abused women report that prior abuse ceased during pregnancy (Brownridge et al. 2011). But in case the violence continued, women were more likely to be victims of more severe forms of violence. They were more likely to report adverse post-violence indicators such as physical injury, psychopathology in different forms, and abuse of alcohol, drugs, and/or medication to be able to deal with the violence (Brownridge et al. 2011). It is suggested that, while physical abuse is reduced during pregnancy, emotional abuse may increase (Daoud et al. 2012).

13.4   Why Is Violence Against Women So Widespread?

Violence against women and girls is rooted in gender inequality and male dominance and control over women (World Health Organization 2013c). When violence against women, especially physical violence by an intimate partner (wife-beating), is accepted or justified, it can be hard to change norms, attitudes, behaviours, and practices. For women, it can be hard to speak out and ask for help.

Violence against women and (strict norms on) women's disadvantaged position in society seem to reinforce each other, by alternatingly being a cause and a consequence. For example, while their lack of power is a risk factor for violence, violence against women can (further) restrict their participation in society.

At least 144 countries have laws on domestic violence and 154 on sexual harassment in public places and workplaces (World Bank Group 2018). Less widespread are the laws on marital rape ($n = 52$) (U Nations - Affairs DoEaS 2015). FGM is outlawed in more than 40 countries (UNFPA 2019). However, to have any effect, the response to women who seek help needs to be adequate. The laws need to be properly implemented, to be sustainable, participatory, and linked to broader policies and programs which support victims (UN Women 2013).

Violence Against Women or Gender-Based Violence?

- Violence against women is an umbrella term and also referred to as sexual violence and gender-based violence. The different wordings are not completely interchangeable.
- Data on violence show that women are more likely to be a violence victim than a violence perpetrator (i.e. being violent against their male partners in a relationship where the male partner was not beating or hurting them).
- By using the term gender-based violence, the main focus is on the gendered aspects of the violence. It is based on the socially established sexual and gender norms, status, and differences between males and females, especially the subordinate status of women and girls in society (IAWG 2019).
- Established sexual and gender norms, which increases women's vulnerability to violence, can also lead to gender-based violence targeting lesbian, gay, bisexual, transgender, queer, questioning, intersex, and asexual (LGBTQIA) persons. Gender aspects can play a role in violence against boys and men as well, for example, in sexual abuse, torture, or abduction and recruitment to serve as child soldiers (IAWG 2019).

13.5 Protective and Risk Factors

Risk factors for intimate partner violence can be identified on four interacting levels: individual, relationship, community, and societal (Heise 1998; Stewart et al. 2017) (Fig. 13.1).

Both victim and perpetrator bring their own history into the relationship, in which the violence takes place. This relationship is formed by and embedded in communities such as social networks (both formal and informal), peer groups, workplace, and neighbourhoods. The societal level represents the economic and social environment, including cultural norms on gender, power, (in)equalities, and support/condemnation of violence (World Health Organization 2005).

Heise et al. (2015) showed that the risk on and acceptance of current partner violence are associated with gender-related norms and laws:

- Norms related to male authority over female behaviour.
- Norms justifying wife-beating.
- Law and practice on resources, such as access to land, property, and other productive resources, that favour men over women.
- Family law on guardianship and rights to child custody, inheritance (land and money), right to marry, or divorce, which discriminate against women.

In regions with high acceptance of wife-beating, individual variables, such as being educated and being older, are protective against violence. Socio-economic development seems to dampen partner violence, with lower prevalence in high-income countries than in low-income countries. This is probably due to changes in

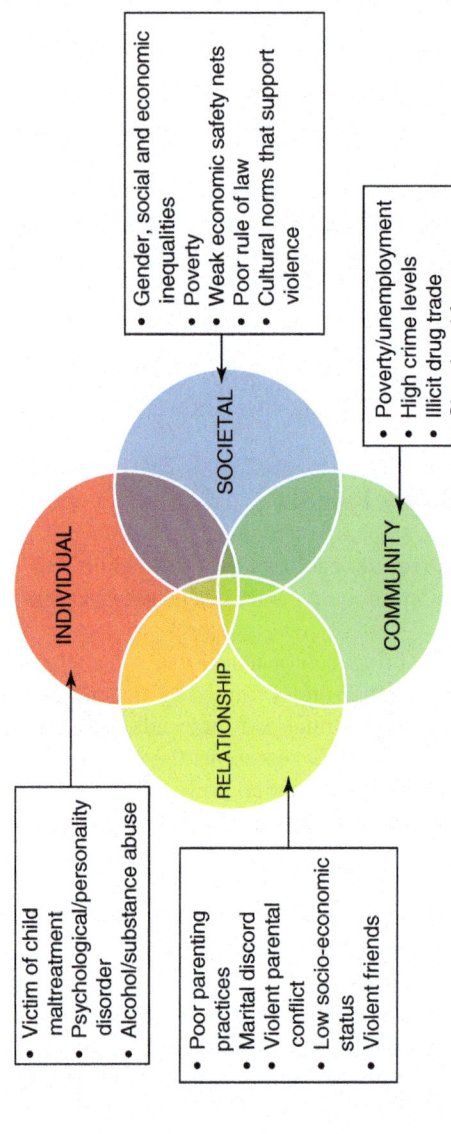

Fig. 13.1 The World Health Organization ecological framework for intimate partner violence. Some examples of risk factors (which may apply to both the victim and perpetrator) at each level. Adapted from WHO, 2002 (Stewart et al. 2017). Copyright © Springer Science+Business Media New York 2017. Permission form: https://s100.copyright.com/AppDispatchServlet#formTop

the roles of women during the economic growth, with more access to education and the paid workforce, and a change into more gender-equitable norms. But, changing norms and empowering women by microfinance or job creation programs for improvements on the long term might perversely increase the violence in the short term. This is the case for women who are enrolling in the paid workforce in an environment in which few women do so (Heise and Kotsadam 2015).

Some risk factors do contribute to becoming either a victim or a perpetrator of violence, such as alcohol/substance abuse, low levels of education, or witnessing domestic violence as a child. The underlying pathways are not always clear: Is violence in later life a 'learned response' due to growing up in a violent home, or a result of a disturbed emotional and psychological development due to the trauma of witnessing violence?

Violence against women is interconnected with other forms of discrimination and exclusion, based on gender, race, class, migrant status, religion, customs, social status, indigenous status, poverty, and other distinctions or identities. This interconnectedness influences the risk on being targeted. It also influences women's possibilities to report abuse and to seek protection and support, as well as the responses they will get on doing so (U Nations - Affairs DoEaS 2015; Michau et al. 2015). Furthermore, it contributes to the persistence of violence against women. For a breakthrough, cross-sectoral coordination between groups, communities, and sectors (such as healthcare, education, justice) is essential.

This interconnectedness puts some women more at risk than others (Deliver for Good 2017):

- Women living with disabilities.
- Migrant women and women from minority communities (ethnic, racial, or indigenous).
- Lesbian, gay, bisexual, transgender, queer, questioning, intersex, and asexual (LGBTQIA) persons.
- Women living in remote, rural communities.
- Women who have been trafficked.
- Sex workers.
- Domestic workers.
- Women with drug abuse, especially if they inject drugs.
- Women living with HIV.
- Women living in humanitarian emergencies, conflict situations, refugee camps, or who are displaced due to the conflict. While living in an environment with no or little functioning social systems, law enforcement, and services, rape, and sexual abuse are being used as weapons of war.

13.6   Impact of Violence on Women's Health

The adverse outcomes and potential health effects of violence are broad and far-reaching, both for the short and long term (Fig. 13.2):

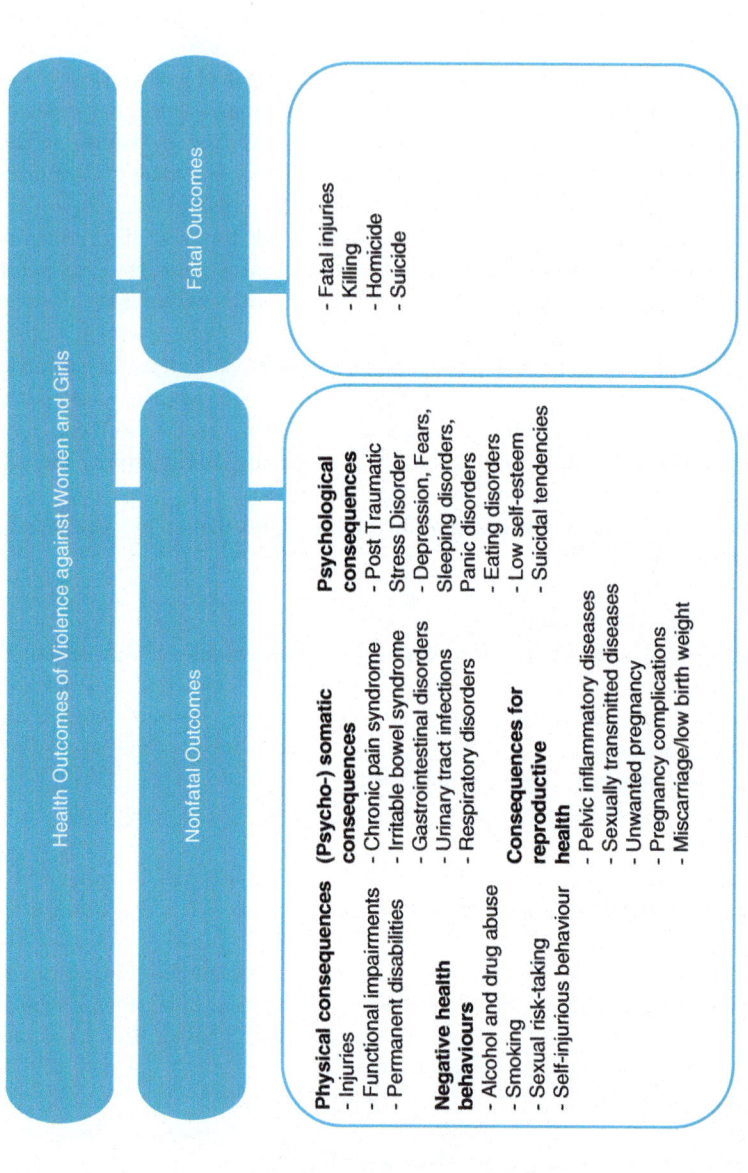

Fig. 13.2 Health consequences of violence against Women and girls. (WAVE-UNFPA 2014). Copyright © UNFPA & Wave 2014 with permission

- Adverse physical health outcomes, such as acute injuries, chronic pain, neurological problems, abdominal pain, and other gastrointestinal illness.
- Gynaecological problems, such as intrauterine bleeding and infertility.
- Mental health consequences, such as depression, anxiety, post-traumatic stress disorder, and substance abuse.
- Sexual and reproductive health problems, such as sexually transmitted infections, HIV, unwanted pregnancy, and lack of control over their reproductive choices.
- Maternal and perinatal outcomes, such as abortion, low-birthweight babies.
- Intergenerational effects, such as negative child health and development outcomes.

13.7 Pathways Between Violence and Health Outcomes

Understanding the pathways between exposures of violence on women's health is essential for prevention and a proper response to women who seek support. But the pathways are not yet fully understood. It is assumed that they are complex, context specific and can be both direct (injury, health problems, death) and indirect (such as biological and behavioral stress). The different mechanisms might reinforce each other and might in turn increase health risks (World Health Organization 2013c).

In response to the stress, different parts of the brain can be structurally changed. This can lead to mental disorders, immune system failures, chronic pain, cardiovascular disease, hypertension, and insulin-dependent diabetes (World Health Organization 2013c). These stress responses have been linked with premature birth and low birthweight of the newborns.

The increased risk on negative health outcomes can also be mediated/increased by behavioural stress responses such as the need for and use of alcohol, prescription medication, tobacco, or other drugs to deal with the violence. But they are not necessarily a precondition for the adverse health effects (World Health Organization 2013c). Another pathway can be caused by controlling behaviours of the male partner. If this behaviour co-occurs with (physical and sexual) violence against her, women might be (extra) limited in her access to healthcare and her sexual and reproductive decision-making (World Health Organization 2013c).

> **The Impact of Violence Against Women in Numbers (WHO Study Group 2006; World Health Organization 2013c)**
> - Women who have been abused by their partner, sexually or physically, are 1.5 times more likely to acquire HIV (or another sexually transmitted disease).
> - Women who have been abused by their partner, sexually or physically, are more than twice as likely to have an abortion.

- Women who have been abused by their partner, sexually or physically, are 16% more likely to have a low-birthweight baby.
- Women who have been abused by their partner, sexually or physically, are 41% more likely to have a preterm birth.
- Women who have been abused by their partner, sexually or physically, are twice as likely to experience depression.
- Women who have experienced non-partner sexual violence are 2.3 times more likely to have alcohol use disorders.
- Women who have experienced non-partner sexual violence are 2.6 times more likely to experience depression or anxiety.
- Women with female genital mutilation are 28% more likely to have a child that dies before or shortly after birth (data are limited to the period in which the women are an inpatient.).

Note that most research is done on the consequences of partner and non-partner violence.

Impacts of violence on women's sexual and reproductive health include the following:

- Fertility control: controlling behaviour by the violent partner within a relationship does not only lead to sexual violence and coercion but to control over fertility and planned parenthood as well. Disapproval or sabotage of birth control contributes to the higher prevalence of unintended pregnancies (unless long-acting reversible contraceptives are being used that are not partner dependent). Probably half of unintended pregnancies are terminated, often by illegal and unsafe abortions which, again, put the woman's health at an extra risk.
- Safe sex: women in violent relationships, or women who fear intimate partner violence, are often faced with limited control over their sexual intercourse, have little say in the use of condoms, and are often with a partner who is more likely to engage in HIV-risk behaviours.

On top of the aforementioned impact of violence on women's physical and mental health, violence during pregnancy is associated with adverse outcomes such as low-birthweight and/or preterm birth. Figure 13.3 shows the health outcomes of intimate partner violence during pregnancy. The results for intrauterine growth restriction/small for gestational age were not that clear, possibly due to differences in data collection. One of the studies (Coker et al. 2004) in the review, although small, showed a dose-response relationship between the frequency of violence and the increase in the risk on low-birthweight and/or preterm birth (Hill et al. 2016).

Women who experience intimate partner violence around the time of pregnancy are seen to be limited in their care for their newborn children. Violent partners might not be willing to lessen their (physical and sexual) demand on women during the postpartum period or might be jealous (Silverman et al. 2006). An American study

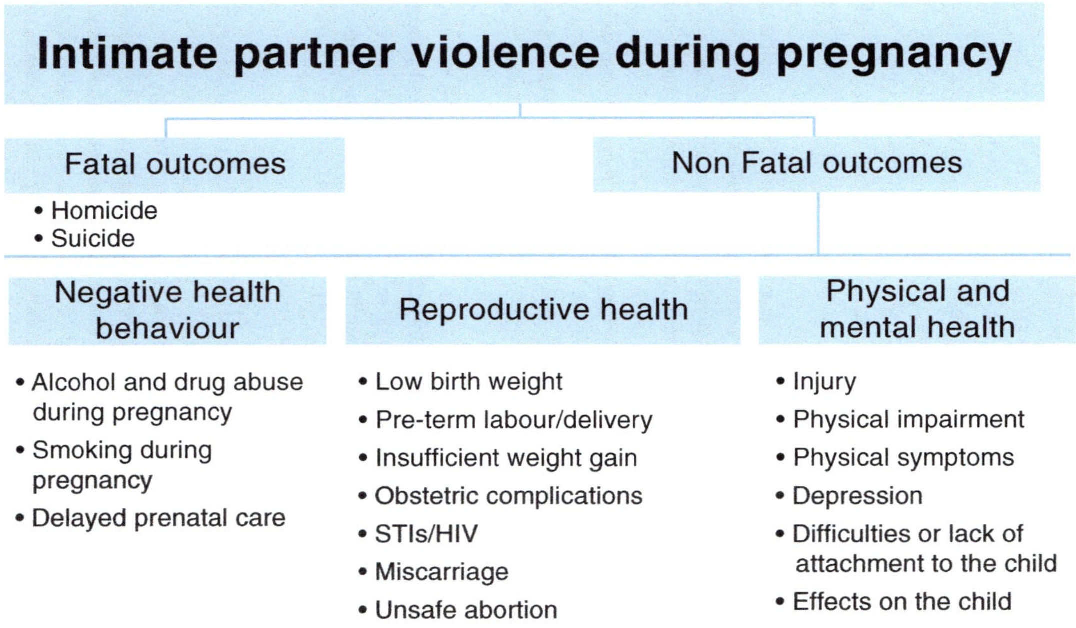

Intimate partner violence during pregnancy

Fatal outcomes

- Homicide
- Suicide

Non Fatal outcomes

Negative health behaviour

- Alcohol and drug abuse during pregnancy
- Smoking during pregnancy
- Delayed prenatal care

Reproductive health

- Low birth weight
- Pre-term labour/delivery
- Insufficient weight gain
- Obstetric complications
- STIs/HIV
- Miscarriage
- Unsafe abortion

Physical and mental health

- Injury
- Physical impairment
- Physical symptoms
- Depression
- Difficulties or lack of attachment to the child
- Effects on the child

Fig. 13.3   Health outcomes of intimate partner violence during pregnancy (World Health Organization 2011). Copyright WHO. With permission

showed that women experiencing intimate partner violence are overrepresented amongst women who do not breastfeed, or do so for a short period only. This over-representation seems to be caused by risk factors that also increase the risk for intimate partner violence. Silverman et al. argue that 'identifying and providing assistance to new mothers experiencing intimate partner violence may also represent a critical intervention to promote child health.' (Silverman et al. 2006)

The adverse effects on maternal and perinatal health outcomes are caused by both direct and indirect pathways. Stress is a known, indirect factor for low-birthweight and/or preterm birth, caused by physiological responses to stress, such as the release of prostaglandin, vasoconstrictors, or cortisol (Hill et al. 2016). The first can lead to premature contractions, and the others can contribute to intrauterine growth restriction. Furthermore, stress can increase chronic health problems (such as diabetes, hypertension, or asthma) and unhealthy behaviours (such as the use of tobacco, alcohol, and illegal drugs) which are associated with adverse pregnancy outcomes as well.

Women in violent relationships often lack the autonomy to decide upon their own health or to make use of healthcare and other services, resulting in extra risk factors such as poor nutrition and inadequate prenatal care (Hill et al. 2016).

Violence against women is known to have intergenerational effects, including:

- Growing up in a home with intimate partner violence increases the risk of physical abuse of children.
- Children who witness intimate partner violence are more likely to become perpetrators (especially boys) or experience violence in their own relationships (especially girls).
- Being exposed to violence as a child is an adverse childhood experience with major influences on health and wellbeing, both in the short and long term. The exposure has detrimental effects on the development of a child's brain, which can increase the risk of social, emotional, and behavioural problems. This experience might lead to behavioural problems in childhood and later in life, poor school performance, and risk-taking behaviours such as addictions.

Due to the adverse health outcomes caused by violence, abused women make more use of health services than non-abused women, especially more use of mental health services, emergency department, hospital outpatient, primary care, pharmacy, and specialty services. Therefore, healthcare professionals often encounter women with present or past experiences of abuse. These encounters are often early in the life cycle of abuse and providers (Michau et al. 2015). Abused women see healthcare professionals as trustworthy in disclosing the abuse. However, healthcare systems often don't recognize that they are the entry point to other providers and sectors and therefore 'favourable positioned' to refer women to social, economic, and legal support.

Care for women who experience violence leads to extra expenses on medical, mental, and other services for the women themselves. The physical and mental health problems of violence against women, including long-term disabilities, can lead to loss of productivity, wages, and income. Their active participation in and contribution to society can be hindered. This includes domains such as education, self-actualization, or livelihood/employment prospects. Less income and less productivity lead to economic costs for the survivors/victims, their families, future generations, and society as a whole.

> **Costs of Gender-Based Violence and Return Investments**
> - Elimination of violence against women is ethical imperative, as well as practical and financially sound. Estimations by the World Bank on the direct and indirect costs of intimate partner violence, which include costs for healthcare, costs for other services, and lost productivity and income range from 1.2 to 3.7% of gross domestic product. This equals the spending on primary education (Klugman et al. 2014).
> - In selecting cost-effective Sustainable Development Goals targets, a group of the world's leading economists and Nobel laureates concluded that investing in the elimination of all forms of gender-based violence is one of the (19) most cost-effective (Post-2015 Consensus 2019).

13.8 What Is Needed

Women who have experienced violence often feel there is nowhere to turn to. Help and support might not be available, or the services might not be known or accessible due to different, multiple constraints (distance, finances, language, cultural differences). They might fear retaliation by the offender, their next of kin, or their community for disclosing the abuse. Shame, embarrassment, wish to keep the incident(s) private, fearing weak responses by the police or the judicial system, and fearing the legal consequences such as losing custody of children can be other barriers for seeking help. These barriers can be even bigger in societies where it is difficult for women to leave their partner/family and live on their own (U Nations - Affairs DoEaS 2015).

To address violence against women, and the abovementioned barriers, a comprehensive approach is needed, which has to include raising awareness on the magnitude of violence against women; awareness on the lifelong effect of violence on health and mental wellbeing of the victims; education on violence against women; prevention; provision of safe places and shelters; counselling; health, legal, and social services; and improved follow-up on reported cases (U Nations - Affairs DoEaS 2015).

Colombini et al. (2012) and García-Moreno et al. (2015) have presented an overview of the core components of the necessary services by healthcare professionals within the broader health systems and societal systems. This overview highlights that all elements, from the individual to the structural level, should be taken into account when addressing violence against women (Fig. 13.4).

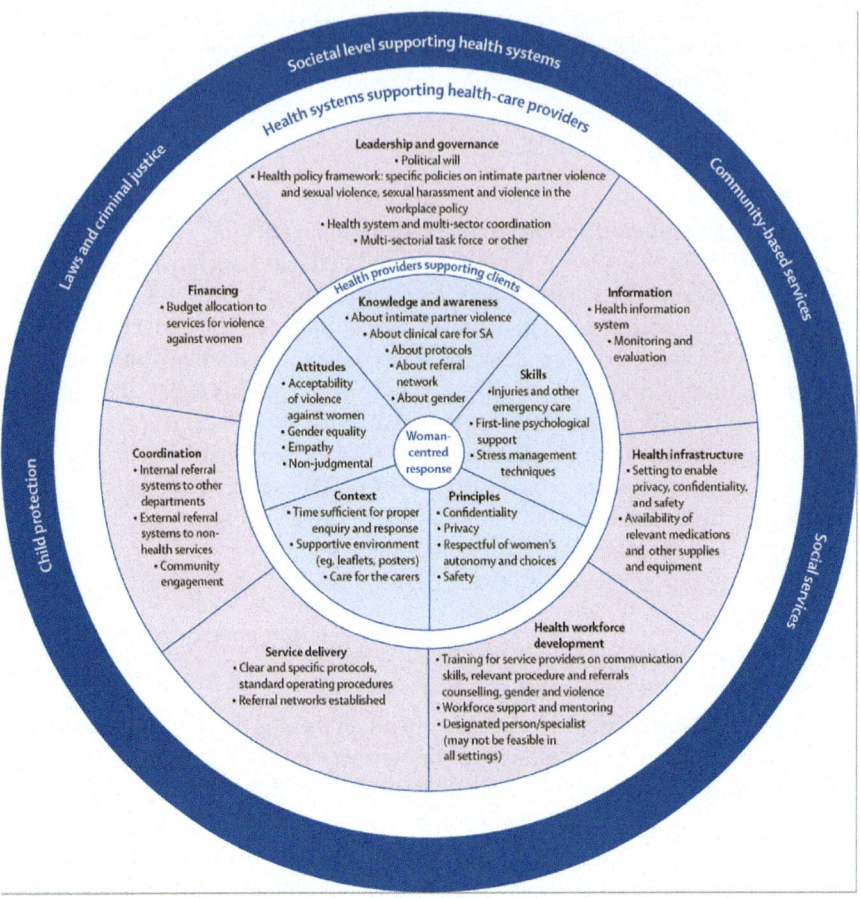

Fig. 13.4 Elements of the health system and healthcare response necessary to address violence against women. Adapted from Colombini and colleagues (Heise 1998), by permission of BioMed central. *SA* sexual assault (García-Moreno et al. 2015)

13.8.1 What Is the Role of the Health System?

Since 2013 violence against women is seen as a health priority (García-Moreno et al. 2015). The health sector plays a key role, both in the prevention of violence against women and as a first responder to women who experienced violence. Different health services can function as such an entry points, such as accident and emergency services, family planning, maternal health or paediatric health. Services for violence against women should be included in all settings: sexual and reproductive health settings, family planning, routine checks, and health services for elderly, adolescent health, mental health, health responses to humanitarian crises, and maternal and child health.

To do so, the readiness of the health system and the skills of providers are essential, as are referrals to and linkages between health, justice, and social systems (World Health Organization 2013c). According to the WHO (García-Moreno et al. 2015; World Health Organization 2016, 2017), health systems need to strengthen:

- Health services, its capacity, and the skills of healthcare professionals to provide comprehensive health services within and outside of the health system for women who experienced violence.
- Information collection to share data on prevalence, risk factors, health burden and the burden of the associated problems, and costs of violence to use for improvement of the services and advocacy.
- Leadership by public commitment to address and condemn, disclose, prevent, and respond to violence against women, within the healthcare sector and with other sectors.
- Prevention of (recurrence of) violence by fostering and informing prevention programmes – in schools, at health facilities, in communities, and through home visits – on parenting, consent, and respect within relationships; on challenging norms that 'justify' violence; and on risk factors such as alcohol abuse for violence.

In order to do so, the WHO has provided clinical and policy guidelines (World Health Organization 2013a) and a clinical handbook (World Health Organization 2014a) to enable policymakers, healthcare professionals, and healthcare managers to respond to women's needs. Countries can make use of the 'Essential Services Packages' to develop, implement, and evaluate services for women and girls experiencing violence. It identifies the essential services, the essential providers (health, social services, police, and justice sectors), and the essential resources and coordination to make things work (UN Women, UNFPA, UNDP 2015).

Women want a supportive response from a well-trained provider, who is able to listen attentively, who enquires about their needs, and who can provide support and help to access other services such as social support, economic security, housing, and legal protection ensuring safety for the woman (and her children).

Identification of intimate partner violence is the starting point for proper treatment, care, and referral to specialized care if needed (and where available). For this approach, health systems have to support the professionals with different issues (García-Moreno et al. 2015):

- Awareness and knowledge: healthcare professionals should be aware of and understand (norms and values on) gender equality and violence against women and recognize mental and physical health signals or problems which are associated with violence. They should know how to respond in a sensitive, compassionate, and non-judgmental manner. They should know the protocols, procedures, and pathways for referral to the relevant services women might need (such as hotlines and safe accommodation/shelters, psychosocial counselling, specialist care, police, and justice or social services).

- Attitudes: healthcare professionals should be sensitive on gender equality, violence against women, and their own role and possibilities to encourage women to disclose and seek help for the violence they experience(d). A sensitive approach can help women to recognize what is happening to her, to name it as abuse, and to empower her to take action.
- Context: providers need time and resources for proper enquiry and response and to allow women to take their time for appropriate disclosure. Time and care for the carers is needed as well, as they might feel undertrained and poorly supported to help women (Colombini et al. 2012).
- Principles: a safe and private space, where confidentiality can be protected, is essential to enable women to disclose the violence. 'Safe' means a physically safe place, without the abusive partner.
- Skills: healthcare professionals should have the skills for the respectful provision of clinical care, such as injuries and post-rape care or first-line psychological support.

> Because of the regular contact with healthcare professional, pregnancy and prenatal care are seen as a window of opportunity for detecting and addressing violence (Devries et al. 2010; Van Parys et al. 2014; Hill et al. 2016). For some women, antenatal care providers are the only healthcare professionals with whom they are in contact.

13.9 Preconception and Interconception Interventions

The impact of violence against women has different forms, with short- and long-term consequences. Witnessing violence as a child, having experienced violence earlier in life as well as experiencing present violence, can result in (multiple) risk factors for adverse maternal child, for child health, even for intergenerational health. The risk factors and violence might even reinforce each other: violence might increase the tendency to a particular risk behaviour (e.g. alcohol abuse), and that risk behaviour, in turn, increases the likelihood of an adverse health outcome (World Health Organization 2013c). Therefore, violence against women is one of the areas that should be part of preconception care (World Health Organization 2013b; Lassi et al. 2014), by recognizing and responding to the risk factors for violence against women; signs of violence against women; intrusive partner or husband present at all consultations; physical health consequences which are caused or complicated by violence, for example, traumatic injury, repeated sexually transmitted infections, or genitourinary symptoms; mental health consequences which are caused or complicated by violence, for example, symptoms of depression, anxiety, self-harm, or suicidality; behavioural stress responses such as the need for and use of alcohol, prescription medication, tobacco, or other drugs to deal with the violence; and adverse reproductive outcomes, multiple unintended pregnancies, and/or terminations.[1]

---

[1] Note that the WHO does not recommend universal screening or routine enquiry for (intimate partner) violence.

In case of any of these risk factors and indicators, providers should enquire about past or present violence. As long as the provider is well trained on first-line response and other minimum requirements are met (World Health Organization 2013a) (Fig. 13.4). The aforementioned is not limited to professionals who provide pre−/interconception care. As is the case in general preconception care, other services such as social services, child services or service to treat alcohol and drug misuse, etc. should be involved as well.

13.10 Prevention of Violence Against Women

Violence against women and girls is deeply rooted in gender inequalities and gender-power imbalances by which boys and men have more access to resources than women and girls. Therefore, and as stated before, prevention needs to include programs and policies at all levels, addressing both the individual, interpersonal, community and societal drivers of violence against women (Fig. 13.1). For example, if women are economically dependent on their intimate partner, reporting the abuse might lead to poverty due to the conviction and imprisonment of the breadwinner (Heise 2011; World Health Organization 2013c, 2019; Michau et al. 2015; Deliver for Good 2017).

In 2019 the WHO has launched the RESPECT approach. This public health and human rights approach aims to strengthen the prevention of violence against women through 7 strategies:

- Relationships skills strengthened
- Empowerment of women
- Services ensured
- Poverty reduced
- Environments made safe
- Child and adolescent abuse prevented
- Transformed attitudes, beliefs, and norms

These strategies should not be seen separately. Interventions mentioned earlier in this chapter often fall in one or more of these strategies.

13.11 Conclusion

Violence against women and girls denies and violates their human rights and can have lifelong negative effects on women's physical, mental, sexual, and reproductive health. It hinders their ability to study, work, and care for themselves and their family. Their children might be affected as well, with negative child health and development outcomes.

Violence against women and girls is rooted in gender inequality and male dominance. Therefore, a comprehensive approach is needed, in which health, legal and social services and local communities work together to address and identify the violence. This approach ranges from creating awareness on the magnitude and life-long effect of the violence, to proper treatment, care and referral for women who seek help and support, from changing norms and enforcing protective laws to supportive response from well-trained professionals.

Because violence against women can occur during any stage of the life cycle, services for violence against women should be included in settings such as sexual and reproductive health settings, family planning, routine checks and health services for elderly, adolescent health, mental health, health responses to humanitarian crises and maternal and child health.

Violence against women is one of the areas that should be addressed by preconception care, using the opportunity for timely recognition and response to risk factors for and health consequences caused by violence.

13.12 List of Key Findings/Recommendations

- Violence against women and girls is a worldwide problem and can occur during any stage of the life cycle, from prebirth to old age. One in three women have experienced sexual or physical violence at least once in her life. Less than 40% seek help for their experience with violence. Less than 2% of all women seek help from the police.
- Risk factors for violence against women include low education, a history of child maltreatment, exposure to domestic violence against their mothers, alcohol/substance abuse, gender norms and attitudes, including the ones on accepting violence and abuse.
- Some women are more at risk for violence than other, for example, women living with disabilities; women living in isolation; and displaced women living in conflict situations or refugee camps.
- Violence against women has different forms ranging from female infanticide to intimate partner violence and abuse and neglect of older women, from genital mutilation of young girls to forced prostitution and trafficking, domestic violence, bullying, or sexual harassment at work.
- Violence by an intimate partner is the most reported and researched form of sexual or physical violence against women. It affects 30% of women worldwide and accounts for at least 60 up to 80% of all the experienced and reported violence in a lifetime.
- Established sexual and gender norms can also lead to violence against boys and men and against gender-based violence targeting lesbian, gay, bisexual, transgender, queer, questioning, intersex, and asexual (LGBTQIA) persons.
- Violence can have a negative effect on women's physical, mental, sexual, and reproductive health. It can lead to adverse maternal and perinatal outcomes, such as abortion or low-birthweight babies. Violence and lack of control over their reproductive choices often go hand in hand, which hinders seeking care and support.

- To address violence against women, a comprehensive approach is needed, including awareness on the magnitude of violence against women; awareness on the lifelong effect of violence on health and mental wellbeing of the victims; education on violence against women; prevention; provision of safe places and shelters; counselling; trained professionals in health, legal, and social services; and improved follow-up on reported cases.
- Services for violence against women should be included in all health services for girls and women of all ages.
- Violence against women is one of the areas that should be addressed by preconception care. Because of the regular contact with healthcare professionals, pregnancy, prenatal, and postnatal care are a window of opportunity for detecting and addressing violence. For some women antenatal care providers are the only healthcare professionals with whom they are in (regular) contact.
- Prevention of violence against women needs to include programs and policies at all levels, addressing the individual, interpersonal, community and societal drivers of violence against women. Therefore, the WHO has recently introduced the RESPECT approach: Relationships skills strengthened, Empowerment of women. Services ensured, Poverty reduced, Environments made safe, Child and adolescent abuse prevented, and Transformed attitudes, beliefs and norms.
- Women want a supportive response from a well-trained provider, who is able to listen attentively in a non-judgemental way, to enquire about their needs, and to provide support and help to access other services such as social support, economic security, housing, and legal protection ensuring safety for the woman (and her children).

References

Brownridge DA, Taillieu T, Tyler KA, Tiwari A, Ling Chan K, Santos SC. Pregnancy and intimate partner violence: risk factors, severity, and health effects. Violence Against Women. 2011;17:858–81. https://doi.org/10.1177/1077801211412547.

Coker AL, Sanderson M, Dong B. Partner violence during pregnancy and risk of adverse pregnancy outcomes. Paediatr Perinat Epidemiol. 2004;18(4):260–9. https://doi.org/10.1111/j.1365-3016.2004.00569.x.

Colombini M, Mayhew SH, Ali SH, Shuib R, Watts C. An integrated health sector response to violence against women in Malaysia: lessons for supporting scale up. BMC Public Health. 2012;12:548. https://doi.org/10.1186/1471-2458-12-548.

Daoud N, Urquia ML, O'Campo P, Heaman M, Janssen PA, Smylie J, Thiessen K. Prevalence of abuse and violence before, during, and after pregnancy in a national sample of Canadian women. Am J Public Health. 2012;102:1893–901. https://doi.org/10.2105/AJPH.2012.300843.

Deliver for Good. Dramatically reduce gender-based violence and harmful practices. facts, solutions, case studies, and call to action. 2017. https://womendeliver.org/wp-content/uploads/2017/09/Deliver_For_Good_Brief_5_09.17.17.pdf. Accessed 22 Apr 2019.

Desmarais SL, Pritchard A, Lowder EM, Janssen PA. Intimate partner abuse before and during pregnancy as risk factors for postpartum mental health problems. BMC Pregnancy Childbirth. 2014;7:132. https://doi.org/10.1186/1471-2393-14-132.

Devries KM, Kishor S, Johnson H, Stöckl H, Bacchus LJ, García-Moreno C, Watts C. Intimate partner violence during pregnancy: analysis of prevalence data from 19 countries. Reprod Health Matters. 2010;18:158–70. https://doi.org/10.1016/S0968-8080(10)36533-5.

Finnbogadóttir H, Dykes A. Increasing prevalence and incidence of domestic violence during the pregnancy and one and a half year postpartum, as well as risk factors: -a longitudinal cohort study in Southern Sweden. BMC Pregnancy Childbirth. 2016;16:327. https://doi.org/10.1186/s12884-016-1122-6.

García-Moreno C, Jansen HA, Ellsberg M, Heise L, Watts S. WHO Multi-country Study on Women's Health and Domestic Violence against Women: initial results on prevalence, health outcomes and women's responses. Geneva: World Health Organization; 2005. www.who.int/reproductivehealth/publications/violence/24159358X/en/. Accessed 10 Oct 2018.

García-Moreno C, Hegarty K, d'Olivera AFL, Koziol-Maclain J, Colombini M, Feder G. The health-systems response to violence against women: an overview. Lancet 2015;385:1567–1579 (published online Nov 20, 2014). https://doi.org/10.1016/S0140-6736(14)61837-7.

Heise LL. Violence against women: an integrated, ecological framework. Violence Against Women. 1998;4:262–90. https://doi.org/10.1177/1077801298004003002.

Heise LL. What works to prevent partner violence? An evidence overview. London; Strive, 2011. http://strive.lshtm.ac.uk/resources/what-works-prevent-partner-violence-evidence-overview.

Heise LL, Kotsadam A. Cross-national and multilevel correlates of partner violence: an analysis of data from population-based surveys. Lancet Glob Health. 2015;3:e332–40. https://doi.org/10.1016/S2214-109X(15)00013-3.

Hill A, Pallitto C, McCleary-Sills J, García-Moreno C. A systematic review and meta-analysis of intimate partner violence during pregnancy and selected birth outcomes. Int J Gynaecol Obstet. 2016;133:269–76. https://doi.org/10.1016/j.ijgo.2015.10.023.

IAWG. Inter-agency field manual on reproductive health in humanitarian settings. New York (NY): IAWG; 2019. https://resourcecentre.savethechildren.net/library/imported-file-87-sc-toolkit-children-and-adolescents-sexual-and-reproductive-health-rights-0. Accessed 25 Mar 2019.

James L, Brody D, Hamilton Z. Risk factors for domestic violence during pregnancy: a meta-analytic review. Violence Vict. 2013;28:359–80. https://connect.springerpub.com/content/sgrvv/28/3/359.

Klugman J, Hanmer L, Twigg S, Hasan T, McCleary-Sills J, Santamaria J. Voice and agency: empowering women and girls for shared prosperity. Washington, DC: World Bank, 2014. https://doi.org/10.1596/978-1-4648-0359-8. Accessed 22 Apr 2019.

Lassi ZS, Dean SV, Mallick BZA. Preconception care: delivery strategies and packages for care. Reprod Health. 2014;11:S7. https://doi.org/10.1186/1742-4755-11-S3-S7.

Martin S, Mackie L, Kupper L, Bacchus L, Maracco K. Physical abuse of women before, during, and after pregnancy. JAMA. 2001;285:1581–4. https://doi.org/10.1001/jama.285.12.1581.

Michau L, Horn J, Bank A, Dutt M, Zimmerman C. Prevention of violence against women and girls: lessons from practice. Lancet 2015;385:1672–1684 (published online Nov 21, 2014). https://doi.org/10.1016/S0140-6736(14)61797-9.

Miller S, Lalonde A. The global epidemic of abuse and disrespect during childbirth: History, evidence, interventions, and FIGO's mother-baby friendly birthing facilities initiative. Int J Gynaecol Obstet. 2015;131:S49–52. Epub 2015 Feb 24. Review. https://doi.org/10.1016/j.ijgo.2015.02.005.

Muehlenhard CL, Peterson ZD, Humphreys TP, Jozkowski KN. Evaluating the one-in-five statistic: women's risk of sexual assault while in college. J Sex Res. 2017;54:549–76. https://doi.org/10.1080/00224499.2017.1295014.

Murray Gáson C, Misunas C, Cappa C. Child marriage among boys: a global overview of available data. Vulnerable Child Youth Stud. 2019;14:219–28. https://doi.org/10.1080/17450128.2019.1566584.

OECD. How's life in the digital age?: opportunities and risks of the digital transformation for people's well-being. Paris: OECD Publishing; 2019. https://doi.org/10.1787/9789264311800-en Accessed 22 Apr 2019.

Post-2015 Consensus. Nobel Laureates Guide to Smarter Global Targets to 2030. www.copenha-genconsensus.com/post-2015-consensus/nobel-laureates-guide-smarter-global-targets-2030. Accessed 22 Apr 2019.

Raymond JG. The new UN trafficking protocol. Women's Stud Int Forum. 2002;25:491–502. https://doi.org/10.1016/S0277-5395(02)00320-5.

Silverman JG, Decker MR, Reed E, Raj A. Intimate partner violence around the time of pregnancy: association with breastfeeding behavior. J Women's Health. 2006;15:934–40. https://doi.org/10.1089/jwh.2006.15.934.

Stewart DE, Vigod SN, MacMillan HL, Chandra PS, Han A, Rondon MB, MacGregor JCD, Riazantseva E. Current reports on perinatal intimate partner violence. Review Curr Psychiatry Rep. 2017;19:26. https://doi.org/10.1007/s11920-017-0778-6.

UN Women. Ending violence against women and girls: Programming essentials. 2013. https://evaw.unwomen.org/en. Accessed 4 Apr 2019.

UN Women, UNFPA, UNDP. Essential services package for women and girls subject to violence. New York: UN Women; 2015. http://www.unwomen.org/en/digital-library/publications/2015/12/essential-services-package-for-women-and-girls-subject-to-violence. Accessed 2 Nov 2018.

UNFPA. Bending the curve: fgm trends we aim to change (Infographic). 2018. www.unfpa.org/sites/default/files/resource-pdf/18-053_FGM-Infographic-2018-02-05-1804.pdf Accessed 21 Apr 2019.

UNFPA. Female genital mutilation (FGM) frequently asked questions. 2019. http://www.unfpa.org/resources/female-genital-mutilation-fgm-frequently-asked-questions#banned_by_law. Accessed 8 July 2019.

UNICEF. Child Marriage. 2018. https://data.unicef.org/topic/child-protection/child-marriage/ and Database https://data.unicef.org/wp-content/uploads/2015/12/Child-marriage-database_Mar-2018.xlsx. Accessed 8 July 2019.

United Nations, Department of Economic and Social Affairs, Statistics Division. The World's Women 2015. Trends and statistics. New York: United Nations; 2015. https://unstats.un.org/unsd/gender/downloads/WorldsWomen2015_chapter6_t.pdf. Accessed 2 Nov 2018.

United Nations General Assembly. Declaration on the elimination of violence against women. A/RES/48/104. New York: United Nations; 1994. https://www.securitycouncilreport.org/un-documents/document/wps-ares-48-104.php. Accessed 2 Nov 2018.

UNODC. Global Report on Trafficking in Persons 2016. New York: United Nations; 2016. www.unodc.org/documents/data-and-analysis/glotip/2016_Global_Report_on_Trafficking_in_Persons.pdf Accessed 21 Apr 2019.

Van Parys AS, Verhamme A, Temmerman M, Verstraelen H. Intimate partner violence and pregnancy: a systematic review of interventions. PLoS One. 2014;9:e85084. https://doi.org/10.1371/journal.pone.0085084.

WAVE-UNFPA. Strengthening health system responses to gender based violence in Eastern Europe and Central Asia: a resource package. Turkey: UNFPA Regional Office for Eastern Europe and Central Asia, Turkey & Vienna: WAVE Network and European Info Centre against Violence. 2014. https://eeca.unfpa.org/sites/default/files/pub-pdf/WAVE-UNFPA-Report-EN.pdf

WHO Study Group. Female genital mutilation and obstetric outcome: WHO collaborative prospective study in six African countries. Lancet. 2006;367:1835–41. https://doi.org/10.1016/S0140-6736(06)68782-5.

World Bank Group. Women, Business and the Law. Washington, DC: World Bank; 2018. http://documents.worldbank.org/curated/en/926401524803880673/pdf/125804-PUB-REPLACE-MENT-PUBLIC.pdf. Accessed 4 Apr 2019.

World Health Organization. WHO Multi-country Study on Women's Health and Domestic Violence against Women: initial results on prevalence, health outcomes and women's responses. Geneva: WHO; 2005. www.who.int/reproductivehealth/publications/violence/24159358X/en/. Accessed 10 Oct 2018.

World Health Organization. Intimate partner violence during pregnancy. Information sheet. Geneva: World Health Organization; 2011. https://apps.who.int/iris/bitstream/handle/10665/70764/WHO_RHR_11.35_eng.pdf?sequence=1. Accessed 22 Apr 2019.

World Health Organization. Responding to intimate partner violence and sexual violence against women: clinical and policy guidelines. Geneva: World Health Organization; 2013a. http://apps.who.int/iris/bitstream/10665/85240/1/9789241548595_eng.pd. Accessed 10 Oct 2018.

World Health Organization. Preconception care: Maximising the gains for maternal and child health. Geneva: World Health Organization; 2013b. www.who.int/maternal_child_adolescent/documents/preconception_care_policy_brief.pdf. Accessed 10 Oct 2018.

World Health Organization. Global and regional estimates of violence against women: prevalence and health effects of intimate partner violence and non-partner sexual violence. Geneva: World Health Organization; 2013c. https://apps.who.int/iris/bitstream/handle/10665/85239/9789241564625_eng.pdf;jsessionid=F133CBFFD6970FCE8F99976C8886165C?sequence=1. Accessed 10 Oct 2018.

World Health Organization. The prevention and elimination of disrespect and abuse during facility-based childbirth. Geneva: World Health Organization; 2014. http://apps.who.int/iris/bitstream/10665/134588/1/WHO_RHR_14.23_eng.pdf?ua=1&ua=1. Accessed 4 Apr 2019.

World Health Organization. Health care for women subjected to intimate partner violence or sexual violence: a clinical handbook. Geneva: World Health Organization; 2014a. www.who.int/reproductivehealth/publications/violence/vaw-clinical-handbook/en/. Accessed 4 Apr 2019.

World Health Organization. Global plan of action to strengthen the role of the health system within a national multisectoral response to address interpersonal violence, in particular against women and girls, and against children. Geneva: World Health Organization; 2016. http://apps.who.int/iris/bitstream/10665/252276/1/9789241511537-eng.pdf?ua=1. Accessed 15 Mar 2019.

World Health Organization. Strengthening health systems to respond to women subjected to intimate partner violence or sexual violence: a manual for health managers. Geneva: World Health Organization; 2017. www.who.int/reproductivehealth/publications/violence/vaw-health-systems-manual/en/. Accessed 15 Mar 2019.

World Health Organization. RESPECT women: preventing violence against women. Geneva: World Health Organization; 2019. www.who.int/reproductivehealth/publications/preventing-vaw-framework-policymakers/en/. Accessed 31 May 2019.

Global Strategies for Change

14

Salimah R. Walani and Kelle H. Moley

14.1 Introduction

Under the auspices of the United Nations (UN) Millennium Development Goals (MDGs) to reduce maternal and child mortality rates, significant resources were invested to save the lives of women and children, during pregnancy, labor, delivery, and in the immediate postpartum period. Families, communities, funders, governmental agencies, and civil society organizations made targeted efforts to ensure that a woman received adequate antenatal care, delivered her baby with the help of a skilled birth attendant, and in a setting where her life and that of her baby could be saved. These investments paid off well. Overall maternal and child mortality rates dropped significantly between 1990 and 2015 (World Health Organization 2018).

Toward the end of the MDG era (2000–2015), it started to become clear, however, that to continue to improve birth outcomes, intervening only after a woman announced her pregnancy was too late to maximize prevention. Hence, the notion of preconception health, the health of a couple prior to pregnancy, started to gain attention. Globally, preconception health discussions and interventions have been most influenced by a 2013 policy brief by World Health Organization (WHO) that outlined a preconception care package, with 13 broad areas of interventions, to serve as a guide for national policy makers (World Health Organization 2013a). This publication set into motion regional- and national-level discussions on the importance of preconception care and how and when to deliver it. One example of this new direction was the establishment of regional guidelines following expert consultations and presentations by WHO's regional offices in Southeast Asia and Eastern Mediterranean (World Health Organization 2013b, 2015).

S. R. Walani (✉) · K. H. Moley
March of Dimes, Arlington, VA, USA
e-mail: SWalani@marchofdimes.org

© Springer Nature Switzerland AG 2020
J. Shawe et al. (eds.), *Preconception Health and Care: A Life Course Approach*,
https://doi.org/10.1007/978-3-030-31753-9_14

Presently, with the campaign for Universal Health Coverage across the life course as part of the UN's 2016–2030 Sustainable Development Goals (SDGs) agenda (United Nations 2019), there is an opportunity to accelerate and strengthen advocacy for preconception health interventions. This chapter proposes strategies for advancing the utilization of preconception care globally by discussing who to target, what interventions to promote, and how to advocate for needed services and resources.

14.2 Global Strategies

As the experience in population-level delivery of preconception care has been increasing, there is some debate in the literature about what is the ideal time frame for achieving one's optimal preconception health status (Stephenson et al. 2018). One perspective is to do away with a time bound concept of preconception health and focus more broadly on improving the health of men and women throughout their life, with particular emphasis on advancing the health of women and girls as individuals and not as potential mothers. This approach is logical since globally 44% of all pregnancies are unintended, with even higher rates experienced in Asia and Africa (Bearak et al. 2018).

In many societies, it is unusual for men and women to plan their pregnancies. Seeking healthcare advice and taking steps to optimize health status before conception is not the norm. Further, the challenge with advocating for starting preconception care during the pregnancy planning period is that even if healthcare providers succeed in getting all couples to seek counseling, screening, and care before conception, issues such as obesity, hypertension, stress, domestic violence, and unhealthy health practices may take years to correct. It is therefore essential to use a life-course approach to preconception care with population-level measures that empower boys and girls and men and women to improve their health, irrespective of their pregnancy plans (Stephenson et al. 2018).

14.3 Target Groups

Many barriers exist in the delivery of preconception care at the population level. Strategies to improve preconception health need to take a multifaceted approach to target three groups. First, the focus needs to be placed on increasing the interest and motivation of individuals in taking steps to improve their health. Studies from around the world have repeatedly shown that there is a lack of awareness among men and women about the importance of preconception health (Ayalew et al. 2017; Shawe et al. 2019). Public health education programs for adolescents and adults of reproductive age about the risk factors for adverse pregnancy outcomes and the importance of seeking care and counseling before pregnancy may increase the demand for preconception care.

Second, it is important to influence national policies and leverage financial support for population-based programs. One barrier to the adoption of preconception care at national levels has been the indifference of policy makers and financiers of healthcare delivery systems in investing in primary care and health services for young adults. One example of this lack of leadership support is the issue of preconceptional folic acid intake for prevention of neural tube defects. Two most common neural tube defects are spina bifida and anencephaly, and there is solid evidence that adequate intake of folic acid by women before pregnancy prevents neural tube defects, yet many countries still have a high prevalence of neural tube defects associated with lack of folic acid intake (Blencowe et al. 2018). It has been known widely that countries which have implemented effective mandatory folic acid fortification programs have lower rates of neural tube defects. Countries such as Chile, South Africa, Canada, and Costa Rica have documented significant decline in their rates of neural tube defects through fortification. Globally, over 50% of the 300,000 estimated cases of neural tube defects can potentially be prevented by expanding national efforts for folic acid fortification (Centers for Disease Control and Prevention 2015).

Moreover, fortification of staples with micronutrients has been shown to be a cost-effective public policy intervention that can help improve the nutritional status of women and girls preconceptionally. Yet, due to lack of national fortification efforts globally, a recent study estimated 57,000 preventable cases of spina bifida and anencephaly occur worldwide, annually (Kancherla 2018). Policy makers and financiers (public and private) of the healthcare delivery systems must recognize and embrace preconception care as a way to achieve major improvement in the health of a population at a relatively low cost.

Third, health professionals need to be empowered to deliver effective preconception care. Preconception care delivery needs to occur before a woman becomes pregnant to help her and her partner reach their optimal health status, plan their pregnancy, and develop healthy behaviors. Therefore, healthcare workers who work with women and girls in community settings must be engaged in improving access to preventive care. Traditionally, primary care providers and general practitioners have played a key role in the delivery of disease prevention and health promotion services; immunizations, screening for infections and chronic diseases, and family planning services are some examples of such population-based interventions delivered in primary care settings. A few specific interventions currently integrated into primary care services of some countries are actually included in preconception care packages. For instance, vaccination against rubella, HIV testing, treatment and counseling, and screening and treatment for other sexually transmitted infections are currently offered in community health centers in many countries. Preconception care needs to be viewed as a primary care service and must be embedded in the healthcare delivery system at district and community levels. Unfortunately, there exists a general lack of awareness about the importance of preconception health among health providers in primary care settings (Ojukwu et al. 2016; Kassa et al. 2018). Many healthcare workers in low- and middle-income countries are unable to differentiate between preconception health and antenatal care. Any strategies for promotion of preconception care need to target healthcare workers, so that they are equipped with knowledge, skills, and resources to respond to the public demand for preconception care counseling and interventions.

14.4   Programs and Interventions

Over the last decade or so, organizations such as the US Centers for Disease Control and Prevention, World Health Organization, and March of Dimes have emphasized improving access to preconception care as a means for preventing adverse maternal and newborn outcomes. This has influenced implementation of preconception healthcare interventions at institutional, local, national, and regional levels, worldwide. The scope of preconception interventions has ranged from small school-based health education programs to country-level policies for implementation of prepregnancy screening and counseling. For example, between 2011 and 2012, the American University of Beirut with support from March of Dimes implemented 30-min preconception health education sessions in 70 high schools in Lebanon reaching over 7000 male and female students (Charafeddine et al. 2014). At national levels, there are examples of programs in low- and middle-income countries such as the one in Sri Lanka, where the Ministry of Health in 2011 launched a preconception health package for newly married couples with the aim to improve reproductive health outcomes nationally (World Health Organization 2013b). In high-income countries, the rising awareness for integrating preconception heath in the public health systems is evident from a recent publication by the government of the United Kingdom; the document titled *Making the Case for Preconception Care* aims to not only highlight the impact of improving preconception health on birth outcomes but also propose ways to embed preconception health in the nation's prevention agenda (Public Health England 2018).

The above examples of preconception health efforts have been informed by published literature on evidence of interventions for preconception health that has been increasing. However, there are significant gaps in our knowledge of the full impact of preconception care interventions at population levels. According to a review of published reports between 2005 and 2016, most preconception interventions focussed on assessment and education or counseling. The interventions usually aimed to change specific behaviors (e.g., smoking, alcohol use) and used before, after designs to assess behavior or knowledge change. Most preconception education or care-related interventions have been on small scale and have not measured actual birth outcomes, such as birth defects and preterm birth (Hemsing et al. 2017). Preconception care projects at a population level can benefit many groups and result in significant health and social benefits with a potential to reduce a variety of adverse maternal and newborn outcomes and improving the overall well-being of communities (Mason et al. 2014).

Preconception interventions at a population level should take a multifaceted approach, focusing on creating a demand through public health education programs and enabling healthcare workers to meet that demand. Simultaneously, national governments must support preconception health agenda through policies that fully incorporate preventive care into healthcare delivery systems. In many countries, there is a disjointed approach in the delivery of services, whereby primary care clinics, antenatal and maternity care centers, family planning services, adolescent health services, HIV and other sexually transmitted screening and treatment programs, and chronic disease management programs all work independently so that there is no opportunity for comprehensive and continuous care for a person with multiple risk factors for poor health and future adverse birth outcomes. This fragmented and disease-oriented model of healthcare results in a tremendous missed opportunity for prevention of adverse birth outcomes, which could be addressed by embedding preconception and preventive health into these services.

Furthermore, there is a need for advocacy programs to engage stakeholders at national and global levels in order to gain financial support for preconception care. Global organizations and foundations working to improve maternal and child health outcomes and in-country consumer-led organizations must be engaged in advocating for support for preconception care. Health education programs for promoting health can occur in workplaces, in schools, and in community centers and can reach a much wider audience digitally through use of technology.

14.4.1 Workplace Interventions

According to an analysis commissioned by the March of Dimes, preterm birth costs employers over \$12 billion in the United States due to lengthy hospital stays and specialized care that premature and low birth weight babies need (March of Dimes 2014). Not all adverse neonatal outcomes can be prevented, but the likelihood of certain conditions can be reduced by improving the health and well-being of young adults through healthy workplaces. Men and women of reproductive age spend significant portions of their days in workplaces, and their overall psychosocial and physical health and health practices are impacted by their work environments. According to a World Health Organization proposed healthy workplace framework and model, in addition to ensuring that a workplace promotes physical and psychosocial health, employers need to make personal health resources available in workplaces (World Health Organization 2010). Although we could not find any published research studies showing the direct impact of workplace wellness programs on improving birth outcomes, workplaces may serve as an avenue for improving individuals' preventive, preconception, and interconception health awareness and behaviors. Workplace wellness resources and education materials can be delivered in many forms from discussion groups and structured health education sessions to online access to knowledge and support for promoting health knowledge and behavior. A March of Dimes workplace wellness program known as Healthy Babies, Healthy Business® is available to companies to help improve access to health knowledge of their workforce. This fully online educational resource includes information for before, during, and after pregnancy through a personalized user dashboard (March of Dimes 2019).

In addition to health education, employers can offer workplace wellness programs that include access to on-site health resources (facilities and services) to their workers, particularly those in their reproductive years. Services on-site or covered by the employers may include exercise facilities, weight and diet management programs, healthy food options and nutritional counseling, stress management supports, family planning counseling, behavioral health services, and, most critically, access to primary care. Employers have a lot to gain from investing in health promotion of their workers; in addition to helping workers have healthy pregnancies and birth outcomes, a healthy workforce means less sick days, less turnover, and improved job satisfaction which are all essential for improving productivity (World Health Organization 2010; Office of Disease Prevention and Health Promotion 2017).

14.4.2 Schools

Adolescence is an important period for addressing lifestyle and nutritional behaviors. Lifelong habits (e.g., smoking) and nutritional deficiencies, such as anemia during adolescence, have an adverse impact to not only the health of adolescents as they grow older but that of their future generations. Investing in improving the health of young people has tremendous benefit for families and societies. It is essential to ensure that youth have the knowledge that empowers them to make healthy lifestyle choices. Many health education programs that target youth occur in school settings. One approach to making preconception health education widely available to young people in school settings would be to broaden the focus of sexuality education programs in countries where they exist. Sexuality education programs have been integrated into school health curricula of many high-income countries, mainly for prevention of sexually transmitted diseases and teenage pregnancies. In European countries, these programs are often supported by national and regional policies and in some cases even mandated by law and are generally well-accepted (International Planned Parenthood Foundation European Network 2018).

School-based health centers, usually managed by nurses, may also serve as an avenue for imparting preconception health education and care. School-based health centers, particularly in the United States, have traditionally provided an array of services from meeting the immediate health needs to provision of mental health services, chronic disease management, and on-site access to contraceptives in some cases. Many school-based health clinics provide sexual and reproductive health services to help adolescents avoid unintended pregnancies (Guttmacher Institute 2015). Leveraging the established sexuality education programs and school-based health services to include information and services aimed to address behavioral and nutritional risk factors for adverse pregnancy outcomes is a cost-effective and feasible way to deliver preconception health education to young people. In countries where there are no existing programs for health education in schools, there are examples of targeted efforts for delivering health education in classrooms and universities and engaging youth in peer-to-peer health programs, such as the one described above in Lebanon (Kassa et al. 2018).

14.4.3 Community

At the community level, integrating preconception health education and services into healthcare delivery systems is an effective method, particularly in primary care systems. A comprehensive approach to well-being for young adults may produce tremendous gains for society at large. One example of such a program is China's National Preconception Health Care Project, which was launched by the Chinese government in 2010 to provide free preconception care in rural areas with the aim of reducing conditions such as birth defects and maternal mortality and morbidity in China. The project is integrated into primary health and family health delivery system and includes free preconception health examination to identify risk factors, followed by appropriate advice and appropriate medical services for those with genetic, behavioral, nutritional, or disease (chronic or infectious)-related risk factors. Within 2 years of implementation of the program, over 22 million married couples planning a pregnancy benefited from the program (Zhou et al. 2016). This program is an example of a unique preconception health promotion model at population level, supported by investments from a country's government. If adopted by other countries with modification as appropriate, this approach to integrating comprehensive preconception healthcare may have tremendous benefits for populations in low- and middle-income countries.

14.4.4 Digital Access

By the end of 2018, about 60% of households worldwide had access to the Internet, and almost the whole world now has access to web-based information through mobile phones (International Telecommunication Union 2018). Rising access to information online has provided opportunity for dissemination of health services and knowledge to large populations cost-effectively and conveniently. A wide variety of information and communications technology (ICT) innovations, aiming to improve maternal and child health outcomes, have emerged in the last decade, including mobile health (mHealth) technology-based health messaging, use of smartphone applications for mapping supports such as family planning resources, web-based support groups, and eLearning platforms. Although most of these ICT-based programs have focused on targeting women during pregnancy and postpartum period, there are a few examples of web-based preconception health promotion programs, particularly from high-income countries. One such online program is a public-private partnership initiative in the United States, known as Show Your Love (www.showyourlovetoday.com), which aims to provide preconception health knowledge resources to men and women.

In low- and middle-income countries, use of mHealth technology for delivery of preconception health knowledge and services may gain effectiveness as majority of adults around the world own at least a basic mobile device. A systematic review of mHealth interventions to advance reproductive, maternal, newborn, and child health, published between 2011 and 2016, noted that of the 245 studies reviewed, only about 10% ($n = 26$) of the studies offered interventions in the prepregnancy period (Chen et al. 2018). Although underutilized currently, if implemented at population level, mHealth is a cost-effective way to reach men and women of reproductive age with health information that can help optimize their health before pregnancy.

14.5 Advocacy for Preconception Care

As a result of MDG targets to reduce maternal child mortality, significant advocacy efforts were made at all levels for increasing funding and support for care during pregnancy, labor, and delivery and in the immediate postpartum period. Moving from the MDG era to the SDGs, advocacy efforts for funding and policy support to save newborn and maternal lives continue. Publications such as the *Every Newborn Action Plan* (World Health Organization 2017) and the *Global Strategy for Women's, Children's and Adolescents' Health (2016–2030)* (Every Woman Every Child 2015) have served as roadmaps for mobilizing action and investments for the health improvements of women and children globally. Stakeholders interested in advancing a preconception agenda may use these publications to make a case for preconception care. However, since the 2013 policy brief on preconception care by WHO (World Health Organization 2013a), no landmark documents have been published to help nations move their preconception agenda forward.

Advocacy to advance preconception care and its integration into primary care can use the momentum created by the push for healthcare financing for universal health coverage under SDGs. There is a need for the global health leaders to develop roadmaps that specifically address prevention of adverse birth outcomes by making preconception health a part of universal health coverage strategy, which calls for all people to have access to quality prevention and health promotional services along with curative and rehabilitative services (World Health Organization 2019). There is an opportunity to mobilize resources for preconception care as a prevention strategy that has the potential to go beyond what has been achieved through care programs under MDGs. Civil society organizations, particularly parent and patient organizations, must be engaged. Preparing for Life (www.preparingforlife.net), a parent-patient organization, is an example of a civil society organization in the Netherlands that promotes preconception care for women and their partners globally by promoting cooperation among public and private organizations. Global campaigns that use social media-based advocacy efforts to reach millions of individuals also provide opportunities for raising awareness. Two such yearly global campaigns are World Prematurity Day, observed on November 17th, and World Birth Defects Day observed on March 3rd. World Birth Defects Day, started in 2015, has engaged hundreds of organizations through its web-based platform www.worldbirthdefects-day.org. It is a major uniting force for advocating for preconception care for prevention of birth defects.

14.6 Conclusions

Preconception care is about prevention. As with most prevention programs, especially in low-resource settings, where healthcare is driven by disease-based services, the uptake of preconception health interventions has been slow. A comprehensive preconception care agenda includes efforts that reach men and women, with education and services, that can help promote their overall well-being. This can be achieved by helping them improve their physical health, mental health, nutrition, and pregnancy planning. The first step in advancing preconception care is to raise the public demand. Health education programs, regardless of the setting or the modality (online or in-person), should aim to promote the overall health of individuals. Considering a life-course perspective, health education should be made available to boys and girls from adolescence and should continue for men and women through their reproductive years with a focus on the importance of being healthy, regardless of their intention to have children. For individuals with intentions of becoming pregnant, more direct content on risk factors of adverse pregnancy outcomes, such as birth defects and preterm birth, can be included. Preconception care must be viewed as a disease prevention and health promotion strategy that needs to be integrated into primary healthcare systems, supported by national policy and investments from public and private sectors.

Advocacy for preconception care can begin at grassroots level by engaging youth and parent-patient organizations. Moreover, campaigns for promoting preconception care must take advantage of the social media movements and platforms that can reach millions of individuals in raising awareness and demand for preconception care. In support of a 2018 preconception health series published in the Lancet, the editorial board of the magazine wrote "There should be no obesity strategy, no undernutrition strategy, no non-communicable diseases strategy, and no adolescent health strategy without including preconception health" (Editorial Comment 2018). Promoting preconception care globally has potential social and economic benefits for a society, beyond simply advancing the health of women and children. Gains from ensuring access to preconception care continue beyond a couple's lifetime and extend to their future generations.

References

Ayalew Y, Mulat A, Dile M, Simegn A. Women's knowledge and associated factors in preconception care in adet, west gojjam, Northwest Ethiopia: a community based cross sectional study. Reprod Health. 2017;14(1):15.

Bearak J, Popinchalk A, Alkema L, Sedgh G. Global, regional, and subregional trends in unintended pregnancy and its outcomes from 1990 to 2014: estimates from a Bayesian hierarchical model. Lancet Global Health. 2018;6(4):e380–9. https://doi.org/10.1016/S2214-109X(18)30029-9.

Blencowe H, Kancherla V, Moorthie S, et al. Estimates of global and regional prevalence of neural tube defects for 2015: a systematic analysis. Ann N Y Acad Sci. 2018;1414:31–46.

Centers for Disease Control and Prevention. Folic acid and neural tube defects, an overview. 2015. https://www.cdc.gov/ncbddd/birthdefectscount/basics.html. Accessed 13 Aug 2019.

Charafeddine L, El Rafei R, Azizi S, Sinno D, Alamiddine K, Howson CP, Walani RS, Ammar W, Nassar A, Yunis K. Improving awareness of preconception health among adolescents: experience of a school-based intervention in Lebanon. BMC Public Health. 2014;14:774. https://doi.org/10.1186/1471-2458-14-774.

Chen H, Chai Y, Dong L, Niu W, Zhang P. Effectiveness and appropriateness of mHealth interventions for maternal and child health: systematic review. JMIR Mhealth Uhealth. 2018;6(1):e7. https://doi.org/10.2196/mhealth.8998.

Editorial Comment. Campaigning for preconception health. Lancet. 2018;391(10132):1749. https://doi.org/10.1016/S0140-6736(18)30981-4.

Every Woman Every Child. The global strategy for women's, children's and adolescents' health (2016–2030). 2015. http://globalstrategy.everywomaneverychild.org/. Accessed 16 Aug 2019.

Guttmacher Institute. Meeting the sexual and reproductive health needs of adolescents in school-based health centers. 2015. https://www.guttmacher.org/gpr/2015/04/meeting-sexual-and-reproductive-health-needs-adolescents-school-based-health-centers. Accessed 26 Aug 2019.

Hemsing N, Greaves L, Poole N. Preconception health care interventions: a scoping review. Sex Reprod Healthc. 2017;14:24–32.

International Planned Parenthood Foundation European Network. Sexuality education in Europe and Central Asia, state of the art and recent developments. 2018. https://www.ippfen.org/sites/ippfen/files/2018-05/Comprehensive%20Country%20Report%20on%20CSE%20in%20Europe%20and%20Central%20Asia_0.pdf. Accessed 25 Aug 2019.

International Telecommunication Union. Measuring the information society report. 2018. https://www.itu.int/dms_pub/itu-d/opb/ind/D-IND-ICTOI-2018-SUM-PDF-E.pdf. Accessed 9 July 2019.

Kancherla V. Countries with an immediate potential for primary prevention of spina bifida and anencephaly: mandatory fortification of wheat flour with folic acid. Birth Defects Res. 2018;90:956–65. https://doi.org/10.1002/bdr2.1222.

Kassa A, Human SP, Gemeda H. Knowledge of preconception care among healthcare providers working in public health institutions in Hawassa, Ethiopia. PLoS One. 2018;13(10):e0204415. https://doi.org/10.1371/journal.pone.0204415.

March of Dimes. Premature babies cost employers $12.7 billion annually. 2014. https://www.marchofdimes.org/news/premature-babies-cost-employers-127-billion-annually.aspx. Accessed 12 June 2019.

March of Dimes. Healthy babies, healthy business. 2019. https://www.marchofdimes.org/professionals/healthy-babies-healthy-business.aspx. Accessed 20 Aug 2019.

Mason E, Chandra-Mouli V, Baltag V, Christiansen C, Lassi ZS, Bhutta ZA. Preconception care: advancing from 'important to do and can be done' to 'is being done and is making a difference'. Reprod Health. 2014;11(Suppl 3):S8. https://doi.org/10.1186/1742-4755-11-S3-S.

Office of Disease Prevention and Health Promotion. Five reasons employee wellness is worth the investment. 2017. https://health.gov/news/blog/2017/05/five-reasons-employee-wellness-is-worth-the-investment/. Accessed 8 July 2019.

Ojukwu O, Patel D, Stephenson J, Howden B, Shawe J. General practitioners' knowledge, attitudes and views of providing preconception care: a qualitative investigation. Upsala J Med Sci. 2016;121(4):256–63. https://doi.org/10.1080/03009734.2016.1215853.

Public Health England. Making the case for preconception care. 2018. https://www.gov.uk/government/publications/preconception-care-making-the-case. Accessed 15 Aug 2019.

Shawe J, Patel D, Joy M, Howden B, Barrett G, Stephenson J. Preparation for fatherhood: a survey of men's preconception health . knowledge and behaviour in England. PLoS One. 2019;14:e0213897.

Stephenson J, Heslehurst N, Hall J, et al. Before the beginning: nutrition and lifestyle in the preconception period and its importance for future health. Lancet. 2018;391:1830–41.

United Nations. About sustainable development goals. 2019. https://www.un.org/sustainabledevelopment/health/. Accessed 12 Aug 2019.

World Health Organization. WHO healthy workplace framework: background and supporting literature and practices. 2010. https://www.who.int/occupational_health/healthy_workplace_framework.pdf. Accessed 20 Aug 2019.

World Health Organization. Preconception care: maximizing the gains for maternal and child health. 2013a. https://www.who.int/maternal_child_adolescent/documents/preconception_care_policy_brief.pdf. Accessed 10 May 2019.

World Health Organization. Regional Office for South-East Asia: Report of a regional expert group consultation, 6–8 August 2013, New Delhi, India. 2013b. http://www.searo.who.int/entity/child_adolescent/documents/2014/sea-cah-16/en/. Accessed 8 June 2019.

World Health Organization. Regional Office for the Eastern Mediterranean: Summary report on the meeting on promoting preconception care in the Eastern Mediterranean region. 2015. http://applications.emro.who.int/docs/IC_Meet_Rep_2015_EN_16333.pdf?ua=1. Accessed 8 June 2019.

World Health Organization. Reaching the every newborn national 2020 milestones: country progress, plans and moving forward. Geneva: 2017. Licence: CC BY-NC-SA 3.0 IGO.

World Health Organization. Millennium development goals (MDGs). https://www.who.int/news-room/fact-sheets/detail/millennium-development-goals-(mdgs) (2018). Accessed 12 July 2019.

World Health Organization. What is health financing for universal coverage? 2019. https://www.who.int/health_financing/universal_coverage_definition/en/. Accessed 27 Aug 2019.

Zhou Q, Acharya G, Zhang S, Wang Q, Shen H, Li X. A new perspective on universal preconception care in China. Acta Obstet Gynecol Scand. 2016;95:377–81.

Advancing Preconception Health Globally: A Way Forward

15

Sarah Verbiest, Jill Shawe, and Eric A. P. Steegers

Preconception health is a simple yet comprehensive concept that provides a significant opportunity to prevent chronic disease, reduce the risks of maternal and infant mortality and morbidity, and improve the health of two generations. At its most basic definition, preconception wellness is the biopsychosocial health of a person before they conceive a child. Given that well-being begins early in life and is important for all people to achieve their full potential, preconception interventions are just one part of a larger call for a life course approach to population health. The global inequitable distribution of access to medical and mental health care, housing, education, economic mobility, rights, safety, nutritious food, and other needed resources to achieve health and wellness presents a major challenge to this work. At the same time, the two-generational potential offered by focusing on the sensitive period of development that preconception health represents provides a unique forum for taking key steps forward in advancing preventive health and care for people of reproductive age.

To support this work, chapter authors have contributed their expertise across an array of topics, offering a general overview, current research, and recommendations specific to preconception health and care. Early chapters make the case for the importance of focusing attention on health and well-being before pregnancy,

S. Verbiest (✉)
Center for Maternal and Infant Health, UNC School of Medicine, Chapel Hill, NC, USA

Jordan Institute for Families, School of Social Work, University of North Carolina at Chapel Hill, Chapel Hill, NC, USA
e-mail: sarah_verbiest@med.unc.edu

J. Shawe
Faculty of Health, School of Nursing and Midwifery, University of Plymouth, Plymouth, UK

E. A. P. Steegers
Department of Obstetrics and Gynaecology, Erasmus MC - Sophia Children's Hospital, Rotterdam, The Netherlands

© Springer Nature Switzerland AG 2020
J. Shawe et al. (eds.), *Preconception Health and Care: A Life Course Approach*,
https://doi.org/10.1007/978-3-030-31753-9_15

including a description of the biological pathways involved in ovum and sperm health and early fetal development. Genetics, likewise, plays a role in the health of a couple's offspring. Creating opportunities for couples to learn about and discuss their unique backgrounds provides them with the knowledge they need to make informed decisions for themselves and future family. In order to make sure that all people have access to the technology available to learn about potential genetic risks and act on ways to reduce risks, more investment is required. A similar focus on equity was elevated in the chapter about fertility, as many people do not have access to the full complement of services that they might need to achieve or prevent a pregnancy. Likewise, limited knowledge of reproduction and fertility combined with a variety of economic and societal pressures and untreated health conditions can lead to challenges for people in achieving their desired future family.

Experts shared research and clinical guidance on topics including chronic disease, substance use, weight, nutrition, infections, tobacco, and alcohol. While all people benefit from having healthy lifestyles and well-controlled (or prevented) disease, there are some unique considerations for people contemplating a pregnancy that were presented. Mental wellness can be influenced by physical health, and likewise depression, anxiety, and other conditions can make it difficult for people to achieve the health status they desire. While mental health is a topic touched upon in many chapters, a unique chapter on this topic was included to underscore the importance of addressing this topic in clinical practice, policy, and community services. The evidence presented in the chapter on environmental exposures—at home, at work, and in the community—elevate connections to climate change, worker safety, and environmental justice. This is a prime example of the need to form partnerships with environmentalists and advocates as many people exposed to toxins may not have the resources or power to protect themselves and families. Likewise, violence is another social determinant of health that causes physical, psychological, and economic harm to millions of people globally, often women. Healthcare professionals and other service providers need to screen for violence and offer evidence-based support and trauma informed care. Overall, advice on preconception health provided to people who may not have the ability or resources to act on that information is likely to augment stress and anxiety.

While the chapters are organized by distinct topics, in reality the various issues are often intersecting and interrelated. For example, exposure to interpersonal violence can impact a woman's access to services, ability to stop using tobacco products, and reproductive choice. Women who live with chronic conditions may also be facing fertility concerns and have mental health needs. People do not lead single issue but complex lives and true health and well-being including physical, emotional, social, financial, and spiritual wellness. Further, each chapter highlighted areas where more research and investment is needed. From a clinical perspective, specialists and primary care providers must consider their patients in context and not assume that they are receiving advice or support from other sectors. Innovating approaches such as adding lawyers and community advocates to healthcare settings can help meet complex needs. Cross-sector collaboration, economic investment, and community capacity building are necessary to achieve preconception and population wellness for all people. While addressing all of these factors falls outside the scope of this book, improving the health of the world's future families requires a significant paradigm shift.

Chapter 12 provided examples of emerging global strategies that are taking steps toward raising awareness about preconception health and building coalitions and programs to improve well-being. International collaborations like the Preconception Period Analysis of Risks and Exposures influencing health and Development (PrePARED) consortium (Harville et al. 2019) and the Health in Preconception, Pregnancy, and Postpartum (HiPPP) global alliance (Hill et al. 2019) are emerging groups that are advancing research and conversations in this arena. Community-driven, consumer engaged research is needed to develop evidence-based strategies for improving health and wellness. The remainder of this chapter offers several potential directions for advancing preconception and preventive health for people of reproductive age.

15.1 Provide Access to Continuous, Quality, Culturally Appropriate, Comprehensive Care Across the Life Course

All people should receive quality medical and behavioral health services. Some nations have policies that clearly center health as a human right and provide services to everyone. Other countries do not insure that all people can access needed healthcare services. In addition to economic barriers to health care, people may experience geographic barriers to accessing services. Nine-to-five weekday clinic hours are provider focused not necessarily consumer aligned. People may also face cultural and language challenges and suffer from inequitable treatment by healthcare providers due to the color of their skin, gender, ethnicity, ability, gender expression, education, and income. Women may also not understand what a preventive visit should be, how to schedule one, and what to expect (Preconception Health and Health Care Initiative 2019). Comprehensive clinical care is an essential component of preconception and general health and wellness.

Healthcare systems across the globe are largely designed to attend to sickness instead of to promote health. For example, significant healthcare resources are spent to treat chronic conditions, including substance use and obesity, instead of providing supports to people and communities to prevent these conditions. A shift in focus to early life course medicine that advances preventive care and programs has the potential to reduce healthcare spending and improve intergenerational health (Steegers 2019). An intentional focus on preventive care means making sure investments are made in providing screening and supports early in the life course to reduce the risk of chronic disease and proactively managing conditions at an early age. It may lead to living longer lives without major disabilities. Mental health services, nutrition counseling, healthy lifestyle coaches, stress management techniques, occupational and physical therapy, bias-free full-service family planning care, and routine preventive visits could help young people lead their best lives. Healthcare providers need a mindset change to shift from managing disease to managing health.

The specialization within medicine has further splintered care with some providers focusing only on one health concern without context or continuity of care for the whole patient. While some primary care practices are beginning to integrate behavioral health and social work services, there is much work to be done to care for the complete and interrelated needs of the person. The 2019 Technical Report from the US Department of Health and Human Services, Health Resources and Services Administration's Global Maternal Mortality Summit recommended improving access to patient-centered, comprehensive care for women before, during, and after pregnancy (U.S. Department of Health and Human Services Health Resources and Services Administration 2019). The findings highlight the importance of increasing the types and distribution of healthcare providers who serve women, including midwives, and providing continuous team-based support using a life course model of care.

Work in the United States and Europe calls for identifying then capitalizing on missed opportunities for care. For example, the Every Woman, Every Time campaign in California suggested that preventive care be provided each time a person encounters the healthcare system. In the UK preconception, health initiatives are still developing, and Public Health England has provided strategic oversight of opportunities for embedding preconception care in practice (Amrita Jesurasa 2018). Similarly, in Europe, initiatives which aim to join up care across services and communities (Sijpkens et al. 2019) are being evaluated. Some examples of more integrated care suggest that family planning and sexually transmitted infection care should include wellness messages and screenings as well as access to community resources and behavioral health care. Pediatric visits could include some screening of parents, especially new mothers, and warm referrals to services as needed. Specialty care providers should ask about the reproductive goals of the people they serve and be ready to provide condition specific advice and referrals for care as needed. Mental healthcare providers should ask about the physical health of their clients and assess for stressors related to violence, housing, and other social drivers of health. In providing adequate care, medical and social domains should work together, moving toward context driven medicine instead of evidence-based medicine only.

A life course approach to health underscores the importance of starting early in providing quality, comprehensive care to children and adolescents and into young adulthood. Youth should be screened for tobacco, alcohol, and drug use as well as for risky sexual behaviors and provided trauma-informed, realistic, and evidence-based services from a trusted provider as needed. Young people should learn about nutrition, food preparation, and exercise in schools along with money management, reproductive health and function, and communication skills. Adolescent mental health should be well-funded and widely available as helping youth manage stress, anxiety, learning and developmental differences, and other challenges early can better equip them for their life. More attention needs to be paid to transitions from pediatric care to adult care and during key points in development such as moving away from home. Adolescent care should create value and build health-seeking behaviors at an early age. Likewise, young adults in their early 20s tend to be both healthy and more likely to engage in risky behavior. They may have less interest in accessing preventive care even though this is important. Systems of care need to be created to provide comprehensive care to young adults who may engage in the healthcare system only for contraceptives or emergent care.

Finally, within the healthcare system, steps should be taken to create trusting and continuous relationships between patients and providers. Recent studies have identified that some women experience fear and anxiety when accessing healthcare services. Community-based research by Garbers et al. underscored the fact that providers must focus on the way they talk with their patients if they are to be able to accurately assess their needs (Garbers et al. 2020). Others may question if providers have alternative agendas when making recommendations for care. Clinics should be welcoming spaces where people feel respected and safe.

15.2 Advance Reproductive Justice and Equity

Patriarchal societies across the globe have advanced norms, policies, and even medical care that have sought to control women's sexuality and reproduction for centuries. Women of color, particularly in the United States, have a history of being forced and unwilling participants in research, victims of eugenics programs, and having their bodily autonomy denied by the very systems that were supposed to be providing them with care. While many advancements have been made, there is still significant work ahead to create full gender equity and acknowledge and repair centuries of harm. The reproductive justice framework as defined by Black women activities in 1994 as "the human right to maintain personal bodily autonomy, have children, not have children, and parent the children we have in safe and sustainable communities" (Reproductive Justice—Sister Song 2020) offers a strong foundation or preconception and general wellness work. This framework explicitly defines women's rights to make decisions about when and if they wish to have children and to have access to a full scope of reproductive services from infertility care to the full range of contraceptive methods as well as access emergency contraception and abortion care.

There has been a growing interest in the United States and in Europe in asking people about their interest in becoming pregnant in the next year at the start of a clinical encounter as a way to provide better care. As such, women who are certain they wish to avoid becoming pregnant can receive a contraceptive method and women who are seeking pregnancy or open to pregnancy should it occur can receive preconception health information. In many cases this question may be difficult for women to answer as they hadn't given this consideration, may be conflicted, and/or may be living in circumstances that make the concept of planning feel foreign. This question opens the door for a guided conversation and the provision of resources so women are supported regardless of where they fall in this spectrum. These conversations while important also run the risk of perpetuating bias unless providers are trained in having person-centered conversations and are able to put aside their own judgment about a person's decision and instead provide the care, information, and resources needed to support autonomy and well-being.

Normalizing conversations about reproduction and family formation could help address bias and stereotypes by elevating the many different ways that people think about having a family as well as the different barriers that might keep them from being able to achieve their goals. Many people are uncertain about when and if they wish to become parents and might benefit from listening to and engaging in discussions with others. Likewise, young adults who have decided they do not wish to have children should feel fully respected in that decision. Conversations in community and online spaces also decenter the power of physicians as gatekeepers to knowledge and advice. At the same time, this also takes a burden from providers who are currently being tasked with leading on this sometimes challenging and charged conversation. Talking about the desire to become a parent should happen regardless of identity, health condition, age, race, immigration status, or income.

The general population also needs a better understanding about the basics of human reproduction across the life course. There is a need for better information provided at multiple points in time about fertility, puberty, sperm health, menarche, pregnancy, postpartum, and menopause. Education on how to protect and understand fertility has to be guaranteed at different ages—not just one class at one age with parental permission. Likewise, women need resources to support their well-being across these changes—from sanitary supplies for girls to be able to go to school and work to basic hormonal therapies to cope with symptoms of premenstrual syndrome, menopause, and everything in between. Focusing only on the 9 months of pregnancy as has been done to date leaves many knowledge gaps which can have significant impact on people's health and ability to make informed choices.

15.3 Foster and Fund Creative Strategies

The rapid rise of technology, including global access to smart phones and expanded access to the Internet, provides new opportunities to put tailored information and resources into the hands of young adults. New online programs and resources such as ShowYourLoveToday.com, the Gabby Project (Boston University Medical Center Family Medicine 2020a) and Gabe Men's Health Project (Boston University Medical Center Family Medicine 2020b), the mHealth program Smarter Pregnancy (van Dijk et al. 2017), and a Dutch Internet questionnaire for preconception risk assessment (Landkroon et al. 2010) are being developed and shared to democratize access to health information. The development of apps and wearable devices to track fitness, diet, hydration, and sleep remind people to take their contraceptive pill and other medications, and more has the potential to provide individualized support (Preconception Health and Health Care Initiative 2020). Gamification of learning for people and professionals should be also explored. For example, the SIMS games allow people to design virtual lives, homes, and families. How might messages around safe sex, fertility, and positive relationships be integrated into the creation of these fantasy worlds? More work is needed to partner with new industries to continue to design, test, and evaluate health promoting strategies, but the possibilities in this new decade are truly endless.

Sometimes the "old" really is "new." Community health workers, doulas, midwives, and community health associations have long been the closest to really understanding local culture and need. Much of the information shared by experts in this book doesn't, in fact, require a healthcare provider or specialist to deliver. The Hesperian Foundation in the US (hesparian.org) has championed books and resources for decades tailored to provide community health workers with medical information and techniques to care for each other when a physician isn't available. When people understand and own accurate, culturally appropriate health information, they can liberate strategies within their own communities for sharing this knowledge and caring for each other. Resources need to shift to support this important workforce and to democratize access to health information and support.

Human-centered design, community-based participatory strategies, and an array of engaged research methods and program development approaches should be used to co-create health and wellness programs with the people who need care. Historically, experts with academic training have looked at published peer-reviewed research to identify and test solutions to problems. Trends are shifting, and equity-aligned researchers are recognizing their own bias and blind spots. Co-designing with patients, consumers, women, frontline health workers, local community leaders, and policy makers opens the door for better and more feasible approaches to long-standing challenges. This may help address perennial concerns about program recruitment and sustainability.

15.4 Invest in Healthy and Economically Sound Communities

Healthcare providers will not have the resources or capacity to fully support their patients' wellness until policy makers and society at large are willing to prioritize and invest in strategies aimed at improving health at the community level. Current medical and healthcare recommendations center the person with expectations that he/she/they will figure out how to act on clinical advice. A life course approach seeks to shift some of that burden from the individual to the larger population and society recognizing that each stage of life is important across generations. Attention needs to be payed to the social determinants of health and equity. As described in many sections of this book, this includes focusing on the environment—air, water, workplace, and food should be toxin-free. Advocates and scientists must consider the impact of climate change on reproductive health. People face fewer barriers to achieving a healthy weight and balanced diet when nutritious food is easily available and affordable, making the healthy choice the easy choice.

Violence is a public health issue and requires attention to not only interpersonal safety and relationships but attention to country-specific threats and challenges. For example, gun violence in the United States and the mass incarceration of black and brown people has an impact on stress, reproductive health, and preconception health and general wellness. Young people need access to economic opportunity as financial status is closely connected to health.

Policies need to be put in place at the organizational, system, community, and national level to advance gender equity and address structural racism and other forms of discrimination. While these are daunting challenges, a discussion about preconception health in the context of the life course and the developmental origins of disease would be incomplete without identifying the larger work that needs to take place. Further, as described above, a reproductive justice framework requires attention to issues such as community safety, quality childcare, and economic security.

15.5 Measure Change

Traditionally, infant mortality and morbidity rates have been used as a marker of the health and well-being of a society. Childhood nutrition and disease and access to prenatal care are also common indicators. Tracking and reporting on maternal mortality and morbidity is becoming more common. While important, a life course approach to preconception health calls for the identification and routine reporting of measures that can report and benchmark the health of young adults in a society.

Population-wide measures proposed by the Centers for Disease Control and Prevention in the United States identify a number of areas that could be monitored including smoking, diabetes, depression, folic acid intake, heavy alcohol use, hypertension, weight, physical activity, and contraceptive use (Kroelinger et al. 2018). Stephenson et al. proposed that an annual report card on preconception health be issued in the United Kingdom to hold governments and other relevant agencies to account for delivering interventions to improve preconception health (Stephenson et al. 2019). Clinical measures are also required to hold providers, healthcare systems, and healthcare payers accountable for quality comprehensive care. Frayne et al. developed a series of proposed metrics that could in theory assess preconception wellness at the beginning of prenatal care.(Frayne et al. 2016) The measures are similar to the population measures described above with the addition of prescription of teratogenic medications and untreated sexually transmitted infections. Research is needed to identify how these indicators could be extracted from electronic medical records, potentially prioritized, and then used in practice to improve prevention in a healthcare system. The Women's Preventive Services Initiative supported by the American College of Obstetricians and Gynecologists recently released updated guidelines for well woman care across the life course.(Women's Preventive Services Initiative—WPSI 2020) The project included recommendations and proposed performance measures for use in practice.

Indicators that identify the percent of women at different ages who receive an annual preventive visit could benchmark basic access to healthcare services. Larger surveys such as the *Listening to Mothers* series(National Partnership for Women and Families 2020) could be conducted with diverse populations to assess content of preventive care and women's perceptions of the care they receive. Medicaid and insurers could regularly review and report the preventive care provided to people of reproductive age. National surveys could be conducted in different countries with women and men of reproductive age and healthcare providers to assess general knowledge and understanding of fertility, reproductive, and the factors that influence healthy birth outcomes for women and babies.

Community health indexes and data from other fields on housing, violence, access to child care, and employment could be leveraged to address the non-medical risks to the health and well-being of young adults. Further local government data that describes how community resources are allocated could inform this work. Health equity impact assessments could assist policy makers in considering the impact and consequences of spending and policies in their communities. The impact of deprivation and poverty is significant contributing to the persisting and in some parts of the work rising inequalities in both perinatal and adult health.

Demographic information including race/ethnicity, socioeconomic status, and geographic location must be included to assess for and assure equitable outcomes. Without careful attention to monitoring disparities and promoting programs that aim to create equity, it is possible that outcomes for some populations will improve while others fall behind. Further, care should be taken when reporting data to place it within a larger social context so as to avoid perpetuating individual stereotypes and bias and to highlight the true levers of change at the societal level.

15.6 Just the Beginning

As Merry-K Moos noted in the forward, *As should occur with all new paradigms that impact multiple interest groups, the work should be constantly interrogated and be able to shift and evolve.* Over the past two decades, the preconception health movement has continued to expand, recognizing the role of the social determinants of health, men, and diverse populations and realigning to better center on reproductive justice and women's health equity. While some professionals might find this overwhelming, in truth the new decade holds exciting opportunities to see improvements in health and wellness.

The majority of people on the globe become parents with the shared hope that their child will be born healthy. There are large disparities in birth outcomes, which demonstrate that not all parents and children have the same chance for achieving this goal. There is a role that everyone can play in shifting this paradigm to close generational health disparities and create a place where young adults and the future generation they will produce can thrive.

References

Amrita Jesurasa AJ. Public Health England. Making the Case for Preconception. PHE Publications; 2018 July.

Boston University Medical Center Family Medicine. Project Preconception Care [Internet]. Boston University Medical Center Family Medicine. [cited 2020a Jan 18]. https://www.bu.edu/familymed/programs-and-research/project-preconception-care/

Boston University Medical Center Family Medicine. Gabe Men's Health Promotion Program [Internet]. Boston University Medical Center Family Medicine. [cited 2020b Jan 19]. https://www.bu.edu/familymed/programs-and-research/gabes-mens-health-promotion-program/

van Dijk MR, Oostingh EC, Koster MPH, Willemsen SP, Laven JSE, Steegers-Theunissen RPM. The use of the mHealth program Smarter Pregnancy in preconception care: rationale, study design and data collection of a randomized controlled trial. BMC Pregnancy Childbirth. 2017;17(1):46.

Frayne DJ, Verbiest S, Chelmow D, Clarke H, Dunlop A, Hosmer J, et al. Health care system measures to advance preconception wellness: consensus recommendations of the clinical workgroup of the national preconception health and health care initiative. Obstet Gynecol. 2016;127(5):863–72.

Garbers S, Falletta KA, Srinivasulu S, Almonte Y, Baum R, Bermudez D, et al. If You don't Ask, I'm Not Going to Tell You': using community-based participatory research to inform pregnancy intention screening processes for black and Latina women in primary care. Womens Health Issues. 2020;30(1):25–34.

Harville E, Mishra G, Mumford S, Schisterman E, Jukic AM, Hatch E, et al. The Preconception Period analysis of Risks and Exposures Influencing health and Development (PrePARED) consortium. Paediatr Perinat Epidemiol. 2019;33(6):490–502.

Hill B, Skouteris H, Teede HJ, Baily C, Baxter JP, Bergmeir HJ, et al. Health in preconception, pregnancy and postpartum global alliance: International Network *Preconception* Research Priorities for the prevention of maternal obesity and related pregnancy and long-term complications. J Clin Med. 2019;8:2119.

Kroelinger CD, Okoroh EM, Boulet SL, Olson CK, Robbins CL. Making the case: the importance of using 10 key preconception indicators in understanding the health of women of reproductive age. J Womens Health (Larchmt). 2018;27(6):739–43.

Landkroon AP, de Weerd S, van Vliet-Lachotzki E, Steegers EAP. Validation of an internet questionnaire for risk assessment in preconception care. Public Health Genomics. 2010;13(2):89–94.

National Partnership for Women and Families. Listening to mothers reports and surveys [Internet]. National Partnership for Women and Families. [cited 2020 Jan 19]. https://www.nationalpartnership.org/our-work/health/maternity/listening-to-mothers.html

Preconception Health and Health Care Initiative. Preconception Health and Health Care Initiative May2019 newsletter: National Preconception Health + Health Care Initiative [Internet]. Preconception Health and Health Care Initiative. 2019 [cited 2020 Jan 18]. Available from: https://myemail-constantcontact-com.libproxy.lib.unc.edu/PCHHC-May-2019-Newsletter-.html?soid=1110472552145&aid=UUI7pc_pDpE

Preconception Health and Health Care Initiative. Preconception Health and Health Care Initiative June/July 2019 newsletter—Building Women's Health Equity [Internet]. Preconception Health and Health Care Initiative. 2019 [cited 2020 Jan 17]. https://myemail-constantcontact-com.libproxy.lib.unc.edu/PCHHC-June%2D%2D-July-2019-Newsletter-.html?soid=1110472552145&aid=GKSD9rst4P4

Reproductive Justice—Sister Song [Internet]. [cited 2020 Jan 22]. https://www.sistersong.net/reproductive-justice

Sijpkens MK, van Voorst SF, de Jong-Potjer LC, Denktaş S, Verhoeff AP, Bertens LCM, et al. The effect of a preconception care outreach strategy: the Healthy Pregnancy 4 All study. BMC Health Serv Res. 2019;19(1):60.

Steegers EAP. Understanding preconception health for early life course medicine. Paediatr Perinat Epidemiol. 2019;33(6):503–5.

Stephenson J, Vogel C, Hall J, Hutchinson J, Mann S, Duncan H, et al. Preconception health in England: a proposal for annual reporting with core metrics. Lancet. 2019;393(10187):2262–71.

U.S. Department of Health and Human Services Health Resources and Services Administration. HRSA Maternal Mortality Summit: Promising Global Practices to Improve Maternal Health Outcomes. U.S. Department of Health and Human Services Health Resources and Services Administration; 2019 Feb.

Women's Preventive Services Initiative—WPSI [Internet]. [cited 2020 Jan 22]. https://www.womenspreventivehealth.org/

The manufacturer's authorised representative in the EU is Springer
Nature Customer Service Centre GmbH, Europaplatz 3, 69115 Heidelberg,
Germany. If you have any concerns regarding our products, please
contact ProductSafety@springernature.com

Printed and bound by CPI Group (UK) Ltd, Croydon, CR0 4YY
24/04/2026
02096338-0001